Tom
with Grati

MW00462413

Intuition Technology

100 ᴺᴴ
2008

John Living, Professional Engineer

Dedicated to the memory of

Dan Wilson

With Deepest Gratitude

For his Wisdom and Advice

And with Sincere Appreciation of

the Great Help freely given by so many

Other Leaders of the Dowsing Community

'True Holy Love, Namaste'

"I see in you myself;   I recognize in you my image;
I will do my best to help you in your life for good intent.
Without hurt or harm to others."

Intuition Technology

Copyright © John Living, 2008
All rights reserved.

No part of this book may be reproduced or transmitted in any form or by any means, electronic or mechanical, including photocopying, recording, or any information storage and retrieval system, without the written permission of the Holistic Intuition Society.

Permission is hereby granted for reproduction of extracts in articles and web sites providing that full reference is made to this book title and the Holistic Intuition Society to include the web site www.in2it.ca

For more books by John Living see:

www.in2it.ca/Books.htm

The Holistic Intuition Society

c/o Executive Secretary, John Living, Professional .Engineer

RR# 1 Site 9 Comp 6, Galiano Island,

British Columbia, V0N 1P0 Canada

Phone (250)539-5807 Toll Free Canada & USA: 1-866-369-7464

Check www.in2it.ca for any change in address

ISBN 978-0-9686323-4-5

UNDERSTANDING OURSELVES

Locational Dowsing   Continued

Earth Energies   197

HEALING

The Holistic Intuition Society
www.in2it.ca

"Who Done It ?"

This is the standard question of all detective stories ! We are investigating the biggest mystery of all. This is one detective's report.

First let us look at the detective himself.

Teaching staff at Southend High School, the Royal Military Academy, Sandhurst, the School of Military Engineering, Chatham, and the Royal Military College of Science, Shrivenham, all attempted to give John Living an education.

He was one of the first officers commissioned by Her Majesty Queen Elizabeth II into the Corps of Royal Engineers, and is believed to have been the first British commander of a nuclear armed vessel - which is another long story !

Perhaps due to some mix-up, he was awarded an Honours Degree in Civil Engineering by London University, and has been a Royal Engineer, a Chartered Civil Engineer, and a Professional Engineer.

John has had experience in the Military, in Real Estate, as a Town Councilor, and has worked as an engineer as the Resident Engineer in charge of major projects, as a Consulting Engineer, as an Engineer in a major city, and in a senior position with a National Government.

Born in London, England, he has lived in Jamaica, and now resides in Canada - living in a cabin overlooking the golf course of Galiano Island, midway between Vancouver and Victoria in British Columbia, where he is watched by eagles, swallows, humming birds, deer, and golfers.

John is currently employed as the servant of two dogs, does Intuitive Healing work on the side, and writes in his spare time.

He can be seen wandering around looking rather lost, puffing a Peterson Pipe and wearing a Deerstalker Hat (like Sherlock Holmes), while he searches for clues as to the meaning of Life.

'True Holy Love, Namaste'

"I see in you myself;   I recognize in you my image;
I will do my best to help you in your life for good intent.
Without hurt or harm to others."

Failing to Succeed is not Failure;
Failure is not Doing your Best to Succeed !

Introduction

Thank you for taking an interest in this book - I hope that you will find that it gives you a few good ideas of how you can access your 'Soul Senses' and your Intuition to improve your own life - and that of others.

I am an engineer - not trained as a literary person; so the style of this book is more akin to an instruction manual than a novel. I have tried not repeat myself too much, so to get the most out of this book you may have to read it more than once.

I believe that there is a Power greater than us, a Power that is benign and wants to help us; but there are a few big problems - often we are not aware of this help, we do not listen when help is offered, we fail to show our gratitude when such help is given - and we have given so much of our own power away to others.

It seems to me that this Power can do many things that we cannot do - especially in the non-physical realms. In the same way, often we can do things in the physical realm more easily than 'Upstairs' - my label for this Power.

When we work together with 'Upstairs' for the good of all creation, most things are possible ! But they may take time to happen.

This is best accomplished when we regain the powers of our own that we have given away to, or had taken by, others. So much of what we do is governed by our beliefs - mostly things that we have been told or taught by others.

Often these were not for our own good, although that is what we were told - but for control. This includes what we told by our parents, our religious leaders, our school authorities, and our governments.

In many of these cases, what we were told were the honestly held beliefs of others, who believed that they were doing good. But were such beliefs the real truth ?

Are we, as human beings, capable of understanding the real truth ? Many things are beyond our comprehension, and we may only be able to grasp a few of them. Imagine telling a person from a thousand years ago about electricity, radio, germs, or nuclear warfare.

My strongest belief is that we must keep an open mind. Hold the things that we have been told as if they were pieces of a jig-saw puzzle that we are trying to complete. We assemble groups of pieces, but when we try to fit those groups together there are mis-matches - so we have to re-assemble parts of these groups.

I have not yet got all my jig-saw pieces to give a complete finished pictures - but perhaps the hints that I give in this book may help you to form your own picture better.

Remember that some of the pieces in my puzzle may not belong in yours - we all have our own puzzles to solve, and yours may already have pieces that belong to others, not you.

When working to make your puzzle be finished correctly, it is important to be working on a firm base - otherwise the pieces will keep falling apart.

Perhaps the strongest base to use is Love. Especially 'True Holy Love' - best described by 'Namaste':

> *"I see in you myself; I recognize in you my image;*
>
> *I will do my best to help you in your life for good intent.*
>
> *Without hurt or harm to others."*

The key here is not to help if harm would ensue to any life form - to help manifest only that which is beneficial to all.

Perhaps LIFE is given by 'Upstairs' in LOVE - and perhaps 'Upstairs' does not want worship - but help in creating and spreading more LOVE.

If so, let 'LOVE' and 'LIFE' be interchangeable in all that you think, all that you do !

Remember, what you give out usually comes back to you, often more strongly and in different, unexpected ways.

That is my sermon - now let the lessons be read !

Namaste *John*

Intuition is NOT our sixth sense !

Intuition uses all our senses to give the message !

Naturally, We ARE Intuitive !

Have you ever felt 'something is not right' - and, forewarned, avoided a problem ?

Have you met someone for the first time and felt something about them - and been correct ?

Have you lost something and then thought 'it is there' (in an unexpected place) and so looked and found it ?

Have you felt apprehensive before eating something, eaten it, and had a stomach ache ?

If any thing like this has happened to you, then you have been Intuitive.

We are all Intuitive to some degree - and can all improve our Intuitive abilities; and it helps to understand more about the Intuitive process, so that we can choose the method that suits us best.

A Simple Exercise

Stand up, and form a simple YES/NO question in your logical mind, such as *"Am I wearing clothes ?"*

Next, being sincere (as in prayer) ask your Heart (as if it were another person !) this question - and be aware of any slight body movements.

If you bent or swayed forward, the answer is YES ! A backwards movement would indicate NO.

Practice on a few more simple questions, such as:

"Am I over [or under] the age of XX years ?"
"Am I male [female] ?"
"Have I visited [a country ot city] in the last [20] years ?"
"Is my name [one of your correct names] [incorrect name] ?"
"Do I enjoy [hobby/sport] ?"
"Do I regret any actions that I have done ?"
"Are there improvements that I can make to my life ?"

What is Intuition ?

Winston Churchill is understood to have said *"in truth, all people are offered help by their intuition - but most pick themselves up and escape as fast as possible".*

Those of us who accept this help become convinced that it is a 'Force for Good', and wish that it could be accessed 'On Demand'.

Guidance from 'The System' is a fair definition, 'The System' being the total environment in which we operate in life, including our memories, our sub-conscious self, our Guides, our 'Higher Self', and our 'Guardian Angels' and Deities as representatives of 'God' (or whatever labels we choose to use), and the total knowledge banks and information centres of 'All that Is' in the past, present, and (to some extent) the future.

In 'Awakening Osiris' - the beautiful and topical translation of the 'Egyptian Book of the Dead' by Normandi Ellis - it tells about the first human: Horus, the son of Osiris and Isis ...

"He was born out of death, carrier of his Fathers wisdom, he was the living emblem of Love. He was the Light triumphing over darkness, the first man, the miracle of nature - and he was followed by magic. A pair of hawks circled above him ... They dropped two plumes which he placed on his forehead, two gifts that fell from the sky - Intuition and Love, gifts from the Goddesses - that he might walk towards Heaven and his Father, and never lose his way".

Intuitive Examples

It is recognized that humans have five senses - seeing, hearing, feeling, tasting, and smelling. Many people have called Intuition our 'sixth sense' - having direct input into our conscious thoughts.

It is more correct to understand that Intuition is at a level above our physical senses, and uses them to get messages to us.

Usually we recognize our Intuition only when an especially important message is received such as not feeling 'good' about a person or situation, or we get an impulse to take a particular action.

There have been a number of well publicized cases when a person has felt that a particular flight or journey was 'not good' and so cancelled or changed their reservation - and avoided death or serious injury when their original plane or train crashed.

Mothers are well known to have a special 'connection' to a baby - automatically knowing if their child is in trouble, and racing to prevent a tragedy.

Some notable investors who are most successful admit to relying heavily on their intuition, and revising their investments when they feel that that a stock is 'troubled'.

Scientists and inventors may get a sudden idea - and it often leads to a successful solution of the very problems that they have been concerning them.   Einstein has told that his understanding of relativity occurred in this way.

Perhaps the biggest difference between top executives is their attitude to Intuition - those who use it as a helpful indicator tend to be more successful.

Our Real Sixth Sense

In fact we do have a sixth physical sense, but most people are so accustomed to it that they overlook it as a separate sense - it is our sense of balance.

We have balance sensors associated with most of our joints - hence the skill of tightrope walkers, of steeplejacks who build high structures, and of waiters who carry loaded trays through crowded restaurants without spilling their loads.

They have developed a greater awareness of the 'feedback' from these receptors than most people; but we can all improve such awareness - and the first part of this is to realize that we do have this sixth sense, the sense of balancing.

When you asked your Heart the questions in our first experiment, you received an answer by a body movement; this was your Heart-Mind-Brain team working with your nervous-muscular system to give you a signal - by adjusting your 'balance system' so that your body swayed forward to indicate YES, or backward to indicate NO.

How does Intuition Operate ?

It seems that Intuition has three modes:

1. Forcing a message in some way if the matter is really important - and doing this even if the recipient is not normally open to Intuition.

2. Giving messages of various descriptions to people who are normally open to Intuition.

3. Responding to questions that are asked by those who actively seek the help of their Intuition.

In this book we are concerned with the third mode - that of asking questions and getting correct answers 'On Demand'.

Awareness is Most Important

The more that we are aware of our environment, the easier to note any changes in our perception. Seeing not just an object, but all the contouring, shading, and variations in colour (and carefully noting the surrounds and background) gives us a better appreciation of 'what we see'.

When we ask our Intuition for help on a subject, we can also define that 'all that we see' in the next few minutes has a meaning relating to the subject.

We will still perceive the same views as would have otherwise been seen, but our sight now may emphasize certain shapes, colours, contrasts, or even objects.

When ready, be fully aware of your environment, ask your question, and then note all the changes to your environment - a memory of a person or situation that comes to mind, a change of taste in your mouth, the shivers, a funny smell, hearing a noise that you did not notice before, or a picture flashing into your mind.

You may walk down the street and notice a particular colour, shape, or object; perhaps certain flowers in a garden 'call' to you; or your attention may focus on something in a shop window. Yes, all these things were there before, but your Intuition is now drawing your attention to them to 'get a message across'.

You seek guidance on a situation, and a memory of a person or a happening comes to mind - could your relationship with that person, the memory of how they behaved (to you or to others), or the outcome of that happening be an indication regarding your present situation ?

Laura Day, who has written a number of books on Intuition, suggests another way in her 'Practical Intuition': ask the question, and then check - How do I feel ? What am I thinking now ? What taste is in my mouth ? What am I smelling ? What am I seeing first when I close and then open my eyes ?

Also write down the first thing that comes to mind when you think of a place, person, colour, time, town, river, food, weapon, fear, memory, etc.

You can write each of these on a card, and go through them to get immediate answers; do each one quickly - and if you do not get an answer then make one up !

Sounds stupid ? But there is a good reason - your mind is lazy, so it is far easier to use what is available in memory, etc., than to 'make something up'. So you may well be 'getting the truth'.

And since it is the 'first thought' then it probably comes from your Intuition.

Understanding Intuition

It pays to immediately record all your intuitive experiences. Often you will find a pattern that indicates the way that your intuition works.

Certain symbols seen (or persons popping into your mind) may have special meanings, even appearing in dreams.

By recording these, you may find the key to deciphering such meanings.

Then we have to 'make sense' of these impressions - a job for the logical part of our thinking team !

It helps to ask for further clarification, and a thought may 'pop' into your mind.

That 'first thought' is probably from your Intuition, and should be taken seriously; any second thoughts are likely to be from your logical mind, and may best be disregarded.

This is probably because one's ego seems to operate from the logical part of the mind; being egoistic, it thinks that it 'knows it all' - and tries to imply that any other thought must be nonsense !

This would also explain why asking questions of your mind will tend to tell you the answers that you want to hear - by asking your Heart, you will be getting a more correct answer.

Knowledge Base

When you ask a question the answer can only be understood within the limits of your knowledge. The more knowledgeable that you are, the greater the range of contexts that can be used to give a true answer.

Imagine a nuclear physicist trying to explain sub-atomic particles to a class of young children, a scientist talking about television to people living in the Amazon jungle, or an astronaut telling of his trip to Europeans in the fifteenth century who believed in a flat earth.

You do not have to be a nuclear physicist to understand atomic theory, but you do have to understand the basic principles of chemistry and physics - and the more depth of knowledge, the more than can be understood.

We know about atoms, and can understand molecular chemistry. But have we seen an individual atom ?

We rely on what we can see and believe some of what we are told. This forms the contextual framework that we use in our own life.

We can see light, and the things that it illuminates; we know that they are 'real'. Who has seen an X-ray or a radio wave ? We can observe an X-ray picture and listen to a radio - so we now know that they are real. But imagine trying to explain these energies to someone from a few centuries past !

Perhaps there are many more energies that we do not recognize, or do not understand. Our own reality is guided by our own belief system. If we have a fixed belief system then we cannot change.

Most of our belief system has been constructed from things that we have seen or been told - and what we were told may not be the real truth, only a belief that has been passed on.

It is important to keep an open mind, to accept that all that we are told may be believed by others - but may not be correct. We can include (or exclude) things in our own belief system as we decide.

Having an open mind enables ourselves to grow, to increase our knowledge and understanding of all things.

It may be that another person has 'hit on a truth' but finds it difficult to express correctly; by accepting that there 'may be some truth' in what you hear, your Intuition may 'feed you' the actual truth in a way that you can understand.

Prophecies

One of the big problems with prophecies is that prophets who could see pictures of the future had to understand what they were shown, and then try to explain their prophecies in terms that their contemporaries could understand.

Nostradamus saw pictures of wars in the 20th century - he told of Hitler (as Hisler - the German way of writing ?) and was precise about the death of Mussolini.

He described a submarine periscope as 'the eye of a dog' and a helicopter as 'oars against the wind'.

Nostradamus was a brilliant prophet, but due to fear of persecution he scrambled the time lines, which makes most of his prophecies useless as forecasts tied to any period of years.

Mother Shipton, who lived in northern England about the same time, kept the sequence correct - and most of her prophecies up to date have come true; use Google to see her work, and to get a forecast for the near future.

Have you ever heard the phrase *"It's a bunch of malarkey"* ? The Irish Church had St. Malarkey (1095-1148) (note spelling was not formalized in those days) who made a prophecy - he gave an identifier of each Pope to come in the future. For this and some other prophecies see **www.crystalinks.com/papalprophecies.html**.

Naturally the Church of Rome was not amused, doing its best to discredit the prophecy - even though the identifiers have proved correct in most cases. So any thing else which was discreditable was called *"a bunch of malarkey"*.

The last three elements of the prophecy (Pope John Paul II, his successor, and the end of the Church) are:

- **De Labore Solis** (Labour of the Sun) Pope John Paul II was born during a total eclipse of the sun.

- **De Gloria Olivae** (Glory of the Olive) the penultimate Pope. Pope Benedict - the colour olive is associated with the Benedictine Order.

- **Peter Romanus** (Peter of Rome) *"During the final persecution of the Holy Roman Church there will sit upon the throne Peter the Roman, who will pasture his flock in the midst of many tribulations. With these past, the city of the hills will be destroyed, and the awful judge will judge the peoples."*

Note that 'awful' is often used to describe something that is terrible (full of terror) or extremely bad; perhaps it also means 'full of awe' or 'to be held in awe, in high esteem'.

Many of the prophecies in religious books are probably correct, but told in language that could be understood at the time of writing, trying to describe what (at that time) was indescribable.

As shown above, the meaning of words has often changed with time; many works were passed down verbally, only to be in written form centuries later - and then translated into various languages.

Such translation often misses the nuances used in older times, and is subject to the bias of the translator who, for various reasons, may 'adjust' the context to conform with beliefs held.

ABOU BEN ADAM - Son of Adam

Abou ben Adam, may his tribe increase
Awoke one night from a dream of peace
And saw in the moonlight of his room -
Making it rich, like a lily in bloom -
An Angel writing in a book of gold.
Exceeding peace made Ben Adam bold
To the presence in the room he said
"What writest thou ?" - The Angel raised his head
And replied, with a look of sweet accord,
"The names of those who Love the Lord".
"And is mine one ?" spoke Abou. "Nay, not so"
Replied the vision. Abou spoke more low,
But cheerily still, and said: "I pray thee, then,
Write me as one who loves his fellow men"
The Angel wrote and vanished. The next night
It came again with a great waking Light
And showed the names whom Love of God had Blessed.
Lo ! Ben Adam's name led all the rest.

It is much Easier to Establish a New Science
Than to Change any Existing Scientific Belief.

Science and Beyond

Let us look at the basis of science. Later we will look at technology, which is different from science. In technology we accept that something works without having to prove how, and concentrate upon improving our skills of use.

Religious Influences

One of the major tragedies due to the extent of the authority throughout the western world of the Roman Catholic Church is the split between Science and Spirit. This is due to a battle between the 'flat earth people' and the 'roundheads'.

Although the wisdom of the East had always known that the earth was roundish and orbited the sun, in Europe the belief was that the world was flat - and that if you went too far you would fall off (which helped to explain losses of ships).

The Roman Catholic Church subscribed to the theory (actually their strong belief, not just a theory !) that the earth was the centre of the universe, and that all planets, suns, and stars revolved around the earth - in the heavens.

Young Galileo had a telescope, and was using it to look at the stars - which were in the heavens, the domain of the Church ! And this dreadful fellow was telling everybody who would listen that the Church was wrong !

Of course, with the threat of eternal damnation and lesser penalties, not too many did listen. But there were enough to start a movement to check this new fangled idea - and soon the evidence became overwhelming.

So much so that the Roman Catholic Church had to admit that Galileo was right (not, of course, that the Church was wrong).

Finally a deal was negotiated between the Church and these mad scientists - they could delve further into physical matters, so long as they did not poke their noses into anything spiritual.

All the European universities at that time (and for many succeeding centuries) were founded with close ties to the Church - and so this deal was enforced within these places of learning. If you wanted tenure, you 'toed the party line'.

This included supervising all research, so all became subject to 'proper scientific validation' - confined to the physical dimension.

Even today, if a scientist dares to explain things by associating them with the non-physical then he is subject to revile and his papers are not published. The 'peer review' system keeps present beliefs entrenched - changes could lower the prestige of the established leaders. 'Radical' leads to 'Ridicule'.

It is interesting to realize that many key inventions were made outside of university influence - Stephenson and his railway engine, the Wright brothers in flight, Edison and light bulbs, Marconi and radio waves, the Kirlians and auric photography, and many more.

Science needs to have everything explained - but scientists and physicists have been searching for the 'theory of everything' without success for many years. At the present time they are now realizing that they must look beyond the physical world, but have yet to accept that everything has intelligence.

Few people realize that although scientists (and 'the establishment') tell that they require 'scientific proof' before accepting any thing as 'existing', they fail their own criteria when dealing with electricity and magnetism.

They have to accept that the effects exist, and they know how to make magnets and electricity - but they do not know how this actually occurs within an atom; they do not know the detailed construction of an electron or the effects within an electron.

Scientists cannot find the 'Life Force' which is in all living creatures. They cannot examine or quantify God or the Angels, or the hidden forces of nature - except by Intuition. Albert Einstein (a self-confessed Dowser) tells how he came upon his special theory of relativity through Intuition.

We believe what we see. We see a piece of metal and know that it is made of solid matter. But when we use a microscope we see far more detail - not visible to our naked eyes. An electron microscope shows us the atomic level. The matter is not solid, but mainly space.

Perhaps changes are now in progress; physicists delving into sub-atomic particles are finding that they are having to investigate other dimensions to explain their observations - including the now established fact that their observations and beliefs affect the outcome of experiments !

Other Dimensions

One such well known experiment is the splitting of a photon by an electron - reforming it into 2 photons. Photons travel at the speed of light; when a photon is split, the two new photons are each travelling at the speed of light, but in opposite directions away from their original position.

A photon can be measured as a wave or as a particle. If either of the 'splits' is measured as a wave or as a particle, then it has been found that the other split can only be measured as the same wave or the same particle.

Somehow a message is passed from the first split to the second split *"I am measured as a wave (or particle)"* and determines the state for measurement of the second split.   And this message is received almost instantaneously.

The relative speed between the two splits is twice the speed of light - so the message, the thought of 'how I am measured', must travel at many times the speed of physical light !

So to investigate sub-atomic physics requires an acceptance that there are other dimensions. Electrons are found to 'be there' and then 'not be there' - perhaps moving between dimensions.

Mathematicians, trying to build a mathematical model of the universe, have found that at least 10 dimensions are needed. In the physical world we are aware of four - length, width, height, and time. They calculate that in a cubic centimetre of space there is the energy equivalent of 10^{94} (10^{94}) grams.

Speeds of Light

It is possible that the missing dimensions have higher wave speeds - for electrons, for light, and for thoughts. Perhaps each dimension has an influence on all that is in those dimensions that operate at slower speeds - and that the reverse is also true.

Lorenz's equation for the speed of light (the speed of all the electromagnetic spectrum) has two solutions - the one recognized as the speed of physical light, and one which incorporated the 'imaginary number' $\sqrt{-1}$, the square root of minus one.

Physicists have found that sub-atomic particles do not always follow the 'normal' rules of mathematics - and that some of them seem to use this $\sqrt{-1}$ as their normal mode of operation.

This second equation gives a speed of 'other light' as about the square of the speed of physical light (perhaps there is a factor of Π involved) - perhaps we do not see this spectrum because our eyes cannot cope with it. This may be the key to Einstein's equation $E=MC^2$ - where C has been accepted as the speed of physical light.

Because we cannot see it we cannot presume that it does not exist. This may well be the speed at which thoughts travel, and would account for electrons being there (or not there) as their constituent sub-forms move between dimensions.

Our minds, not found in the physical body, may well 'reside' in this higher dimension - operating at this higher speed - or even in higher dimensions having even greater 'speeds of light'.

Is this an explanation for 'Black Holes' ? Their mass attracts all physical matter, and they appear 'black' since no physical light can escape this gravitational pull.

But they may transform the attracted particles into such a higher dimension, having this much greater speed of 'non-physical light' so that they are no longer captive, and transmit them to the stars and space as a form of 'cosmic energy'.

Is it possible that our sun is not 'burning itself up', but acts as a transformer - taking this higher speed of light and transforming it back down to a lower speed that we see it as physical light ?

Earth Changes

If you take the continental shelves and fit them together without any oceans, they fit perfectly to a smaller sphere ! Is it possible that the cosmic radiations that are captured deep in the earth and over millions of years have caused the earth to grow ?

Perhaps the radiation such as sunlight which is captured by plants also contributes to the growth in size of the earth.

It is generally accepted that the end of the age of Dinosaurs was caused at the time of a major earth change - the 'horizon' of the earth at that time is marked by a deposit of chemicals strange to the rest of the earth - probably a deposit from 'space' that had a poisoning effect on life such as the Dinosaurs.

Immanuel Velikovsky was a student of Freud; he decided that the Oedipus Rex complex probably had a basis in the historical past, so set out to examine ancient stories and records.

In his searches he discovered that if the years assigned by archeologists to Egyptian dynasties were 'adjusted' by about 700 years, then the Egyptian records and the stories in the Bible corresponded even to the names of the individuals involved.

The 'opening' of the Red Sea, and the loss of the Egyptian armies by drowning were confirmed as actual happenings !

Velikovsky left his search for Oedipus Rex, and started research into the historical records of other nations of similar date. He found that there were records indicating a major shift in the heavens:

- In a pyramid were pictures of the 'sky before' and the 'sky afterwards' which indicated a shift of about twelve degrees of latitude.

- The Arabian astronomers were meticulous, but data from 'before' was ignored by the western world since it did not 'match' their understandings - so bad, if fact, that there were not any records of Venus ! In fact, 'venus' is the past participle of the latin verb 'to come' - 'it (etc) came'.

- In classical Greek times the people could see the twin moons of Mars, and even gave them names. Quite ridiculous, of course, since they were only discovered in the late 1800's with the development of high powered telescopes.

Velikovsky wrote 'Earth in Upheaval' and 'Worlds in Collision' to publicize his findings - and most of the scientific world laughed at him ! There were a few who had open minds, such as Albert Einstein, who even wrote a preface to one of the books.

These books indicate that a major earth change occurred within historical times ! Perhaps Venus was a moon of Jupiter, a satellite of Saturn, or a major asteroid that came as a twin tailed comet, nearly hit the earth, almost collided with Mars, and then took up an orbit as a planet - and changed the orbits of the Earth and Mars.

In these books Velikovsky gives scientific and historical proof of his theory. If shifts occurred in latitude due to changes in the solar system, then other effects might also be implied.

The geological appreciation of ice ages may not represent spreading and recession of ice caps, but relocation due to repositioning of the poles.

The movement of continents may be due to sudden major attractions of mass by large bodies that approach the earth - and the later gradual movements so be due to the momentum remaining.

Deposits of minerals may have been captured; perhaps oil, almost certainly bauxite - which in Jamaica overlays very recent coralline limestone, with no existing 'geological' source. The deposits of bauxite seem to form a band around the earth, so indicating deposition from 'elsewhere'.

It is also of interest that there are birds in Tasmania that still endeavour to migrate to Antarctica, following an ancient instinct that now only leads to their death.

Archeological finds indicate the presence of very advanced human beings millions of years ago; but since these conflict with accepted archeological doctrines they are hidden away and ignored.

Hindu records have a picture of 'Atlantian Flying Machines' and indicate pre-historical nuclear warfare.

Local records of Siberia and scientific examination of 'ground zero' indicate a nuclear explosion there in the early 1900's.

A map exists from medieval times in the middle east that is a good representation of Antarctica and the American continents - probably a reproduction of a far more ancient map.

So perhaps what people normally accept as the understanding of the world 'ain't necessarily so' - and should keep an 'open mind'.

Matter of Fact - or Fiction ?

When I went to school my chemistry teacher explained that each atom had a nucleus (of protons and neutrons) around which electrons orbited in bands - somewhat similar to the planets orbiting the sun in our solar system.

The early Theosophists, led by Leadbeater and Besant, were able, in the late nineteenth century, to visualize an atom as being a made of a number of smaller units - sub-atomic particles. Their research was published in a book 'Occult Chemistry'.

They were ridiculed, since everyone knew an atom could not be sub-divided; it was only with the advent of the electron microscope that they were proved correct.

Currently physicists favour a 'String Theory', where every sub-atomic particle is made of tiny string-like energies.

The modern 'String Theory' is still a failure (from a mathematical viewpoint) since the calculated mass-energy system of our universe is not in balance.

Perhaps this is because the other forms of energy, such as thoughts, life forces, and life forms in other dimensions have not been accounted.

If the 'String Theory' is even approximately true, it follows that each sub-element in a string must have a certain amount of intelligence - at least to the extent of knowing how to make the correct 'dance' in making its spiralling orbit, of thinking *"Am I doing the correct dance for this element ?"*, of understanding that the dances may change if the element is combined in a molecule, perhaps receiving or even calculating the needed instructions for such a growth or for interaction with other atoms and molecules.

Sub-Atomic Life

Leadbeater, the leader of the investigation by the Theosophists, visualized an atom as being a made of a number of sub-atomic particles, each sub-atomic particle having three Heart shaped smaller particles which they called 'Anu' - Sanskrit word: 'real atom'.

He reported that these Heart shaped Anu had variations of their polarity, in the positions within the sub-atomic particles, and in the directions that they pointed. This variation appears to influence their behaviour.

Each Anu is formed by ten core rings of continually moving and spiraling coiled strings - or whorls.

Each string is made of coiled strings (or spirilla) of even smaller size 'The Koilon' - there being seven layers of spirilla to form one string.

In each Anu, ten sets of strings were found, as shown overleaf. Three of these were slightly larger than the others.

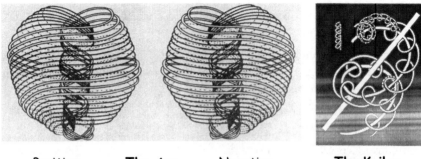

Positive   **The Anu**   Negative   **The Koilon**

In the three whorls flow currents of different electricities; the seven slightly smaller whorls vibrate in response to etheric waves of all kinds - to sound, light, heat, etc.

They show the seven colours of the spectrum; give out the seven sounds of the natural scale; respond in a variety of ways to physical vibration - flashing, singing, pulsing bodies; they move incessantly, inconceivably beautiful and brilliant.

Is it possible that the three slightly larger strings are associated with gravity, magnetism, and para-magnetism ?

A force (or flow of 'Life Energy' ?) pours into the heart-shaped depression at the top of the Anu, and issues from the point, and is changed in character by its passage (maybe it exchanged some 'Life Energy' ?).

This force rushes through every spiral and every spirilla, and the changing shades of colour that flash out from the rapidly revolving and vibrating Anu depend on the several activities of the spirals; sometimes one, sometimes another, is thrown into more energetic action, and with the change of activity from one spiral to another the colour changes.

Each of the Anu have three proper motions of its own, independent of any imposed upon it from outside:

- it turns incessantly upon its own axis, spinning like a top;
- it describes a small circle with its axis, as though the axis of the spinning top moved in a small circle;
- it has a regular pulsation, a contraction and expansion, like the pulsation of the heart.

When a force is brought to bear upon it, it dances up and down, flings itself wildly from side to side, performs the most astonishing and rapid gyrations, but the three fundamental motions incessantly persist.

If it be made to vibrate, as a whole, at the rate which gives any one of the seven colours, the whorl belonging to that colour glows out brilliantly.

An electric current brought to bear upon the Anu checks their proper motions, i.e., renders them slower; the Anu exposed to it arrange themselves in parallel lines, and in each line the heart-shaped depression receives the flow, which passes out through the apex into the depression of the next, and so on.

The advances in modern physics have not yet reached this level of understanding - it is accepted that sub-atomic particles have differences, and these have been measured; but no understanding has yet been achieved at the level of the Anu.

HYDROGEN H_2

Electrons

Although Leadbeater could see these fine coils of energy, he could not see an 'electron' - and yet this is the prime unit used in physics, chemistry, and science generally, and is measured in all electrical applications and investigations.

Leadbeater could see the effect of passing an electrical current (a flow of electrons) through matter - the Anu all 'lined up' in the direction of the flow.

As reported by physicists, electrons are found to 'be there', then 'not be there', and re-appear (or a replacement is found) somewhere else.

Using my 'message chart' (which is fully explained later in this book) I gathered some information about electrons.

I understand that an 'electron family' comprises in the order of 1,000,000,000,000 tiny 'Lights' - extremely small life forms that may form all space.

Their speed of movement as Lights is far greater than any other speed, so cannot be seen in the physical dimension - or in other auric dimensions, since they are above those levels.

It is only when they form larger 'groupings', as 'families of Lights', that their speed slows and enables them to be found.

This may help account for the 'black light' of physicists, and the missing parts of the equations formed by mathematicians when trying to define the universe.

The basic atomic weight of hydrogen (and other elements) as found by Leadbeater based on his exploration of the Anu is slightly different from the scientific value; is this due to him not including electrons ?

He describes a barrier (or bubble-like wall, similar to that of a bubble of air in water) that surrounds each atom, or each combination of atoms that are formed into a molecule.

My own understanding is that each Anu is associated with a 'free electron family'; I have the idea that electron families do the dances to form the spirilla in the Anu, and that the 'free electron families' of the Anu work together to 'dance' the barrier.

It may be that an 'electron family' does the 'barrier dance' and also goes into one of more of the spirilla (order of this is not known) so that they have experience of 'being' an Anu, of being in an atom, of taking part in the physical world, perhaps even being in an atom which is part of a plant or an 'animate' life form - the ultimate experience !

Atomic Auras

Leadbeater was able to 'see' that each atom had four levels of etheric aura. He describes these for the various elements, and 'Occult Chemistry' shows pictures of the different etheric auric levels - and how they combine from the universal Anu of the Astral plane to do the 'dance' of the element in the physical plane.

"Since observation shows us that each physical atom is represented by forty-nine astral atoms, each astral atom by forty-nine mental atoms, and each mental atom by forty-nine of those on the buddhic plane, we have here evidently several terms of a regular progressive series, and the natural presumption is that the series continues where we are no longer able to observe it."

It seems that all in the physical world is built from energies that exist in faster dimensions - the astral, the mental, the buddhic, and higher planes of existence. So it follows that all that exists in any plane is 'made' of energies from a higher plane.

The implication of this to us as human beings is that our own energies belonging to the higher levels are similar to all other life forms in those planes of existence.

If so, then these energies can communicate with each other ! In other words, our Mind, working within our own different auras, can communicate with all other energies (and Energy Beings) in those planes of existence, those auric levels.

Such other Energy Beings would include other Souls, Spirits, Devas, Angels, Arch Angels, Gods, (remember these are labels that we use - which may not be completely correct) and other life forms such as in the auras of insects, plants, water, minerals, animals, and the cells (and their component parts) within any such life form.

Occult Chemistry

There is much to be learnt from the book by Leadbeater & Besant called 'Occult Chemistry'; it describes each element (some not even known when the book was written, of which a few have since been discovered and accepted by science) including the reasons for their valency and weights, and structural forms - the 'platonic solids' of Sacred Geometry.

Oxygen is an exception; it has the shape of a double helix, like DNA strands: *"On the E4 level the two snakes divide.   The positive and negative snakes each consist of 55 duads (pairs of Anu) and 5 brilliant discs (of 7 Anu) .... "*

It is very interesting to see that there are only a few basic shapes, that the most basic are the form of a particular 'light' element, and that the 'heavy' elements are formed using 'building bricks' of the patterns existing in the lighter elements.

For example, mercury includes the patterns of gold, selenium, chlorine, and tellurium; the dance patterns of the components become part of a larger 'dance set' - to form the structural shape of the new element.

"The elements have definite shapes.   With a few exceptions all the elements fall into 7 groups or forms; the groups were named: Spikes, Dumb-bell, Tetrahedron, Cube, Octahedron, Crossed-bars, and Star.

Valency can be subdivided, that is to say an atom with valency 1 can divide itself into two halves, each exercising 1/2 valency. Hydrogen divides itself into 2 or 6 parts each with 1/2 or 1/6 valency when it enters into combinations. Similarly, elements having valencies 2, 3 or 4 can subdivide.

The valency has some connection, with the shape. Divalent elements are predominantly tetrahedra, trivalent elements cubes, and quadrivalent octahedra.

When one element combines with another the atoms almost always break up. The combination is not of one atom with another as a whole, but the component parts are re-arranged to form a complex structure."

This has much similarity to the formation of molecules comprising different elements: *"In salt, Sodium and Chlorine are interblended in such a manner as to give to the compound the outline of a cube."*

Perhaps the difference is in the stability of the result - a molecule changes with chemical reaction, whilst an element remains unchanged.

When dealing with Phenol (or Carbolic Acid) intelligence was noted:

"Mr Leadbeater touched the top of the bottle with his finger, smelt it, and then touched his gum with it. Evidently there was some point of infection in his gum, for as he touched the spot with the Phenol something happened that made him laugh.

On my inquiring, he said that the Oxygen left the Hydrogen to do its work of disinfection. But, as it left, it experienced a little thrill of delight, for the oxygen had been held as a prisoner in the Hydroxyl group.

But when the opportunity came to break the bondage and be free once again there was a clear sense of relief, of duty done, and furthermore the sense 'Now I can Die in Peace'.

The feeling was slight, but there is an interesting side to all this - the side of the feelings of the chemicals involved."

Note that this intelligence seems to have come from the oxygen atom - the only atom with a double helix form.

Holographic Fields

Rupert Sheldrake suggests that we exist in 'metamorphic fields' where all that has ever occurred is in continual vibration as 'standing waves', which others have likened to a 'holographic universe'.

Is it possible that these 'Lights', having experienced the physical world in 'electron families', return to 'unassigned space' carrying with them memories of their experiences ? Do they form the 'metamorphic fields' of a 'holographic universe' ?

The Periodic Law
(after Crookes)
Showing a progression similar to the swing of a Pendulum

Note that some of these elements have still not been discovered. Some
found since this diagram was made have had different names assigned.

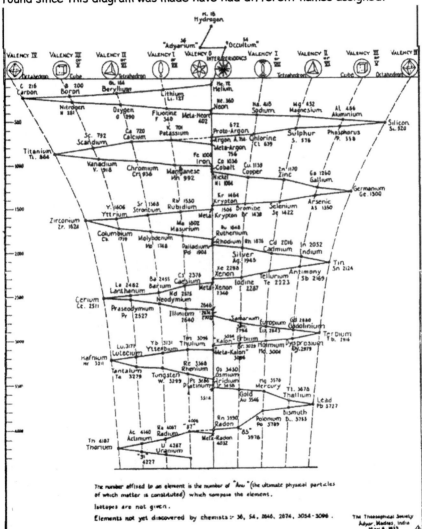

The valency lines show values of 0, 1 or 7, 2 or 6, 3 or 5, and 4; the lower
values relate to the elements on the line from the centre going outwards,
the higher value being for the return swing; They increase from lighter to
heavier - from top to bottom on the diagram.   The intrinsic structural
shape seems to depend on the valency of the element,

THE PERIODIC LAW
A Spiral Representation

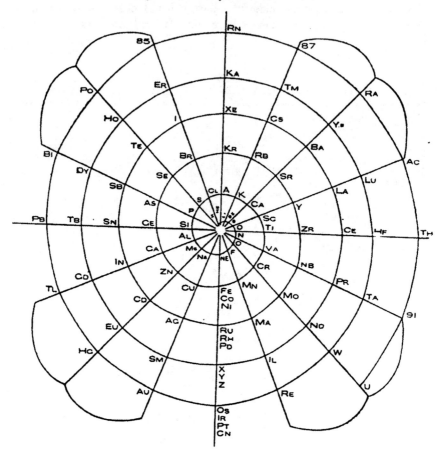

When Kristina Nielsen was shown this diagram, she put her hand over it and exclaimed "It is tremendously powerful - I can feel the energy funnelling into the palm of my hand from the centre !"

Kristina described the energy as coming in at the heavy elements and being channeled to the centre - rather like a rotary pump operating in reverse, to suck water from the outside and force it out of the centre point.

I wonder if the 4 'petals' are like those of a Chakra ! What would this be like in three dimensions ?

It is probable that our Intuition is our own link to such metamorphic fields (remember that this is just a label that we use for description) including the fields formed by the thought patterns of others.

By having a particular thought we may send out such a pattern which then seeks to find other patterns that are similar; this is the 'Like likes Like' behaviour that has been recognized in many ways.

So we may be able to 'tap into' the thoughts (and past thoughts) of other people that have similarities to our own thoughts, without knowing those people, or them being aware of the linkage.

Birds and Bees

It is interesting to consider the action of a flock of birds - they all change direction together, as if one mind was controlling them all. This behaviour also occurs with schools of fish.

Bees are wonderful little insects; the individual bee has a short life, but the memories of the bees have been shown to last for far longer than the life of a bee. This is the 'hive' effect - where the mind is of the whole hive, not just the individual bee.

Ants provide another example of a group mind - even when building an ant hill from both sides, the pieces are put together to give a perfect fit without visual co-ordination.

Perhaps human beings are also subjected to group minds - such as belonging to the family, the community, the work group, and the various organizations with which they are associated.

The group mind may be temporary - such as that generated by a powerful speaker at a mass rally (Hitler was a prime example) or by the spectators at a sports meeting.

Thoughts

When we have a thought, get a feeling, or express an emotion, we broadcast it to 'All that Is', as do all animals, reptiles, insects, and plants.

The strength of the signal sent out may be weak, so that it may best be received locally. It may be directed at a particular recipient, and so go by a more focused path - a casual thought may be weak, but an intense thought can have a profound effect, as is found in Healing work.

Perhaps the unimportant broadcasts are dissipated over time, but those that 'The System' (which seems to be the controlling factor in 'Upstairs', in charge of all actions that are taken) considers to be noteworthy seem to be stored - added to 'The System's' store of knowledge or retained as memories in any stones or crystals affected.

On the basis of 'Like attracts Like' similar thoughts would group together; although memories of a person or incident may dissipate over time, new thoughts of that person or incident may reinforce the existing group and extend its group life.

A thought that is broadcast is like a pebble thrown into a pond - it sends ripples that travel the whole surface, perhaps meeting other ripples and changing to jointly form an interference pattern, similar to that used in a hologram.

We, and 'All that Is', receive these complicated interference patterns; from our interpretation of these interference patterns we formulate our own actions.

Thus each thought that we have (and broadcast) has a potential effect in the future, both our future and that of others.

Any thought, etc., that we broadcast is sent out as a symbol; my thought, if in English, is translated into a set of symbols; a Chinese speaking recipient gets the symbols, and his sub-conscious reacts; if considered to be important to his conscious self then the symbols are probably translated into his Chinese dialect.

However it does seem that our vocabulary and verbal structure do have a great influence on our thinking processes; thus a person who speaks only an alphabetically based language has a different 'context' for thoughts than somebody speaking a language based on symbols.

An alphabetically based language is more precise - a symbolic one relies on associations, perhaps similar to the way our mind-brain team operates.

Thus it is seen that language is not a barrier. Plants and animals also communicate using these same symbols, which helps to explain Cleve Backster's experiments.

Cleve Backster's Experiments

Some years ago the lie detector specialist Cleve Backster became interested in plants.

He decided to test how long it took for water in a plant pot to reach the top leaf in a plant which was dry, so he attached a lie detector to the top leaf.

Backster was amazed to see that the lie detector indicated happiness as soon as it was attached, even though no water had been added.

He then wondered if the plant would give an unhappy signal if he set the leaf on fire - and was astounded that the plant gave that unhappy signal as soon as he had the thought ! This experiment has been well publicized both in books and on television.

Later, detectors connected to his plants in California were able to indicate his emotional state when he visited New York.

In other experiments, detectors connected to blood samples (mainly water) have been shown to fluctuate with the emotional state of their donors when miles away, and continue to do so for a number of hours. See 'The Secret Life of Your Cells' by Robert B. Stone - Whitford Press, ISBN 0-914918-96-6 for more fascinating details !

Water - and Dr Emoto's Crystals

Dr Masaru Emoto in Japan has spear-headed the investigation of water crystals subjected to various thoughts - that they hold the vibrational pattern of the thoughts. See the web site:

www.life-enthusiast.com/twilight/research_emoto.htm

When he took two samples of the same distilled water and wrote 'Hitler' on one and 'Mother Theresa' on the other, the crystal from the Hitler sample was distorted - the one of Mother Theresa was beautifully formed.

He played different music to water as it crystallized - heavy metal and rock music caused mis-shapen crystals, while the music of Bach yielded well formed crystals.

Incredibly, when the water was from cultures of flower essences, the distinctive patterns of the flowers could be seen - their vibrationary patterns !

Crystals were formed from water taken from a large and polluted lake before and after a Japanese blessing service; they changed from being distorted to having a beautiful shape, matching the change observed in the lake itself.

About 70% of the weight of a human body is water; this helps to explain the changes in a human when subjected to various thoughts from other people - and your own thoughts.

Blessing is a variation of a thought - and food is mainly water. So when you Bless 'what you consume' you actually improve its value to yourself. Check how the aura changes !

Hitler   'The Message From Water'   Mother Theresa

Before Prayer   Fujiwara Dam   After Prayer

Dr Masaru Emoto   "Thank You"

All Animals are Equal
But Some are More Equal than Others
George Orwell, 'Animal Farm'

The Human Being

We believe what we can see. When we see another human being we see their face, their clothes, and other parts of the body that are not hidden. We see movements and expressions which we can interpret as signals.

But our sight is limited to a small range of the electro-magnetic spectrum, that which includes the colours of the rainbow; we cannot see infra red or ultra violet light, although the effects of light in these colours can be observed.

Some people can see more - and they report that our bodies are surrounded by auras, and that there are flows and patterns of different colours in the various parts of our auras.

Western medicine considers the body to be a bio-electro-chemical system, with various organs that can be dissected and sometimes exchanged, like using spare parts to repair an automobile or computer.

Eastern wisdom accepts that there are systems that cannot be seen, but are crucial to a person's health and well-being.

Both are correct - but the body is more than even the combination of these views. Life force is recognized as existing, but has never been examined; and many religions believe that we 'have a Soul' without being able to describe it completely.

Perhaps it is more correct to know that each of us is a Soul that is having an experience in a human body.

Ships of 'Being'

How can we describe ourselves ? Are we like ships sailing the oceans of existence ? If so, then our Conscious Self would be the Captain, leaving the routine running of our bodies to the officers and petty officers such as our sub-conscious, our glands and organs, our limbs, and our nervous, muscular, and other systems.

Our Heart, our ego, our sub-conscious, the logical and the intuitive parts of our thinking team - they are like the senior officers; very often they do not 'get on' with each other - or the Captain !

Perhaps they have been trying to get their viewpoint to the Captain without success, so are 'taking action' to get their message noticed, which may be disrupting the operation of our ship (causing sickness ?) and spoiling our voyage through life.

Each ship has a communications centre, which in our case may be the intuitive part of our thinking team, equipped with many radio receivers to listen to numerous broadcasts; but most of these do not concern the ship, or are of general interest.

Imagine the communications officer getting an enormous number of such messages; he has to decide which are important, and to whom they should be sent - and not many end up on the Captain's table. Perhaps the Captain has asked for information or help, and some of these messages may be to guide him, but unknown to the communications officer - so are not forwarded.

Some may be sent to the bridge, but the First Mate (the logical part of our thinking team) may not like them, think that they are not important, or try to deal with them himself - or putting his own 'twist' on the report to the Captain.

It seems that the main priority is to get the ship's crew to work together - in Peace, Harmony, and Love. Balancing the left and right sides of our brain is often meant as getting the logical and intuitive parts of our thinking team to be better 'team mates'.

Telling all parts of our Being that we love them and appreciate all that they do for us is similar to the Captain speaking to all the crew, to help get them all working together for the overall benefit of the ship.

The help and co-operation of the Chief Petty Officer is critical - he leads the crew; perhaps we may recognize him as our Heart.

Having the ship in good order and the crew working well together helps us in stormy weather and when sailing in dangerous waters !

Often the ship sails to new ports, where customs and language differ; and we meet other vessels on the way. We may exchange energies with some, tell them about places we have visited, or let them know of any revisions to the charts used for navigation.

When we set sail we seldom know where we are going in life - we may have 'sealed orders' from pre-birth, or be pushed off course by storms or incorrect charts.

Some other ships may signal that they have messages or supplies for us, and others may be flying flags which tell us to beware.

Occasionally a ship may appear to be friendly, but turn out to be run by pirates; in such cases having good communications can help to get good guidance from the Admiralty - perhaps a   friendly warship for protection, or even a flight of Angels overhead !

'Know Thyself'

Atoms form the cells of our bodies; a body which is alive has more than just atoms - it has a life force which has defied all scientific attempts to locate or define it, perhaps a Grand Form of Love.

In the previous chapter we examined how over one hundred years ago Leadbeater and Besant were able to describe the different atoms and their sub-atomic particles - the existence of these only being confirmed by scientists many years later when electron microscopes were developed.   And we saw pictures of how water responds to thoughts.

Perhaps all that exists is made by very tiny 'Beings' - 'Lights', 'Baby Energies' - each of which can Feel, Love, Think, and Act to a limited degree. Perhaps they form 'All that Is' by doing different dances at selected frequencies of vibration and at various speeds.

The larger the concentration (and the greater the complexity of their organization) of these 'Beings' then the greater their potential ability to Feel, Love, Think, and Act.

If this be so, then it explains the old wisdom that 'We are All the Same' - made by 'dance teams' of the same 'baby energies' in various combinations of inter-related dances.

I may be incorrect in my understanding, but such a hypothesis goes a long way to explaining how plants and pets can communicate with humans and how memories can be retained in objects and used by many 'psychics' to give readings.

It also explains how we, as human beings, can communicate with life forms that operate in different dimensions, including Angelic Energy Beings - to which we apply various labels.

Auras and Chakras

There are many reports from people who are clairvoyant that our bodies have auras, and that there are 'objects' in these auras which can affect a person.

Since these objects can be seen, they have form - and have been described as 'thought forms'; it seems that the shape and associated colours have direct meaning, and that when similar thought forms are seen in different people, the observed effects are similar.

A brilliant thought form has usually been found to be beneficial; intrusions of dark colours (including browns, blacks and grays) usually indicate a problem.

There are many reports that problems are so indicated in the auras of people long before a physical illness occurs; similarities in the location, shape, and colour of non-beneficial thought forms have been found to pre-date later manifestations of similar illnesses.

The ancient wisdom is that each human body has 'Chakras', shaped somewhat like microwave aerials and so acting to receive signals - from auras, our environment, and the cosmos.

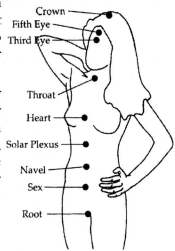

We have personal patterns within our own Being that also help to define our future actions. These may come from past lives, pre-natal impressions, childhood memories, things that we were taught, our analysis of our experiences, and our expressed dreams and hopes. These seem to be stored in our auras and our bodies.

Major Chakras in our Lower Body
from 'Kundalini and the Chakras'
by Genevieve Paulson
Llewellyn New Age
ISBN 0-87542-592-5
A book well-worth reading !

If you send good thoughts to a person, their aura will expand. This happens even if they are thousands of miles away. What you send comes back - so avoid hurting others by having bad thoughts (malice, jealousy, anger, hate, etc) about them.

It is recognized by many that a human is sensitive to the auras of another person, and in some cases to the memories carried in these auras or in the cellular memories of a person.

Sometimes when we meet a person for the first time we move forward in our body towards him (s/he is attractive in some way), or bend backwards slightly to get away (perhaps our Being has found something undesirable or incompatible).

Intuition includes the ability to receive these broadcasts and to respond to these auric interactions, processing them in the intuitive part of our thinking team, and making sense of them with the help of the logical part of our thinking team.

Hidden Energy Systems

Ancient Chinese wisdom is that there are a number of meridians running throughout a body that carry energies around a person. They have found that blockages in the meridian system are causes of ill health, and that most of these blockages occur at junction points.

Using acupuncture (inserting needles) or acupressure (applying pressure) such blockages are removed and the movement of energies is restored - and good health returns.

It may also be that the meridian system is not confined to the physical body - that similar energy paths exist within the auras, and that there are points where these paths enter and leave the physical body.

Kirlian photography of auras has shown that energy discharges do occur at certain places - and that these points are associated with the meridian system.

This meridian system is similar to (but not the same as) the lymph system which is also carrying energies and is subject to blockages - which can be released by tapping the lymph points or 'Sore Spots'; This is described as part of the EFT procedure - see www.emofree.com for full details.

The healing of these hidden energy systems may be temporary; it seems that many health problems are caused by thoughts - such as anger leading to heart and liver problems.

Unless action is taken to release the emotions linked to such thoughts (and their associated thought forms) the ill health will return. When we hold anger, hate, or similar emotions, we hurt ourselves !

The Role of our Sub-Conscious

Very few people really understand the sub-conscious - and how it relates to the rest of our Being. The models used vary between different psychologists and psychiatrists. Many of these are based on the works by Freud and Jung, but nowadays these models have been found to be deficient, and so others are being developed.

One model which is very ancient and has been proven to work over a very long time is the model used in Polynesia in general, and in Hawaii in particular by the Kahunas of Huna fame.

For a detailed explanation read Serge Kahili King's book 'Kahuna Healing'. This tells how we have the Heart aspect, Ku; Mind aspect, Lono; and Spirit aspect, Kane.

The Ku, our sub-conscious self

The Ku is primarily concerned with the human body, with genetic memories stored in the cells, and 'personal' memories stored in the muscles - in those muscles most associated with the action used in the development of the memory.

Serge notes that it is impossible to express emotions, be angry, or have fear if the body is completely relaxed.

The importance of a memory is decided on the amount of emotion generated by the incident, and indexed for retrieval by the type of emotion and the type of incident.

Our sub-conscious self tends to evaluate current situations by comparison with memories stored, and then creates a reaction based on actions occurring in such memories.

In many ways the Ku can be compared to a computer - having its master programs (beliefs and instincts), subsidiary programs (reactions and habits), and access to memories (both for storage and retrieval).

It finds it difficult to differentiate between imagination and fact, so if we have memory of an incident that is causing problems, we can retrieve the memory and change in our memory both what occurred and the outcome - success being accorded by the degree of visualization achieved and the amount of emotion that we now attach to the changed situation.

The Lono, our Thinking Mind

The prime role of the Lono is to make decisions - where to focus attention, evaluate a situation, consider available responses, choose which action to take, and decide the best method of implementation.

It is your conscious self which is aware of all our senses and the events that are happening to us - and what we imagine or forecast may happen.

It has the ability to accept perceptions as facts - and thus form the master program based on beliefs that are accepted as being correct: *"So long as it believes itself to be powerless, it will act according to that belief."*

When a perception is accepted as an unalterable fact, then they are not seen as 'beliefs' which can be changed - and so much effort is needed for them to be amended. Many of these were so accepted before we developed the ability to make judgements - and judgements tend to be based on 'facts' and 'beliefs', so forming a vicious circle.

To amend a program requires persuading the Ku that a change is needed, and to carefully specify the actual change - by thought as creative imagination implemented by visualization and emotion.

The Kane, our Spirit Aspect

Serge describes the Kane as a 'source' aspect, an essence which manifests or projects into reality our physical Being; it is a sub-set of an even greater source or essence.

He gives the primary function as being creativity in the form of mental and physical experience, focused on keeping you 'on track' with your life's purpose. This is accomplished externally by working in co-ordination with other levels to 'make things happen' such as creating situations and opportunities, and internally by Intuition, working through our 'Soul Senses' to help us on our path - if we are open to such guidance.

It does not tell you 'what to do' - but will assist you if you will learn from the experiences offered. In some aspects it is like a 'teacher' - creating a setting for a lesson, giving information if requested, but expecting you to make your own decisions.

Triune Man - An integrated Model

In Kahuna understanding man is a Spiritual Being with the three aspects of Kane, Lono, and Ku; when these are in an ideal state, they work together as one 'Triune Being', able to express the full potential.

For various reasons disunity occurs, with a breakdown in communication, and a lessening of effectiveness. The Kahuna approach is to re-unite the Lono and Ku - and then re-union with Kane also occurs.

It may be that this model should be expanded to five basic levels - the God level, the Higher Self, the Conscious Self, the Sub-Conscious Self, and the physical body, operated primarily by the Sub-Conscious Self.

The God level ('The System') is all-powerful, and can do most things - but is very busy doing the most important things, so does not listen to all the 'chatter' that occurs from individuals.

The Higher Self can be considered to be our Guardian - always aware of what we are doing, but seldom interfering - except (sometimes) in an emergency.

The Conscious Self is our Soul having an experience in a human body. There are a number of reasons why it does not have all its abilities, may not have ready access to some Soul senses, and is heavily influenced detrimentally by ego. Is this the penalty (or the price paid) for being awarded the prestigious gift of experience in a human body ?

The Conscious Self gives lots of orders, some of which are not really understood; it has a major problem in that in many cases it has great difficulty communicating directly with the Higher Self or the God level.

The Sub-Conscious Self (a label for perhaps a motley group of Beings that sometimes do not work together harmoniously !) can be considered to understand things at the level of a four or five year old child.

This may account for it not understanding some of the orders received from the Conscious Self ! But it has one great ability - it is in communication with the Higher Self.

So if we request help from 'The System' we must first of all decide exactly what is wanted and express it in simple and non-contradictory terms.

Next we must then persuade our Sub-Conscious that we are really sincere about getting the help - explaining clearly and precisely what is requested, and 'willing' that our Sub-Conscious ask this help from the Higher Self.

If our Higher Self is 'happy' about the request (that it will help the Human learn a lesson, or be of help to others, for example) then it will ask 'The System' to give the required assistance.

It seems as if our Sub-Conscious, Higher Self, and 'The System' are all so busy doing things that they only act if something is expressed as being done 'now'.

If it is stated in the past then it is ignored. If it is 'in the future' then they consider that no action is needed now - only in some vague and undefined future time ! So it is most important that all this asking is to happen 'NOW'.

All these models are human attempts to understand the 'inner workings' of humanity. They may not be completely correct, and some may not work well. The Huna model has been used for a great many centuries, and has a proven working history.

We are Not Alone !

Most religions preach that there is a God - or more than one; many hold that humans have 'Guardian Angels'; some accept that we have 'Spirit Guides'.

These are all labels that humans use - and the labeling may not be correct, or acceptable to some. But the essence is that all have a belief that there is a power greater than humans, and that there are 'Energy Beings' who work with us in some way.

Many incidents have been reported where help was given in unusual (and sometimes miraculous) ways.

It may also be true that there are energy beings who are not helpful, that are causing problems to us - and also to the rest of creation.

So we need to find ways to get help from the 'Good Guys' and to prevent the 'bad beings' from interfering with our lives - and the lives of those dear to us.

If we try to protect ourselves by just our own efforts, there is a high probability that we will not succeed. When we ask the help of our friends - the Good Guys - then we know that all will be well.

It seems that help is given most readily when we ask help for others; and when we express our gratitude for help given, this encourages more help to be offered !

Our Heart-Mind-Brain Team

Research has shown that the Heart has its own complement of Neurons - not as many as the Brain, but enough to be effective.

There have been a number of reports that people who have received Heart transplants become aware of memories from the donor, even to the extent of changing likes and dislikes, and altering life patterns.

It seems that your Heart is your best access to your Intuition, your link to 'The System' - which includes 'Upstairs' (non-physical influences outside of yourself), 'Downstairs' (the organs and cells within your body), as well as the level at which you normally operate, such as other people, animals, plants, and nature in general.

Little is known about the human Mind; it has not been found within the Brain, in spite of many attempts. Perhaps the Mind is outside the human body, and associated with the auras that surround humans.

The role of the Mind seems to be to operate the higher levels of the Brain - to decide the jobs that should be done, seek resources that are needed, and approve decisions prior to implementation. Perhaps the Soul, the Conscious Self, gives leadership to the Mind.

Sometimes the Mind is by-passed, such as when an emergency occurs and the 'flight or fight' mechanism takes direct control of the Brain; research has shown that such actions originate in the lower levels of the Brain before any response can register in the higher levels.

There are various parts of the Brain, such as the reptilian and animal sections, and the more recently developed 'higher brain' found only in humans and in a few other mammals.

Each part seems to have its own functions, but when damage occurs other parts have been found to take over the jobs of the damaged part in a number of cases.

The most important parts of the Brain (in this study) are the right and lefts parts of the higher Brain - sometimes labeled our logical and intuitive parts.

It seems that the logical part of our Brain is the home of our ego - which believes that it 'knows it all'. So one task when using our Intuition is to prevent interference by the egoistic logical Brain.

Brain Waves

Science has recognized four major ranges of Brain waves; there may be a fifth range, over 24 cps, about which very little is known.

Name	cps	Associated Activity
Delta	0 - 4	Sleep - Deep Inner Conscious
Theta	4 - 7	Sleep - Painless Surgery - Thought - Inner Conscious
Alpha	7 - 14	Sleep - Meditation - Thought - Inner Conscious
Beta	14 - 24	Action - Outer Conscious Level - Physical Senses

It has been observed that as a human, growing from a baby to become an adult, passes through these ranges in sequence.

It seems that a person's intuitive ability becomes enhanced when in the meditative state, having Brain waves in the Alpha range - and that 10 cps, being close to the centre of that range, is a good target to select.

These Brain waves are not exclusive - different parts of a person's Brain can be operating at speeds different from other parts. A Zen Master can be operating in Theta, Alpha, and Beta at the same time, and Spiritual Healers can exceed the Zen Master by operating in Delta as well as all other speeds.

With training, most people can develop the ability to operate in Alpha and Beta at the same time, but it is best to start by getting into Alpha by itself.

A metronome can be used to signal this rate, tapes are sold which guide your Brain to so operate, and musical CD's have been developed to take you directly 'into Alpha'.

Often our Intuition is most active just as we go to sleep or awaken. This is when we pass through the Alpha and other brain wave states. With practice we can 'get into' Alpha state when fully awake - and so be better able to work with our Intuition.

If you are going somewhere you usually prepare first, for example by dressing appropriately.

Similarly if you want to have good Intuition then it helps to get ready - by relaxing, by being sincere, and by getting into Alpha state.

Breathing

Breathing can be most helpful to you. By concentrating on your breath you tend to clear your mind, especially if you take good, deep breaths through your nose.

Dr Marcia Emery in her 'Intuition Workbook' suggests a way of using your breath to improve your intuitive abilities:

- <u>Feel (with your consciousness, your awareness)</u> the incoming breath at the top of your nose while drawing it down deeply into your solar plexus. <u>This is probably the most important part.</u>
- When this area is full, expand your lungs to get more air.
- During all this time say a long 'Hang' while breathing in.
- Slowly move your consciousness down to your solar plexus, and then exhale through your mouth while saying 'Sah'.

The slower and deeper that you breathe, the more relaxed you become; this is an excellent method of helping your self-control in situations that you find to be troublesome.

This breathing technique, especially when done slowly and with deep breathes, can help you relax and get into Alpha.

Choa Kok Sui, in his book 'Pranic Healing', emphasizes that it is important to hold your breath, for a short time, at the end of both inhalation and exhalation - this increases the flow of Prana.

An additional help is to use your visualization while doing this exercise. With each in-breath, imagine that plenty of Pranic life force, with healing energy and all that is good for you, comes in and is distributed throughout your body.

When you reach the ends of your body, start a return journey, imagine collecting all the stress, tension, and problems that beset you; as you exhale, send out all you have collected to be Healed and recycled for good.

Dr Samuel Sagan, MD, in his book 'Awakening the Third Eye', suggests that vibrating your throat just behind and below the Adam's Apple is a great benefit in speeding the transition into a meditative state.

This is similar to the way that many mystic schools teach that when calling on any Spiritual Being by name, you should vibrate that name.

He suggests that this is done by making a buzz like a bee when breathing in and out, and keeping your back straight and head upright.

If you find it difficult to make a buzz on the intake, it may be best to use the 'hang' sound, and use 'zzz' on the out breathe.

Barbara Ann Brennan and others suggest vibrating the top of throat and soft palate. It seems that the more vibration that can be developed the greater the effect.

Variations on breathing include different counts while inhaling, holding, exhaling, and resting - and these are so shown in that order: Choa Kok Sui in 'Pranic Healing' suggests 1-1-1-1, 7-1-7-1, 6-3-6-3.

Jack Schwartz, of the Alethia Foundation, tells how you can use controlled breath to produce specific states of consciousness:

> Beta: 1-1-1-1;
> Alpha: 8-8-8-4;   Alpha/Theta: 4-8-8-4;
> Theta: 4-8-16-4;   Delta: 4-8-32-4

Yogic practice includes nostril alternation, where breath is taken through one nostril and exhaled via the other - and then repeating with the nostrils switched. Thumbs are used to block the unused nostril.

We are Energy Beings !

Physicists have shown that each atom is made of sub-atomic particles, all of which are forms of energy.

Such atoms combine to form molecules - and the properties of molecules differ from that of their components.

For example, hydrogen and oxygen are gases - they combine to form water which has different freezing and boiling points from the constituent elements, and can be drunk and used for cooking. When combined with other elements the properties can change to be acidic or alkaline.

The cells of our body are made from molecules - and controlled by the molecular structures that form our DNA; viruses are tiny sub-sets of DNA portions that can interfere with our own DNA in cells and cause sickness.

It seems that for animate life to exist, a form of DNA is required; conversely the DNA structure itself has a form of life - and this is so for even the sub-microscopic sized viruses.

Our body cells form all our bones, flesh, organs, nerves, neurons, and blood - our physical Being is all made of these energies doing different jobs, like teams of dancers making different dance patterns at varying speeds.

A body may have its full complement of DNA and cellular structures, but may not be alive - so there is more to life than just energy cells and electro-magnetism.

This is confirmed by the auras of people; a person whose aura is badly damaged, misshapen, extremely dark, or missing probably has little 'life force'.

Edgar Cayce was about to enter an elevator, when he noticed that he could not see any aura around any of the other people waiting to descend. He stood back, and so did not get killed with those who rode the elevator to their death when it crashed.

Cayce's record in distant Healing of people that he had never met personally also proves (to all except those who rely totally on the 'must be repeatable' proofs of non-spiritual science) that energies are involved that are not of the physical dimension, although they may operate in it.

Some people, such as Cayce, may be able to see some of these energies some of the time. Most of us do not have this ability - but we cannot see radio waves either, yet know that they exist, because we can hear their effect on a radio receiver.

Currently people know much more than those who lived a hundred years ago about the cosmos, this earth, and how electro-magnetic energies work.

But we do not know it all ! And the biggest gap in our knowledge concerns other dimensions of existence.

We have a choice - we can believe that the physical dimension is the total of all creation, or we can accept that there are other dimensions.

If we choose to have an open mind, we can endeavour to improve our knowledge and understanding of such other dimensions, and find ways to work with the various energies that operate in them.

A good starting point is close to home - so let us have a closer look at ourselves and those with whom we mingle, at home, at work, and at play.

The Illusions of Stage Magicians Fool our Eyes
'All Life is an Illusion' the Heart then Cries !

We are Psychic !

Before you close this book in disgust, are you sure that you understand what is meant by 'Psychic' ?

'Psychic' means 'belonging to, or associated with, the Psyche'.

Looking in Webster's dictionary, Psyche is a Greek word meaning Soul or Mind.

So if you are not Psychic, does this mean that you lack a Soul - or that you are Mindless ?

Since we know that we are a Soul (or some sort of 'other dimensional' Energy Being) that is having an experience in a Human Being in the physical dimension, it is possible that our Soul has some sensing abilities that differ from those of the physical human body.

If the Soul is associated with the Human Being, then perhaps some senses belonging to the Soul are used - even without the Human Being's awareness of such use.

The Human Being may be so accustomed to these senses being used that they do not realize that the senses are those of the Soul, and not those of a 'normal' Human Being.

Successful Teachers

People who are recognized as being successful in teaching or in persuading others to accept their point of view are those who know that some people have a strong sense of 'seeing' (It looks good), of 'feeling' (It feels good), of 'hearing' (Sounds good to me), or of just 'knowing' (I know it is good).

So to get their message to reach all their students they express their teachings in different ways - so that every person that listens has the message told in ways that appeal to them.

Notice that normally the human senses of tasting, smelling, and of balancing are not used - although there are some people who can taste music, or smell colours.

Let us examine the way that such people operate.

Feelers

People who have a strong sense of feeling often get that feeling in the area known as the 'Solar Plexus' - hence the popular expression of 'having a gut feeling about ...'

People naturally turn their body to face objects or people when they want to sense them more deeply; when people feel uncomfortable they often cross your arms in front of their solar plexus area to feel more protected and less vulnerable.

If a Feeler walks into a room where there has been an argument or some other severe discord, the Feeler instantly knows that the 'atmosphere' in the room is 'bad' - and perhaps may get a hint as to the cause.

They will get a 'Danger Ahead' feeling if there are problems with being in a place or with a person that can lead to trouble; they are aware of the 'not good' subtle energies.

Feelers are sensitive to the feelings of others, both good and bad, so they find it hard to remain detached from others. They are 'people people' who give of themselves, and adapt themselves to keep others happy.

They are usually living in the 'now', and so not be too concerned with time; deadlines can wait !

When with a person who is angry about something, a Feeler will know that the anger is there, and often assume incorrectly that the anger is directed at the Feeler.

If a Feeler is in close contact with a person that is sick, the Feeler may often feel the pain - and assume that it is him/her self that is becoming ill.

The biggest problem is learning to understand that many of the feelings that they have are those of others, not their own. Failing this lesson, they can become emotionally overwhelmed.

Hearers

One of the main indications that you are a 'Hearer' is 'talking with yourself' - actually you may be discussing things with thinking life forms that are within your own mind; this is especially so when you hear a response that you did not originate.

Often these thoughts, words, or phrases seem to come from the centre of you head, as an 'inner sound'. A song may keep playing in your mind - perhaps it is hinting at a solution to a problem, or guiding you to take a particular action, either based on the words of the song or circumstances when you previously listened to the song.

When listening to others, the Hearer may hear things 'between the lines' - perhaps hearing the truth that the person who is speaking is trying to hide.

If a Hearer has not decided an issue, the hearer will ask questions continually until a full understanding is obtained. Straight forward answers are best, since the Hearer will take them as being exact; subtleties are seldom understood.

Once a situation is clear in their mind, the decision will be told assertively, with most of the detail needed for implementation - to a Hearer the use of tact and diplomacy only tend to confuse communication !

Hearers can be over-analytical, ask too many questions, often come on too strong, and may radiate too much mental energy.

If you say you will do something, a Hearer expects it do be done correctly - and on time; just 'doing your best' is not enough.

See-ers - or Seers for short !

Men and women who are strong in seeing tend to live their life from a visual perspective. Such a person experiences life as one vivid mental image after another.

Whether planning a meal or one's life work, the ability to see the entire picture is his or her most important reference point and greatest strength.

Seers must have an inner picture; without it they feel lost; they like to have light - and they want it everywhere, sometimes to the consternation of others ! They frequently leave lights on when they leave a room because they want them to be on already when they come back.

A distinctive characteristic of Seers is their initial resistance to change. They have an internal picture of how they expect everything to be, which is their security and reference point.

When someone wants to change that picture, or presents a new idea (no matter how good) that complicates the plan, they will resist strongly. Their whole Being will scream, *"Don't change my picture !"*

This can make Seers seem rigid and inflexible; if you force an immediate answer about a picture change, you will always get a resounding *"No !"*

The secret of success is to introduce the idea calmly and give the person time to reshape his or her inner image. When an idea is introduced without pressure, Seers eventually visualize a way to work the change into the total plan, because they are well able to see problems, can visualize solutions, and are good at seeing fine detail.

If you are a Seer, sleeping on ideas is an excellent policy. Allow yourself time to reshape your perspective. So don't say *"No !"* immediately, but *"Let me think about that and get back to you tomorrow."* Allow yourself to day-dream - you will usually come up with an even better master plan that incorporates the new idea.

Seers like to have a good view, to see other people at a dining table; they are good at packing items and arranging things; they have good colour co-ordination, and an excellent sense of direction.

They can be rigid and inflexible because they do not want their picture changed - and often will not act until they have the whole picture. They are worriers, visualizing all that could go wrong, and so can tend toward perfectionism (wanting a perfect picture); they may be very self-critical (seeing and emphasizing their faults more than strengths).

Knowers - aka Gnostics

Some people just 'know' the answer to a problem, what is going to happen, or what to do at any time. This knowledge may come extremely fast; the impression received may be fleeting, without any substance, reasoning, or supporting information - and so be hard to understand or even accept.

The instant information that a Gnostic receives enables excellent anticipation of problems or difficulties, helps to adjust rapidly to changing circumstances and make better decisions, and be at the right place at the right time. Gnostics do not waste time worrying needlessly ! But they sometimes are easily bored, and frequently don't complete a project.

Because this 'knowing' is so fleeting, so spontaneous, sometimes a Gnostic may not have the full perspective so necessary for mature judgment.

This instant knowing can be a great help in relationships with other people. As a Gnostic you may be surprised at how these insights can improve your understanding of and communication with other people - especially those with whom you have business or personal problems; and how instinctively you know the needs of family members and loved ones.

The insightfulness of the Gnostic can provide information and answers that are otherwise unavailable; it is an unlimited open channel to the universe that can tap a wealth of creative methods and approaches - often not restricted by convention

Gnostics can be scattered by the volume of thoughts and ideas they receive, and may pick up information far in advance - and sometimes too soon, with the result that they are often ahead of other people's timing and are resented for it.

They can speak too quickly, blurting out what comes to mind without thinking it over first.

Interactions

The most complex challenges that face most of us each and every day are our relationships with other people - at home, at work, and at play. Each individual is unique - and sometimes difficult to understand.

How you deal with others is often the key to success - or the cause of failure. Recognizing these differences in sensing can help by giving you new and more creative insights to apply to interpersonal relationships.

Seers must have their inner picture to feel solid, without their pictures they are like Gnostics stripped of their knowingness or Feelers forced to stay in a discomforting environment.

While a Seer needs not only to see the total picture but to see it with all its connections, the Hearer is more concerned with understanding how the current situation can be explained. Just as the Hearer wants to understand why, the Seer want to see how things fit together. Without that complete view the Seer is as unmovable as the Hearer is without his understanding.

In contrast, the Feeler and the Gnostic do not require an inner picture plan. Feelers are wishing to 'go with the flow' - as long as things feel comfortable they will enjoy the moment without much concern for the future. Gnostics know that the plan will come to them in time, so they continue to rely on their instincts to adapt from moment to moment.

There is a logical progression from knowing to hearing. People tend to confuse the two at times because both have an inner mental quality. Hearing can serve as a sort of inner computer, a way to analyze the insights of knowingness.

Your Own Abilities

Now that you are aware of the various Soul-Mind senses, you may have decided which senses are strong for yourself; usually a person will be strong in one sense, and have another sense almost as strong.

Some people have been gifted with a very strong sense, which may even be as strong as their physical senses - such as those people who are naturally clairvoyant.

According to reports some clairvoyants have been surprised to find that other people cannot see the things that they see naturally.

Most people are not so gifted - but can improve their own abilities; the best way to start is to first improve the senses that you know are your own strongest.

Improve your Feeling

Pay special attention to the different feelings that you get when you meet others and go in various places. Especially learn to recognize that many of these feelings are NOT YOUR OWN !

When you feel anger, hate, or even pain on meeting another person, know that you are using your feeling sense to link with them - it is fine to help understand their problems, but do not take them on as your own !

If you get a sudden pain in your stomach, assume that you are linking to the pain in the other person. You may be an empath !

Be aware of the different feelings that you have when you go to a happy celebration such as a wedding, or a sad time such as a funeral.

Cast your mind back to such situations - you will be surprised to find that you can recall your feelings of the vibrations very easily.

Similarly compare the feelings that you get in a crowded shop or market with those that you recall from relaxing on the beach or in a beautiful spot.

The more that you practice your awareness of the different feelings that you get in various places and situations, the better able you will become in recognizing the energy patterns that give you such feelings in other places and situations.

Louder Soul Hearing

If you are aware that you talk to yourself, understand that you are not going mad ! Usually the talk that you hear is very quiet, and seems to be right in the middle of your head.

You may even hear a background noise most of the time; your Heart-Mind-Brain system is like a radio, hearing all transmissions but amplifying only the signal that is chosen by tuning.

But your Soul may be interested in signals that are not just for you as a Human Being; for example, it may be tuning into another person to see if they need assistance or perhaps have intent that would be detrimental to you.

The key with hearing is to listen to the thoughts that come to you, especially those that you did not consciously originate.

As you progress you may find that you can ask your Heart a question and hear the answer ! But be aware that your ego may also be feeding you thoughts - so it pays to check with your Heart whether the thought came from your Intuition or your ego.

People with a strong sense of hearing may have problems when meditating - hearing a constant stream of 'chatter'. It may help to speak to your Heart and ask it to reduce (or to eliminate) all thoughts that are from sources other than your Heart.

How to See More

The better your visualization, the more that you can see; see an apple, cut it and visualize the outside and inside. Now imagine that the colours change - a blue skin and green inside, with yellow pips, and perhaps a red maggot.

Look at the apple from different directions, change the colours, and then 'morph' it into a tomato or cabbage, visualizing all the details.

Visualize your home, and other homes in which you have lived or visited; peer into cupboards, look in the refrigerator, admire the garden.

The most interesting fact is that your Heart-Mind-Brain team is lazy; so rather than go to the great effort of making a pretend picture, it is easier, more fun, and less effort to use the ability of the Soul to visit and then show what is actually there !

Do not expect to get a beautifully coloured picture in full detail. That may happen in dream state, or when you become extremely efficient - but you can expect to just 'know' the overall picture, or somehow have an understanding of what is there.

Your 'Mind's Eye' does not normally use the same procedures as your physical sight, and is usually located in your forehead. If you are looking straight ahead, note where you feel that your eyes are pointing, and then close your eyes - now probably you will feel your sight to be directed via a point in your forehead.

We look at this in more detail in the next chapter.

Knowing Even More

Pay attention to your hunches ! They come and go very fast, and may not be complete in detail. But you can always ask your Heart for more information.

The best way is to formulate a YES/NO question in your logical mind, stand, and ask your Heart - as you did in the very first exercise.

Remember it is the very first idea that 'pops' into your mind that counts - further replies may be ego saying 'nonsense' !

You can play games like 'Twenty Questions' or 'Animal, Vegetable, Mineral ?' to extend your understanding of the hunch.

Practice makes Perfect

If you do not succeed at first, have another go. If you do not keep on making the effort, how can you succeed ? Remember that all the great players (of music, sports, etc) practice - and then practice more !

You may not become perfect in every way, but you will definitely improve your skill and ability - so it is very worthwhile.

Your attitude is critical; believe that you will succeed - and that you deserve to succeed. If you have any doubts, or believe that it is wrong for some reason, then you are sabotaging yourself.

In all these cases, allow your imagination to roam free. Do not force things, just allow things to happen. Be gentle in all your thoughts and actions, and show appreciation and gratitude for every gain that you make - your 'Being-ness' and 'Upstairs' like to be thanked, and when given gratitude will make more effort to help you !

Having even the slightest success is proof that you have the ability, and can improve your skill. Such experience is far more powerful than anything you are told or read in books. Have faith in yourself !

Soul Contracts

If our conscious self is the same as our Soul, then why do so many of us fail to have access to all our 'Soul Senses' ?

Kristina Neilsen (www.clearyourpath.ca) who is a great clairvoyant Healer, has done work with people having very severe behavioural problems, and in some cases she went back to the time when the Soul was preparing for entry into a human body.

It seems that at this time the Soul is 'guided' as to what needs to be done on this particular life; she saw a shining bright 'Light Being' giving such advice - but when she became aware of the content of the 'guidance', she realized that something was very wrong.

The 'guidance' could only cause harm - and in no way be beneficial to any Soul or Being. So Kristina took steps to further examine the 'Light Being' - and found that it was a dark entity wearing mirrors that reflected the true bright light of the Soul !

Now knowing that this was interference, Kristina got the Soul to cancel the Soul Contract - the result was spectacular: the whole behaviour of the person improved immediately !

So if you are having problems in accessing all your 'Soul Senses' (or other problems) then it may help for you to *"Cancel all Soul Contracts that I have made which are not in the Highest and Best Good of my Soul and of my Total Being or were not made with True Holy Love."*

More Information

Much of the above has been summarized from the book 'You Are Psychic !' written by Pete A. Sanders Jr., published by Fawcett Columbine, ISBN 0-449-90507-1; it is the best book that I have read to explain the interaction of Soul and Body senses - and how to work with them to increase your abilities to use these senses.

The book describes the Soul Energy Being to be located above a persons head, with a link down to the brain's control centre (the pituary / pineal glands); a person's 'awareness' (the ability to feel the location of a pain, for example) may be moving (or extending) this link to locations within the body - and, with practice, to places outside the body.

Pete describes the Soul Senses as being guided by funnels. He visualizes a funnel located between the solar plexus and diaphragm as the main input for feelings - which is why so many people place their arms to cover this place when with others.

The other funnels are aimed at the area of the pituary / pineal glands; the Soul Seeing funnel is in the area around the centre of the forehead, the Soul Hearing funnels (one each side) are above the ears, and the Soul Knowing funnel goes upward from the top of the head.

The book gives exercises to recognize these senses and to improve your skills in using them.

Pete Sanders is the leading light in the 'Free Soul' organization, which organizes home-study and instructor-led courses. The web site is www.freesoul.net and their postal address Box 1762, Sedona, Arizona 86339. You can also telephone (928)282-9425.

When you enter into Trance
Another seems to Guide the Dance

Hypnosis and Visualization

Stephen Black describes hypnosis as *"not only the most simple and practical way of proving the existence of the unconscious - which is still in doubt in some circles - but the only way in which unconscious mechanisms can be manipulated under repeatable experimental conditions for purposes of investigation".*

Lyall Watson, of 'SuperNature' fame ('Life Tide' being its sequel), has developed a good understanding of hypnosis; he considers it to be a marvelous instrument, which almost anyone can learn to handle in thirty minutes, although nobody knows exactly what it is.

Simple cues, like the rapid eye movements of active sleep, fail to tell us precisely when someone is hypnotized; sleeping and dreaming can both be differentiated from waking by examining the differences of the patterns that show up on an electro-encephalograph, but the brain waves of a hypnotized person are identical with the waking state - and no change when hypnotization is activated by a code word.

There is no measurable change in cortical potential, pulse rate, skin resistance, or body electrical potentials.

There is nothing in the physiology or behaviour of a hypnotized person that makes it possible for an observer to distinguish someone in this state, yet under certain circumstances, with certain people, it achieves some extraordinary results - seemingly at the unconscious level of the mind.

Leslie LeChron, in his book 'Techniques of Hypnotherapy', says *'the most common misconception is that there will be a loss of consciousness when one is hypnotized ... Actually, unconsciousness never occurs even in the deepest stages - there is always complete awareness'.*

This may be so in a clinical situation - but if misused by a stage magician it could be that if an instruction be given to 'not remember' then the conscious mind may lack access to the memory.

LeChron says *'daydreaming, concentration on a book, a TV program, a motion picture, or any similar focusing of attention may produce spontaneous hypnosis'.* Thus a hypnotist may instruct a client to concentrate on a small moving object, such as a crystal on a chain.

Hypnotic Induction

Charles Tart of the University of California has pointed out that the the process of hypnotic induction vary, but all have certain steps in common.

1. The subject sits or lies comfortably, relaxing as much as possible, to limit anxiety and bodily tension, so that it is easier for consciousness to concentrate on itself.

The kinesthetic receptors - your sensors of balance - which normally tell you what position each of your limbs occupies in space, then fade out as the body withdraws from consciousness, reducing the sense of wakefulness, and your state of being conscious.

2. The hypnotist tells you to concentrate only on his/her voice or actions - to ignore all other thoughts or sensations.

This reduces discrimination between rival patterns of information - deciding relative importance, identifying memory linkages, and preparing responses. Wakeful psychological reactions are dampened.

A very effective method to induce hypnosis without instruction is listen with earphones to magnified breathing sounds from a microphone on your lower throat .

3. The hypnotist tells you not to think about what s/he says, just to listen passively. If s/he says your arm is feeling heavy, just accept that. Stopping evaluation lessens waking attention, and undermines conscious thought.

4. If you still show signs of restlessness you may be told to look fixedly at some single object; this produces retinal fatigue - and unexpected visual effects may occur which disrupt processing centres in the brain, and so help to enhance the power of the hypnotist.

5. When the hypnotist suggests that perhaps you might feel a little drowsy or even inclined to sleep, this recalls memories of sleeping, passivity is reinforced and your body image fades even further.

The hypnotist may tell you that this is not true sleep - because you will still be able to hear him/her, so that you can respond to his/her suggestions.

6. To cement control, suggestions which have built-in physiological responses may be made, such as suggesting that you raise your arm - and suggesting that it feels heavy. Of course it does, it is heavy !

Who is Who ?

Your normal sense of identity is having your own 'inner voice' tell you what to do, but now the hypnotist's voice is taking over this role - and your sense of 'self' has to expand to include him/her as well. He has become a 'Figure of Authority'.

As the complexity of suggestions increases, each new success further blurs your self boundaries - you then enter the trance state known as 'deep hypnosis', weakening the boundaries between 'me' and 'not-me'. To the subject, the hypnotist and subject become identified - one with the other. Perhaps an external authority figure is given more 'credibility' - stemming from the child-parent state.

Lawrence Kubie of the University of Maryland says *"When the demarcation becomes unclear between that which seems to be 'me' and that which seems to be 'you', it is hard to decide who originates any words, criticisms, praises, commands or suggestions"*.

When losing identity and integrity under hypnosis, we may be reverting to some extent to an earlier evolutionary condition, in which we mixed and shared more freely with our environment.

The major problem facing the first organisms was the basic recognition of the material substance of 'self' from the material substance of 'non-self' - the key to an immune system.

Effect on Immune System

One of the effects of hypnotic induction is an ability to bring the immune response under the conscious control of the hypnotist.

Frank Patte, of the Rice Institute, discovered one woman who was able to produce blisters in direct response to just the hypnotic suggestion that an allergen had come in contact with her skin.

A number of people known to suffer from allergic dermatitis when exposed to the leaves of a local tree, were blindfolded and tested both with the leaves of the offending tree and leaves from a harmless common chestnut.

Under hypnosis, all of them produced blisters when touched with chestnut and told it was the allergen; and none of them reacted to prolonged contact with the usual source of their ills.

In the light of experiments of this sort it seems that control of psychosomatic ills such as ulcers, colitis, migraine, eczema and high blood pressure may best be accomplished by relinquishing consciousness altogether.

Key Words

As infants we take so much on trust - even taking orders in our sleep. In one sleep laboratory, experimenters whispered instructions such as: *"Whenever I say the word 'blanket', you will feel cold until you pull up the blanket and cover yourself". "Whenever I say the word 'itch', you will feel uncomfortable until you scratch it".*

Electroencephalograph recordings showed no interruption of the brain patterns of quiet sleep, and the subjects knew nothing of the instruction on waking. But the following night, all responded appropriately to the signals. One even continued to scratch on cue five months later without any reinforcement during the interval.

Certain words or sounds may be more effective than others. Ian Oswald of the University of Edinburgh played a very long tape recording of fifty-six names called out one after the other in various orders, with several seconds between each name.

Electroencephalographic recording of slow wave sleep signals showed most disturbance by the subject's own name, or that of someone important to them. *"While Humphrey slept, the name of Janet would cause a most violent perturbation in his EEC, and a huge psycho-galvanic response, or sudden sweating of the palm".*

Recall of Past Events

Both dreaming and hypnosis seem to be able to draw freely on material not normally available to consciousness - under hypnosis, most people seem to be able to recall almost everything that ever happened to them.

Lyall Watson reports: *"I know that in one session I was able to conjure up an image of the route I used to take while walking to school at the age of six in Johannesburg, and count all the street lights on the way. Two years ago, I returned there and for the first time in thirty years, retraced my steps, and was able to verify a count I don't think I ever consciously made".*

Some therapies involve role playing and the relief of tension by acting out traumas - full recall of the actual experience under hypnosis is better than play acting.

The therapist creates confusion as to the present date, and then talks the subject back down through the years, step by step, stopping at regular intervals to establish ground with comments like *"You are now ten years old.   Where do you go to school ?   What are you wearing ?"*

The replies often show language, logical constructs, and personality traits appropriate for an individual of the relevant age; if asked to write something down the script may have characteristics of a childish scrawl.

In several regressions subjects were taken back to a time when they went through a change of handwriting, and they reverted once again to a style they hadn't used for decades.

This is not a complete change - an American adult regressed to a childhood in which he spoke only German, responded in English to questions asked; a subject supposedly regressed to infancy sat upright in her chair in adult fashion.

Some of the personality seems to remain at the present level and function as a sort of detached observer, but there is equally little doubt that a great amount of actual revivification is taking place.

Robert True of the University of Vermont took fifty students known to be deep hypnotic subjects, between the ages of twenty and twenty four, and regressed them to the apparent ages of ten, seven and four years old.

At each of these points he asked them to pause on Christmas Day and on their birthdays, and tell him which day of the week it was. Then he checked their replies against a permanent calendar and found that at the age of ten, ninety-three per cent of the answers were correct.

At the ages of seven and four the figure fell to forty-one and thirty-five per cent respectively, which is still far greater than the one in seven chance of making a correct guess at random.

Can you remember the day on which your birthday fell last year ?

Getting into a Trance

When you are hypnotized, you get into a trance. I interpret this to mean that there is unrestricted access to the sub-conscious self - so that instructions that are given are taken as being 'the law'.

Guided meditation seems to have this effect - you are not told that you are being hypnotized, but the effect is the same - you get into a trance state, until released by the person who guides the meditation - or by exercising a cue that has been suggested.

Usually, however, you are free to use your imagination in following the guidance, and have control over the actions - and you retain your memory of all that occurred. This includes memory of 'how you got there', so that you can repeat the procedure at any time should you so wish.

Self-hypnosis

Self-hypnosis means that you, yourself, are in command - not any other person. You put yourself into a trance, retaining control over your involvement in all that happens. One method is:

Get comfortable, relax completely - perhaps stressing and then relaxing the various parts of your body, toes to head - pay particular attention to stresses in your chin, lips, mouth, tongue, eyes, eyebrow area, and forehead; these areas are extremely susceptible to tensions.

Define the purpose of the trance clearly and precisely: *"When I reach the violet colour I will be ready for a deep and good night's sleep [until I wake at time]", "When I descend all the steps and reach the bottom I will observe a past life"*, or define another intent in a similar way.

See yourself completely bathed in the colour [RED]; feel the vibrational patterns and energy of the colour [RED] throughout your total body, in all your auras. Note: you must visualize the actual colour, not just think of it !

Repeat with these colours in order: If you have problems in visualizing a colour, hold a CD or DVD disk up so that the light of the sun is reflected - and you will see all the colours needed.

1. Red: Red carnation, Santa Claus coat, traffic light
2. Orange: ripe orange, orange juice.
3. Yellow: ripe banana skin, egg yolk.
4. Green: like your freshly mown lawn
5. Blue: the cloudless sky, the lake in sunlight.
6. Violet: or lilac or lavender - the flower colours.

To deepen the trance - should you decide to investigate a past life, for example, see yourself at the top of a flight of stairs - and <u>see and feel yourself descending</u>, step by step:

You are at the top - 21st step. Down to 20th - 19 - 18 - 17 *Deeper as ever reached before;* 16 - 15 - 14 - 13 *getting Deeper and Deeper,* 12 - 11 - 10 - 9 *going even more Deeper,* 9 - 8 - 7 - 6 - 5: *almost totally Deeper,* 4 - 3 - 2 - 1: *Deeper; at the bottom; Deeper than ever reached before.*

Note: 'Deeper' is a key word, useful to help you get into and deepen the trance. You could use 'Deeperer' as a special word associated only with the trance condition.

See a brilliant golden-white light at the bottom, illuminating some doors. Feel yourself guided to open the door having your specified intent. Feel completely safe as you enter through the door.

When finished, leave through the door, close it, and reverse your numbering as you climb the stairs and then go through the colours violet to red. You are now back in the present time and place *"feeling completely healthy, full of energy and vitality".*

Visualization

Many people seem to have problems in visualization - so it helps to start simple !   Recall a situation from your previous day, remembering what happened, how other people looked. Bring a picture of a loved one to mind.   Think back to a childhood bedroom and gaze around the room.

When you have a clear picture of the bedroom, see an object in it in more detail - you may move your awareness closer to it so that you can see such detail. Repeat with another object, and see it from various angles. See yourself picking it up and feeling it !

Go to the window and look out - what do you see ? Choose something, and then see it 'close-up'. You have now moved your awareness to be outside the room - to be with the object that you saw from the window ! If you saw a flower, recall the smell.

Practice this sequence until you have complete confidence in your ability to bring views of past events to mind. You can then extend this to imagining a future situation - for example, a meeting with someone. Picture what they look like, the clothes that they wear.

Now play-out the situation in your mind - so that what happens is just as you want it to be. You can imagine problems arising, and how you will handle them.   See yourself being successful in achieving your purpose. You can keep repeating this for any very important situation - to 'etch' it into reality !

Exploring

Choose a small plant or flower, and concentrate you gaze on it; see it shape, colours, texture; 'be one' with it; look intensely at a small part, such as a petal or leaf; wonder in your mind what it would be like to be inside the petal or leaf - how it would feel, what you would see. Let any images just come - do not force them ! Just relax into the petal or leaf and be 'with it'.

You may even decide to move within it to explore a different part of the plant system, the 'Beingness' of the plant. It helps to be appreciative of the plant, to send it your love, and express gratitude at being allowed to work with the plant.

Imagineering

When you visualize an apple or banana you can change its colour, and even cut it in two. I find this useful because I can then see the whitish interior, and going for a closer look, the area of white expands.

I can then superimpose other images onto this background - so overcoming a major problem that I found in 'Silva' training. When I visualize an engineering situation or something that I intend to make, I see it in space, without any background.

In 'Silva' you are told to image a white screen on which images will appear - and I have always been unable to do this, until I realized that I could use the inside of a banana or apple as that screen !

In 'Seeing with the Mind's Eye' by Mike & Nancy Samuels (ISBN 0-394-73113-1) they suggest that you relax and deepen (as discussed) then see yourself going into an elevator (the staircase is similar, of course) and going 'Down to a Lower Level'.

At the bottom you open the door and find yourself in a small, comfortable room that is dimly lit - on the wall facing you is a large screen, with a comfortable easy chair in front.

Now visualize yourself sitting in the chair and say *"I am deeply relaxed; my mind feels clear and tranquil; I can visualize vividly and easily. My mind is open to images that will be helpful to me. I can look at the screen and see images come and go. I can hold these images, rotate, or magnify them. I can even influence what type of images appear. I see images which help me to answer questions and solve problems".*

You may see or feel the presence of advisers as well !

When the Table Starts to Walk
Then the Spirits begin to Talk

Other Dimensional Beings

J. T. Richards, in his book 'SORRAT: A History of the Neihardt Psychokinesis Experiments, 1961 - 1981', published by Scarecrow Press, ISBN 0-8108-1491-9, reports on a series of experiments conducted in association with Dr Rhine of Duke University.

These were kept undisclosed because of the increased depth of the experiments and potential for problems in funding for Duke University. It reports his own involvement - 'I' being J. T. Richards.

This is just a small extract - if you would like to know more, get hold of this most fascinating book !

One Episode

I asked, *"Would you write a list of names of those who are to be included in the experiments ? Write it in the Cox Box or in the Mottert Box; don't just rap it".*

These boxes are specially designed to indicate any manual interference.

There was one rap, then three raps, which we interpreted to mean, *"Yes, if I want to".*

Alice put the Mottert Box with its double layer of unmarked aluminum foil sealed inside on the vibrating tabletop. The table, with the box still on it, 'walked' into the study, to the desk, where raps spelled the word 'HAT'.

Alice took the Mottert Box from the table and put it on the dining room table, where it would be less likely to fall to the floor and be stepped upon and crushed. She put Dr. Neihardt's old grey felt hat on the table.

The table promptly levitated about one foot over and slightly to the left of the left front corner of the desk. I took a photograph, and the table fell.

The hat remained levitated about one foot over and slightly in front of the desk corner. I took another photograph, and the hat fell.

When we ended this experiment at 9:50 pm and looked in the Mottert Box; we found that the sealed box had not been opened, but there was a long message, scratched on both sides of the doubled aluminum foil:

"JOHN KING - - MENTOR - - IMPERATOR MESSAGE: LOVE, HELP, DO NOT HOARD OR MISUSE THE PSI POWER WE GIVE YOU.

IT IS MORE POTENT THAN HIGH EXPLOSIVES. LIKE AMMONIUM NITRATE, IT CAN NOURISH AND MAKE GROW, OR IT CAN BE CONFINED AND EXPLODE.

PSI RESEARCH IS NOT A RELIGION OR A SUBSTITUTE FOR A RELIGION.

PSI RESEARCH IS A WAY OF SEEKING TRUTHS.

APPLY THESE TRUTHS FOR GOOD, AND YOU WILL RECEIVE THE BENEFIT OF BENEFACTION.

DO NOT EXCLUDE M. S., M. H., G. M., OR OTHERS WE TRY TO HELP.

EXCLUDE NOT, OR BE EXCLUDED.

WE STRIVE FOR PEACE, LOVE AND HARMONY. MUTUAL CO-OPERATION IS NECESSARY.   OUT REACH!

THINK THOU THE UNCONFINED OF ALL THE UNIVERSES NEEDS MUST ONLY PLAY TABLES AND BOXES AT SKYRIM ? BROADEN YOUR VISION!

YOU HAVE LOVING AND WISE FRIENDS, SO BE LOVING AND HELP OTHERS.

WE WILL SHOW YOU HOW TO USE PSI ON OBJECTS AT YOUR WILL WHEN YOU FULFILL YOUR DUTIES.   J. K.

While we were marvelling at this theoretical message, the raps spelled out the word 'CALL', a precognitive veridical communication, as we soon discovered.

Alice asked, *"Will I get a phone call ?"* - One rap.

Immediately thereafter, the telephone rang. It was Lynn; Alice told her what had just occurred. Sometimes, the raps would urge us to 'trust feelings of love', but on other occasions, a life form would rap out relatively tough-minded advice.

Alice's Dad

As an example, on the same evening that the highest outdoor levitation occurred, Alice was chided for her credulity by raps which she associated with her father's personality.

"Gaki !" she cried. *"Do you still need proof, on the Other Side ?"*

The raps spelled out, "DO NOT THINK THAT I HAVE LOST MY ABILITY TO REASON CRITICALLY".

Alice had often discussed the links between man and the other animals with her father during his lifetime.   Referring to these conversations, she asked, *"Gaki, are there animals over there with you ?"*

There was one rap, then the raps spelled out "PART OF ALL".

Alice asked the next question mentally: *"Is your mind the same as it was here ?"*

Again, there was one rap, and then the word, "GREATER; PART OF THE ALL".   There was a pause, and then the raps spelled "WISDOM".

"What sort of wisdom ? And what do you mean by 'The All' ?"   "GOD".

It was at this time, realizing that the raps had apparently read her mind correctly, that Alice told us precisely what her mental question had been.

Running such a test of the entity was her way of attempting to be as critical and objective as Dr. Neihardt would have been, Alice explained.

Advice Confirmed

Sometimes raps would be quite blunt in pointing out the faults of experimenters.   As an example, when Alice asked a rapping life form whether or not a professor who was an alcoholic should attend the experiments, with the clear implication that she wished to invite him to participate, the entity responded with two vigorous raps, and then spelled the succinct explanation "DRUNK".

On another occasion, the raps described a prospective participant as a "BULL DYKE".   Although we did not know it at the time, we later learned through hearsay that the woman was, indeed, an aggressive homosexual with psychological problems which might have hurt the harmony of the SORRAT group had she been invited to participate.

Margie's Protection

On July 9, 1976, raps advised Margie that her home might soon be broken into by a prowler.   She had been apprehensive about this strong possibility, and asked if she should keep her large dog there for protection.

One rap.   *"Should I also borrow my father's shotgun ?"* she asked.

One vigorous rap resounded.

One of the newcomers to the group expressed her dislike of guns in general, and seemed to expect life forms from a higher plane of existence to share her opinion, but the raps chided this young lady for her hophlophobia.

"DO YOU THINK THAT, BECAUSE WE ARE NO LONGER LIVING IN BODIES, WE ARE NECESSARILY FOOLS ?   YOU MUST DEFEND YOURSELVES AGAINST VIOLENT, EVIL PEOPLE".

This answer was completely in keeping with Dr. Neihardt's philosophy of Pragmatic Mysticism; obviously, good people should not make themselves defenseless and hand over the world to the evildoers, out of a mistaken belief that helplessness in the face of evil is proof of a superior character.

Wisdom

On another occasion, when asked by another altruistic young lady if we should not always be kind and meek to those who are cruel to us, in the hope of reforming them by our good example, the raps replied, "THE MEEK SHALL INHERIT THE EARTH, SIX FEET UNDER IT."

Answers like these, rather than the sort of vague comments on brotherhood and universal love (true though they might be) go far toward convincing one that the messages which 'come through' in psi sessions are not entirely hogwash. Whence they come may be open to question, but pragmatic wisdom is useful, no matter what its source might be.

Usually, the information communicated to us was more gentle and more philosophical than the rather waspish wisdom I have just quoted. As an instance, not long after Margie had been advised to defend herself against attackers, during the same session Alice asked *"Are there trees and plants on the Other Side, as well as people and other animals, Gaki ?"*

One rap responded, and then raps spelled out "ESSENCE. TREENESS OF TREES, ETC."

Upon rare occasions, the raps would continue for over an hour, spelling out lengthy messages.

PSI Activation

There was such a long message spelled out during the session on July 16, 1976.

Alice, Dick, Glenda, Joe, Elaine, and I began this experiment at 9:00 pm, and it did not end until nearly 11:05.

At first, Dick went into a trance, the first which I have ever witnessed on his part, but this was only temporary, and he only made mumbling sounds which we could not comprehend.

Then the long message was rapped out, beginning with the odd word "NAIPON". The gist of this message was that there is a process in the brain which effects psi.

The key area in the brain is the pineal gland. It secretes a chemical, 'naipon' (a term which we could not find in any biological lexicon) which, the life forms said, affects the nodes of the nerve synapses.

The catalyst involved, which is itself non-psi-active but which causes the pineal gland to secrete the psi-active chemical and release it into the bloodstream through capillaries in that area of the brain, can be induced in several ways.

One method is the ingestion of mescaline, the psychedelic agent found in the lepadondria williarnsii cactus, which the raps warned us against, because the side effects (for which most people who ingest this substance eat peyote), the 'cheap drunk' of artificially-heightened consciousness, would interfere with our ability to reason logically.

Another method, we were told, is electrical impulses induced by electrodes into the brain. But the best method, we were assured, is the cultivation of moods which are associated with peace, harmony, and affection.

Apparently, various hormones have effects upon this psi-producing process.

When we touch hands in a circle, there is a passage of energy (of some variety) from person to person.

This may help or hinder the psi effects, depending upon whether one person gets good or bad 'impulses' or 'vibes' from another, and upon the mood of the group.

We were told that there is equipment which would help us to measure and examine reactions, such as the Beckman RM Dynograph used by a 'Dr. Miller' and allegedly described in an (unspecified) psi research journal article.

We searched back issues of all available journals, but did not find such an article.

We were told that a medium normally has a larger and structurally-different pineal gland, but that all people have releases of the psi-active chemical occasionally, and consequently have psi experiences, if other factors are also operant.

The life forms involved in this long rap session claimed to be Dr. Neihardt, John King, Martin Fischer, and thirty-one other 'high levels' who had come to help in the transmission.

In keeping with Dr. Neihardt's belief that we should try to learn something from every experience and, at the same time, not become over-credulous, we did not simply dismiss this long rapped message, and other messages which correlated with it, as nonsense.

Neither did we accept it as a revelation of truth. We recorded it, transcribed it, and passed it along to a prominent brain physiologist who prefers to keep his psi interests a secret.

He later informed me that this information, while seemingly implausible, could easily be true, although he admitted that we do not yet know enough about psi to accurately measure it, and consequently cannot yet correlate it to changes in the pineal gland secretions.

The same objection may be made to some other theoretical information which we have received through various media from the life forms, chiefly through Joe's later trance-talking. If we cannot adequately measure psi, and cannot objectively chart a 'ley line' network on the surface of the earth with equipment which can measure changes in electromagnetic force-fields deep within the earth, then we can only ask for more information.

Levitation and PSI Energy

"What principle is involved in levitation ?" Joe asked, when it was apparent that the raps were able to remain constant long enough to spell out messages.

"FORCE OF ... STASIS. CONSERVATION OF ENERGY".

"Does the mind influence levitation ? Is it really telekinesis ?"

"BETA WAVES".

"Could we ... see those waves ? Is it like ectoplasm ?"

"NOT VISIBLE SPECTRUM".

"What part of the brain produces this phenomenon?"

"PINEAL" the raps replied. "PSI JUNG."

"Is this a reference to Dr. Neihardt's friend, the psychoanalyst Carl Jung, and his theory that psychic energy is related to race memory ... and to the pineal gland, in some way ?" One rap.

"Then at least part of psi is a physical function of the brain, then ? It is, ah, natural to man ?"

"NOT JUST HUMAN. ANIMALS CAN USE PSI ENERGY JUST AS PEOPLE CAN. THIS IS NOT A NEW DEVELOPMENT IN MAN'S EVOLUTION BUT A HOLDOVER ... PREVERBAL ABILITY."

This communicator claimed that the pineal gland emits "JUICES" which cause a series of chemical changes in the brain. In speaking of this catalytic substance (which he did not call 'naipon') he commented that "A LITTLE BIT MAKES A BIG DIFFERENCE TO RAISE ENERGY. BRAIN WAVES PRODUCE MORE PSI ENERGY. THIS IS WHERE WE CAN STEP IN. WE CAN USE THIS, TOO. IT IS NOT MIND OVER MATTER; IT IS MIND MERGING WITH MATTER. WE CAN MAKE USE OF THIS TO RAISE OR MOVE OBJECTS, WITHOUT GOING THROUGH YOUR SYNAPSE PATTERNS OF PACKETS".

"What other factors, I mean physical factors, influence levitation ?"

"THE ROTATION OF THE EARTH SETS UP FORCE FIELDS, SOME HELPING AND SOME INHIBITING LEVITATION. WE CAN COME THROUGH EASIER WHEN THE FIELDS ARE TILTED FOR THE HEMISPHERE, IN FALL, WINTER, AND SPRING, AND YOUR PSI OUTPUT IS HURT BY HOT, MOIST WEATHER'S EFFECT ON YOUR BODIES".

"What about psychological factors ?"

"A VERY SELF-CENTERED PERSON WILL INHIBIT HIS PSYCHIC ABILITY. THE LAST SHALL BE FIRST AND THE FIRST SHALL BE LAST".

"Does this include Uri Geller ?"

"EXCEPTION PROVES RULE".

"What differences are there between us mortals and you, ah, spirits ?"

"YOU ARE SPIRITS, JUST AS WE ARE, EXCEPT THAT YOUR BODIES ARE A DIFFERENT ENERGY FORM. ALL IS ENERGY IN ONE FORM OR ANOTHER. THE MORE YOU ARE IN TUNE WITH THE ALL, THE MORE THIS IS STIMULATED, THE BETTER YOU CAN USE THIS".

"You speak of 'The All'. Can you define this, or do we have to, well, sort of take it on faith ?" After a pause, I added, *"Is this a sort of Cosmic Consciousness like Bucke talked about, or God, or -- -"*

"FAITH IS KNOWING RATHER THAN JUST THINKING. COSMIC CONSCIOUSNESS IS ONE ASPECT OF GOD".

"What do you mean when you use the word 'God' ?"

"GOD IS ALL".

Then the raps ended at 12:35pm., and we terminated the session.

Comment by John Living

This record indicates that there are other dimensional Beings who can communicate with us, given that we are open to their methods.

Just because these life forms are in a different dimension it should not be presumed that their minds are greater than ours. We have access to the same 'greater mind', but in many cases this link has been undeveloped or restricted for many reasons. So they may have access to information not presently available to us.

Having a mind is needed, but it seems that to use it to its best advantage may require a brain - which seems to require some aspect in the physical dimension.

Having knowledge is one thing; understanding the knowledge is another (probably requiring memory) - and putting it to work is a completely different aspect !

My understanding is that 'God' is not any individual life form, but a term for the 'Good Energy' that is in all life, in 'All that Is' - perhaps 'Love' would be a better term.

If so, the term 'God' represents the 'Essence of Love' in all Beings, in all life forms. Various Beings seem to have different responsibilities (and different modes of operation in various dimensions) within this context.

The overall context of a 'Good God System' could be that all these Beings work together in Peace, in Harmony, and in Love - caring for their responsibilities with the intent of what is best for 'All that Is'.

After writing this I found a pair of perfect fuchsia blooms laid carefully on the parapet of my deck - there is no way that they could have broken so neatly without help, or fallen naturally to where they lay ! I believe that this was a sign from 'Upstairs'. Similar occurrences have happened before !

We Compute !

Another way of visualizing a Human Being is as a bio-computer - a self-contained personal computer that can link to a higher level main-frame computer or to the universal/cosmic internet, using modem-like wireless connections. Our Heart is like the CPU (Central Processing Unit).

There are many similarities to an electro-magnetic computer - we have an operating system (our belief system), short term working memory in our mind, medium term memory in our brain, long term memory in our body cells and auras, and mystics tell of memory like a tape backup held in the Akashic records.

When we listen and speak we work at a slow speed - similar to the way that typing on a keyboard is far slower than the speed at which our computer handles data. Even when just thinking, our speed of operation is much slower than when we relax completely - such as when having a snooze.

I have found that if I study the data in the morning, and have a quick snooze at lunchtime, then when I awaken I know the way to process the data efficiently and successfully - this has been a great help in my career as a Chartered Engineer and as a Professional Engineer.

Our sub-conscious keeps things running in the background - even when our input devices (eyes, ears, etc) are switched off when we are asleep.

It does this because it is running programs - installed by the manufacturer, loaded in our operating system, told by others (perhaps virus infected), or formed as the result of our experiences.

We run programs all the time - the most powerful being those in our operating system, based on the beliefs that we hold.

Luckily we can change programs, getting rid of those not now wanted and adding new ones - although we may sometimes need expert assistance to install upgrades to the operating system.

Religions could be likened to proprietary operating systems, having minor variations depending on the cultural and national environments - some may be better than others for various purposes, but often they are not compatible with other systems.

Perhaps the best operating systems are those that are open, not controlled by any one company, or not adjusted for only one environment - similar to having an open mind.

Opening Our Operating System

The best way to have an open mind is to not have any firm beliefs; to categorize all that we have been told, even all our experiences, as being like pieces of a jig-saw puzzle that we are trying to solve.

When we look at a piece, we can see various attributes according to the way that it is seen, the direction our gaze holds, and the effects of different lighting - and what we expect to see !

We may have been told that certain pieces MUST fit together in a particular place; those who gave us these hints helped as best they could, but perhaps did not have an identical puzzle, or understand the complete picture.

We try to fit all the pieces together, but often come across a new piece that can only go in the middle of some collection (a program, perhaps) that has been assembled - so we have to take those pieces apart and re-arrange them to make a better fit.

If we refused to make such re-arrangements we could never improve the picture - the puzzle would never be solved.

The more that we do assemble the overall picture, the more likely that we will find pieces that do not fit at all in our own puzzle - they belong to other puzzles owned by other people, and have got mixed up with our pieces.

Running Programs

There are many different parts to our brain - most well known are our reptilian brain, our animal brain, and our advanced brain with its logical and intuitive halves. These all work together, like the different components in a computer.

It seems that when any new information is received, it is checked by the reptilian brain to see if it corresponds to any previous action, and if any 'fight or flight' action is needed - which takes precedence over all other action.

This has been found to occur before any knowledge is passed to the 'thinking' part of our Mind-Brain system.

Failing 'fight or flight' action, but finding correspondence with a previous situation recorded in our memory banks, the actions then taken may be prepared for re-use.

This is especially so if there is any emotion attached to the memory; then an 'emotional trigger' may be operated - which sets in motion a repeat of the previous actions, even if these are not the best actions to take.

We will examine ways that we can overcome these 'emotional triggers' in later chapters.

Adding and Changing Programs

When we started to ride a bicycle it was hard work, falling off a number of times, because we had not learnt the skill of balancing on a bike.

As we progressed, the skill became an ability that was now natural to us; the program had been installed, so that whenever we got on a bike we ran the 'bike riding program'.

All our life we have added programs in this way - starting to crawl and then walk; learning to talk, read, and write; finding how our behavior was accepted.

As we expanded our contacts, we may have realized that sometimes our behavior had to be modified to work with others and so get what we wanted - and we changed our programs.

Sometimes making a change is difficult; we know what we want to achieve, but perhaps our operating system creates obstacles - or sub-programs are unknowingly involved, and also need to be revised.

To succeed, our conscious mind has to be clear and precise about what is needed - not how it will happen.

This must then be explained in simple language, remembering that most of our sub-conscious mind operates at the level of a four or five year old child - so keep it simple !

Our sub-conscious mind understands pictures better than words, so visualizing the desired effect is important - and emphasizing this by emotions, feelings, and other senses is a great help, since our sub-conscious mind is closely linked to our senses.

Our sub-conscious mind is not well able to differentiate between what we imagine and what is an actual happening in the physical world - especially so if our imagination includes the operation of our various senses.

This is most useful in persuading our sub-conscious to make a change.

It is also important to do all this 'in the NOW' - if it is past, then it is so; if in the future, then it is not to be done now.

Remember that the sub-conscious mind is not logical - it may have its own logic, but it is very different from that of our logical mind, the way that we think with our normal consciousness.

Affirmations

When we have decided the required end result, we can use our logical mind to define an affirmation that represents this result in a clear and precise way, using simple language.

The sub-conscious seems to fail to understand NOT; often it considers this word to be similar to NOW, and so any affirmation which includes NOT is taken to be confirming the opposite intent!

Ways to overcome this included to affirm that you are 'free from' [the unwanted], and that you are [the opposite].

The best time to make affirmations is when we are in that state between being awake and sleeping - as we go to sleep, and as we awake, including any times when we awake temporarily during our sleep period.

It is helpful to repeat any affirmation three times; the first time is an incidence, the second time may be a co-incidence, but the third time indicates that it is really meant!

One problem that has been identified is the verbal structure.

Many times a child may have been told something in the third person such as *"You are stupid !"* - and coming as a judgment from others it is taken to be fact.

To overcome this, it helps to couch any correction in ways that include the third person *"you ..."*, then the impersonal third person, and finally the first person *"I ..."*.

Let us consider an example; you have been told:

> *"You are stupid (or inadequate in some aspect)".*

The basic affirmation could be:

> *"I am intelligent (more than adequate in that aspect) !"*

This may best be expressed (three times as shown):

> *"In each and every moment of each and every day,*
> *You, [your name], are intelligent in every way"*
> *"In each and every moment of each and every day,*
> *You, [your name], are intelligent in every way"*
> *"In each and every moment of each and every day,*
> *You, [your name], are intelligent in every way"*

Then three times more, this time impersonally:

> *"In each and every moment of each and every day,*
> *[your name] is intelligent in every way"*

And finally, three times in the first person:

> *"In each and every moment of each and every day,*
> *I, [your name], am intelligent in every way"*

This may seem tedious, but if you really want the change to occur it may be well worth-while; remember to put lots of feeling and emotion into these statements, and do your best to imagine with all your senses that the results are now existing - they have been achieved already.

How often should this sequence be repeated ?

Opinions vary, but it is probably correct to say for at least three days; if the effect is not manifested, keep on until it does happen.

Do not make any affirmation too long - each affirmation should cover one single aspect, not a whole string of things to be changed.

If there are many aspects to be changed, then do this using separate affirmations.

Donna Eden, in her book 'Energy Medicine', suggests that when you have finished making an affirmation you 'lock it in', by placing your finger on your pelvic bone, and run it up (as if you were doing up a zip fastener) to you lip - this is your 'Governing Meridian', and this action ensures that it is correctly stored.

Her book is an amazing source of information about the non-physical body, on how the physical body responds, and how to work on yourself (and others) for good Health.

Direct Programming

Another way to implement a new or changed program is to write down its details, then ask your Heart if this is correctly understood. If not, revise it until it is understood.

Ask your Heart if this program is in your highest and best interest - if not, then do not proceed, but you can ask your Heart to hint why this is so, and perhaps write a variation that is beneficial.

Otherwise ask your Heart if any changes would improve the program; the very first hint that comes to mind is probably from your Intuition - incorporate this into your program, and ask again.

Repeat this until you do not get any more hints. Then ask your Heart to install and implement the program, and afterwards ask if the installation was successful and will be fully implemented in all cases - if not, ask why.

It takes less time, but more concentrated effort, to install a program this way, but the detailing can be more extensive - you are working with your Heart, not just your sub-conscious.

Another advantage of using this method is that it can build a number of sub-programs which can be re-used in other programs; these can be called in exactly the same way that one computer program can call and link with another.

Programming Example

Perhaps the most important program to load is one that permits direct programming itself - to check that your Heart is willing and able to do the work expected.

First install a key program:

"That my Heart be in command of my total Being at all times, in all 'nows', in all ways, and in all aspects" - so do this as explained above; if any problem is encountered, install this as an affirmation.

Now the base program:

"That my Heart will assist and co-operate with all in my total Being to ensure the correct and satisfactory installation and implementation of all affirmations and programs which I ask to be installed, providing that all changes made are for my highest and best good, shall not cause harm to myself or others, and shall be in effect until revised or cancelled by me".

This is another program that is most beneficial:

"That all calls that I make to my Intuition shall be via my Heart, and that all replies that are given shall be the truth as best I am able to understand, based on information obtained from all possible sources that are reliable as correct, provided that if the information is not available or the reply should not be given then this will be so indicated".

Never, ever, try to impose any affirmation or program on any person except yourself !

Debugging Programs

Any ideas why this is so called ?

In the early days of computers, when instructions were issued by punched cards (which, incidentally, were based on weaving technology !) sometimes a bug would get caught in one of the punched holes - and so change the program.

This has been extended to identifying problems in computers (bugs like warm places) as well as in programs; many of the programs now used (and the computers themselves) are far more complicated than in the old days - as, perhaps, are humans.

Luckily there are some debugging programs available to those 'in the know'.

One of the best for use in 'human computers' is the 'Emotional Freedom Techniques' program developed by Gary Craig - the complete manual can be downloaded from www.emofree.com for free.

Improving Access to Storage

The conscious mind tends to operate on information in a linear fashion, such as reasoning that A+B=C. The sub-conscious mind, however, deals with this as ABC - and it finds the answer to a question based on whether any of these, A, B, or C, are held in a particular storage space.

To take material from short term memory and store it for future use, use the following procedure:

1. Focus your awareness, your attention, between your eyes on the thought or concept that you want to store - you will feel this as energy or pressure in the upper frontal lobes of your brain.

2. Wrap your awareness around the energy, holding the concept very clearly and firmly in your mind until you know it thoroughly; you do not have to think about every detail, just hold the entire concept in your consciousness as one total 'lump' - like holding a mass of cotton-wool balls, without worrying about any individual ball.

3. Now pull the energy downwards towards the base of your head at the rear, and imagine a trap-door opening. This opens the 'reticular formation', and allows the energy of the information to flow down into the cells of the body, to be stored in a holographic way.

4. Keep pulling the energy into your body, until you feel it harmonize and settle into the energy systems of your body.

You can access stored information very simply:

1. Place your awareness on a subject and ask that it be retrieved from memory.

2. Relax - do not put any energy or stress on the subject ! Just 'Space Off' - without thinking intently about anything else.

3. The information will 'appear' in your Mind-Brain system, ready for you to use.

This method, especially the retrieval method, can help you get good marks in an examination !

Like most skills, the more that you use this technique, the easier that it becomes - and the greater your confidence in knowing that you will get information when you need it.

With extended use you may find that just one bit of information can trigger entirely new ways of understanding the information - and lead to new concepts of thought.

Improving Our Performance

Each of us knows one person better than any other - our own self.

We are very aware of all our faults and our problems, and often tend to have a low opinion of ourselves, although we may put on a different face for others to see.

When we meet another person for the first time, it is usual to try to see the best in them; often we may envy their happiness, not realizing that they are worse off than ourselves.

We all have 'ups and downs' in life - the big difference is how we handle the 'downs'.

Life is Full of Lessons

We can choose to learn from the lessons that life gives to us, or we can spend our time complaining about them.

Many illustrious authors, such as Caroline Myss, have written how some very sick people just do not want to be healed.

They spend lots of their time going to Doctors and Healers, and say that they want to be Healed - but deep inside them the story is the opposite.

Perhaps they enjoy telling others of their woes, boasting that their sickness is beyond the skills of Doctor X, getting sympathy from their associates, or even using their illness as a means of getting attention or controlling the lives of family members.

Being a Victim

This attitude is not restricted to health. An individual or group of people may have suffered in various ways at the hand of others.

Any such suffering is to be deplored; but how an individual handles it can vary enormously. Many blame all their problems as the result of such suffering, refusing to take any responsibility even for problems that are not connected to the suffering.

Others realize that what has happened has happened, that it is in the past, and can not be allowed to spoil their life. These people have learnt a big lesson !

They are no longer victims - they have become victors. Victors over their natural 'poor me' attitude. They can get on and enjoy a good life - not forgetting the suffering, but knowing that it can be overcome.

Overcoming Anger

Anger and hate are not necessarily bad. You can hate an animal being mistreated, and have anger at the perpetuator. How you handle this anger is the most important aspect - for you.

Getting into a rage can just cause injury to yourself, and perhaps cause the perpetuator to 'take more' out on the poor animal to relieve the increased emotions that result.

Is it not better to act in a calm fashion to decide how you can act to stop the mistreatment and prevent such actions in the future ?

This may not be easy ! But your intent at self-control is itself a benefit for you - and you may be able to help the mistreated victim as well.

Let us imagine that a bully is beating a dog. What would happen if you take a few calming breaths, and then ask the bully about something completely unassociated with him or the dog, such as the best way to get somewhere ?

Hopefully you will not be told to 'go to hell', but succeed in breaking the chain of action. You may ask a few more similar questions, and perhaps then compliment the bully on having such a nice dog ! Even ask if you can pat him - the dog, not the bully !

The bully may then tell why the dog is bad - perhaps you may be able to suggest a way of training the dog to change its behaviour.

Discretion may be advisable. If you are male, and see a man beating his wife, it may be best not to compliment the man on having a pretty wife - and do not ask to pat (or kiss) her !

Asking questions that do not imply guilt is far better than telling someone that they are guilty - and more likely to change behaviour.

This is so in everyday life - when at home or at work. When you show positive interest in a person, you are more likely to get a positive response.

Holding on to Anger

When you have anger you hurt yourself. It is recognized as being a major contributor to Heart and liver problems.

Holding anger at someone with whom you work, among your associates, or in your family, is most disruptive for others as well - and will result in them doing their best to reduce your influence, so as to lessen the disruption.

This lowering of your influence (in whatever ways are relevant) will also reduce your influence in other ways, which may well reduce your benefits of being in that group. You lose !

When you hold anger at someone distant in place, or at a happening distant in time, you only hurt yourself - not them !

It is imperative to release all anger, hate, and similar negative emotions. Sometimes this can be most difficult - but it is still worthwhile.

Perhaps the most difficult cases involve rape - especially when this occurred incestuously to a young child. In many cases the trauma exists, yet without the knowledge being accessible to conscious memory.

When this is uncovered, or if it is known already, every device possible should be used to enable forgiveness. In many cases this type of hurting runs in families - the father may have suffered similar abuse as a child.

Even draw on the concept of karma, or that some unknown past life incidents may be involved. How does not matter so much as somehow finding the ability to forgive !

There are many instances of women being raped - and this memory is held with emotional triggers that prevent a normal life.

The incident has already happened - you are NOT going to reverse it. But you can accept that it happened and get on with your life. In some cases you may have even contributed in some way to the rape - look inside yourself and forgive yourself, too.

Self Destruction

We know ourselves better than we know any other person. This includes our faults and our problems. When we concentrate our thoughts on ourselves we tend to magnify these faults and problems.

Worrying occurs when we have identified a problem and then go round and round and round thinking of nothing else - except, perhaps, other problems that make matters worse.

This is self destruction - we are sabotaging ourselves.

What is the absolute very worst that can happen as a result of the problem ? How likely is this to happen ? In most cases, it is not likely at all !

Think of the people that you know - or have heard about. Are there any in a position worse than yours ? Did you get a meal yesterday ? Some people have not had a decent meal for many days. You may have shelter - many others do not.

So your situation is not all that bad. How can you improve it ? Be positive ! Some keys to help:

1. Define the problem clearly and precisely - write it down.
2. Identify the factors involved - who, why, when, where, how.
3. Decide if any other influences are pertinent, and their effect.
4. Think of ALL the possible ways to improve the situation.
5. Being realistic, consider which is the most workable way.
6. Plan in detail how you will implement this solution.
7. Do it ! Correctly !

When I first went to the Royal Military Academy, Sandhurst, the Regimental Sergeant Major in Charge explained that if we had decided to make the army a career, we obviously did not have the slightest idea of the thinking process.

Since we were there, to be trained as officers, it would be advantageous to the army if we did learn how to think - and these were the keys that were taught to us.

It was also explained throughout our training that proper implementation was essential.

There were many examples given where excellent implementation of the not-best plan succeeded, whilst the best plan failed when not implemented correctly.

Happiness

Since we know our own faults so well, we find it difficult to be happy about ourselves - or happy in other ways.

The real key to happiness is not to think of ourselves, except to think how we can help others.

This does not mean that we neglect ourselves, since we need to be fit and healthy to be able to do a good job of helping others.

When we help others, we get a great sense of satisfaction - we have 'done good'. And we often find that we get helped ourselves in various ways - not just by those that we helped, but from sources and in ways that we do not expect.

On occasion we may find a person that does not want to be helped. Respect their decision, and do not intrude on their misery. They may have lessons to learn, or enjoy being miserable !

There are always others who we can help - so why waste time and effort where it is not wanted ?

When I lived in Jamaica, a fellow yachtsman took the trouble to tell me that I was drinking far too much and making a fool of myself. I recognized that this took a lot of effort on his part, and showed care - so I listened and took his advice, knowing that he was a real friend.

Joy

Being joyful is different from just being happy - it is a far deeper emotion.

Pete Sanders has written a book 'Access your Brain's Joy Center' in which he describes how the area around the pituitary and pineal glands controls your mood.

Pete instructs how to use your hands to locate and enliven this 'Joy Center'. He warns, however, that if you are too low then you can 'stir up' the reptilian part of your brain with the opposite results.

I have found that I do not need my hands. My 'awareness' intuitively knows where to go, and by sending my awareness to this place and making clockwise circles of the 'Joy Center' I can achieve the result of releasing any negative mood.

This is done with a clockwise movement as perceived when imagining that you are looking down onto your head - passing left to right as you go in front, front to rear on your right side, right to left at the rear, and rear to front on your left side.

For best results, always avoid counter-clockwise movements unless you are intentionally extracting something - as will be explained in later chapters.

Pete explains in his book how this can be of great assistance in working with anger, depression, rejection, and addictions.

This could be a very useful extension of the 'Emotional Freedom Techniques' previously mentioned - they are not mutually exclusive, they actually complement each other.

Sing a Happy Song

There have been many times in my life when I felt deeply depressed and very sad. One way that I found to overcome this mood was to sing a happy song:

I'm Happy, Happy, - Happy all day long
I'm Happy, Happy singing this song.
I'm Happy, Happy, - Happy as can be
I'm Happy, Happy singing merrily.

Remember to sing it to a bright and happy tune - not a dirge ! If in company, you can sing it quietly to yourself, inside you head.

I found it impossible to remain sad and depressed when my reality was that I was singing a happy song !

Try it next time you feel sad or depressed - you may find that it works for you, too ! And it is free ! No doctors prescriptions are needed. No pills to take which may have side effects.

Laughter is Infectious

This is along the same lines. Laughter has been described as the world's best medicine, and there is that old saying:

Laugh and the world laughs with you.
Cry, and you cry alone.

But always remember - laugh <u>with</u> other people, not <u>at</u> other people. If they are sad, perhaps you can help them see the funny side of their troubles, the silver lining to their clouds.

Random Acts of Kindness

No matter how small, the intent is the same - to help another person. If you do this just for your own ego, forget it; the intent to help the other person must be paramount - yes, you will feel good, but this should not be the aim.

Perhaps it is better to give long-lasting help, rather than just a temporary fix - like giving a fishing hook and teaching them how to catch fish, rather than giving them a fish to eat.

Help others to help themselves. Sometimes they may be in dire circumstances and need immediate assistance, and this should be given to the best of your abilities - to help them get on their own feet again.

But beware of those who go from one person to another, asking help, getting it, but never helping themselves; and do not let your family suffer unduly in giving help, except in a real emergency.

Respect and Love

As we grow, our influence grows - similar to the way that ripples in a pond go out to cover the whole pond.

We start with our own self, then our family, next our community, perhaps our country, even the whole world.

One person's idea can change the course of history - like Florence Nightingale's efforts, resulting in wide-spread nursing; the Wright Brothers getting a flying machine to work; Marconi sending messages across the ocean; and many other examples.

Many people often forget that the Holy Creator did not just make humans, but all creatures. Perhaps God is not just the God of humans, but also of the animals, plants, insects, and bacteria.

It may be that we should show respect for, and give love to, all the creations made by the Holy Creator - and not treat nature as just being there for our own convenience.

Life Review

One of the biggest changes in my life came after I realized that instead of waiting to die before having to do a 'Life Review', I could do it now - and benefit now !

As I was going to bed, I made an affirmation: *"As I go to sleep, I will go through my life to review and correct all the 'not good' actions that I have taken, doing so with True Holy Love, Namaste, going backwards in time to each and every moment in my life".*

I would suddenly be thinking of a situation; in most cases I would start by believing that all I did was good - so why bring this up ?

Then I would think *"How was this seen from the view of others who were involved ?"* and realize that I had been at fault !

This is the old adage of 'putting yourself in someone else's shoes', of 'wearing the moccasins of the other person'.

It is best to undertake to do what can be done to correct the actual situation; but in most cases the action had occurred many years past, and there was little that I could do now in the physical world.

So I then stated my apology and asked forgiveness; in some instances there were further points that I had missed, so these were then repeated in my mind, so that these could be cleared as well.

As soon as this was completed, another situation would be brought to mind, and the process repeated.

This continued backwards in time until I reached babyhood. The good things that I had accomplished were not included - so ego was 'kept at bay'.

I did not go further back, to any past lives - but this would not be without gain, if appropriate.

For me the process took two nights - but from that time onwards I felt to be a very different person ! It was certainly a most worthwhile exercise, which I recommend to all who read this book.

To help in this, I have written the following program - which you can use as a guide. Some aspects are explained later.

Healing the Total Being Program

'We ask all parts of our Being, in all dimensions and in all our auric levels, to be open to good suggestions, and that our belief systems do not block our progress. In all creation, in all heavens - all hypnosis is ended; we are free of all hypnosis, and now able to exercise our own free will.

A good team leader identifies the problem, get suggestions from the team about needed actions, places these in context, and develops a plan of action, and persuades all concerned that it is to their benefit to take the required action, which they have helped to select.

We now ask all the parts of our Being, all the members of our team, to consider how their present actions affect the overall performance and well being of our total Being.

We ask all to regress together, day by day and year by year, to when they were formed - and to suggest the changes that they need to make to ensure that they all have a positive influence in re-forming as a really good team, with all members doing their correct job to help our total Being for the Highest and Best Good of All.

We go back together, year by year, stopping at events that had a major impact on our lives - to re-assess our understandings of these events with our present knowledge, and decide any changes that are needed.

We accept the responsibility for our actions, apologizing for thoughts and actions that hurt others, asking to be forgiven, and forgiving those that hurt us - perhaps they taught us a lesson and should be thanked !

We have personal and ancestral memories of events that cause problems with our understanding of our Beingness and how we react to situations and occurrences. We now change our memories of the events to eliminate all such detrimental attributes so that our reactions result in beneficial behaviour, and change the memories of our cells and of our muscular systems to eliminate all memory of hurts and pains.

Thoughts that we sent to others are part of our own 'Energy Being' - we bring them home so that we again become complete. We send the thoughts of others back to them with True Holy Love - so that those others can be complete, and to prevent any interference with our team.

Influences from past lives of ourselves and others may have joined with us to seek recognition and Healing; perhaps some 'not good energies' entered into our being; in some cases we may have been 'possessed' by others; it may be that Soul parts of others have entered our Being. These are 'not wanted on voyage' and must now leave - so in True Holy Love, Namaste, we ask 'The System' that they be taken 'into the Light to be Healed with True Holy Love, Namaste, in the way that is best for All Creation'.

We go back together to our youth, to our childhood, to our infancy, to before our birth, to before our conception - learning all lessons as we regress, and releasing all emotional triggers.

Before we came into this world we may have made 'Soul Contracts' as a result of karma or to work with other to overcome problems, to learn lessons, and to achieve success in missions. We send Healing with True Holy Love, Namaste, to all involved in such karma and Soul Contracts.

Some of these 'Soul Contracts' may have been forced on us, been not for our Highest and Best Good, may involve causing harm to others, or not be applicable to our present circumstances.

We now cancel and void all 'Soul Contracts' and other influences, including those from any other existence of any life form, which are not now for our Highest and Best Good or could cause harm to others.

Let our total Being be cleansed by the Violet Flame, Healed by all needed colours of Light, and protected by layers of Good Gold and Good Silver Light.

Our development may be such that we can now be entrusted with new missions for Good - we check and accept those that we know we can achieve.

Let all needed Healing be given in True and Holy Love to our Spirit, Higher Self, Lower Self, Soul, and other levels of Beingness involved with us even without our conscious knowledge, and be given to all their associates and in their families.

Let all our guides and other helpers always act in the Highest and Best Good of our Being and of All Creation, and that any who act otherwise be immediately removed and Healed in the way that is best for All Creation.

If it be in the Highest and Best Good of ourselves and of All Creation then:

1. Let all constraints on our use of our Soul Senses be removed and that these be fully co-ordinated with our physical senses, let us have full access to all knowledge that will help us in our life, and let our whole Being always be kept free of damage, balanced, and fully operational in all aspects and in all dimensions - so that we are best able to accomplish the tasks given to us, always acting in True Holy Love. This is to include all our Chakras, glands, organs, meridians, grids, assemblage point, auric bodies, personal information fields, and other systems.

2. If any influences have mis-aligned our cells (or any other part of us) let this now be corrected, let all of us align with the 'Master Cell'. Let all of our cells always spiral good and be in communication with the 'Wisdom of our Body'. Let any of our genes that have been damaged be repaired, and all our repair and maintenance genes be made fully operational.

3. For all time to come let all our reactions to others be in Harmony and True Holy Love, and our intuitive abilities be fully operational including the removal of all blockages - by altering genes or by any other method, without causing any effects that are not beneficial to our Being or that cause any hurt or harm to others.

4. Let all hooks and cords that we have used to link to others, and all that have been placed in our Being by others, be removed. Let all implants, all imprints, all control devices, all interference, all thought forms, and all that has been sent to us without True Holy Love be removed. Let protection be placed to prevent any re-installation of these or similar things that are not beneficial to our Beingness.

We now pledge to operate at all times, in all ways, and in all aspects to help others with good intent for the highest and best good of all - to so operate in True Holy Love, Namaste.

All changes are to be for the Highest and Best Good of our Being and of All Creation, and be effective in all planes of existence, in all dimensions, in all domains, in all times, and in all 'nows'.

In all cases our cellular memories are to be adjusted accordingly, and changes in genes are to be imprinted in all genes and re-imprinted as needed.

Now we all agree to come together again in Harmony and True Holy Love, making sure that our Spirit, Soul, Ego, Higher Self, Lower Self, Conscious Self, Sub-conscious Self, Unconscious Self, and Non-conscious Self and all other parts of our Being are doing their correct jobs as members of the team, adjusting our intentions and our ways so that they are compatible with working together as a well co-ordinated team for the Highest and Best Good of our Being and of All Creation.

We come back to conception, to before our birth, to our infancy, to our childhood, to our youth, to being an adult - always stopping at events which had a major impact on our belief systems and memories, and taking the needed time to put these into a correct perspective according to our current knowledge.

We now ask that screens of the required dimensions of good gold and of all other needed colours be placed with True Holy Love within and around our Being, to protect and guard against all energies that are not in the Highest and Best Good of our Being or of All Creation for all our life, and to Heal all such energies in the way that is best for All Creation.

End of program. Thanks.'

Having read the 'Healing the Total Being' program, now check with your Intuition (through your Heart) that it is clear, non-contradictory, and without errors. Make any changes that are indicated, and re-check.

Ask permission to install the program; if granted, ask that it be installed now; check if the installation has been successful and without error - and then run the program on yourself.

Expect that this program will take a few days (and nights) to run and do the needed Healing - depending on the amount of corrective action to be taken. The key is to sincerely desire the corrections to be made and to be open to accepting the errors that you have made.

We all make many mistakes - what is important is to recognize our errors, apologize for harm that we caused (to ourselves and others), forgive others involved, understand the lessons that we can learn from our mistakes - and learn those lessons, so we do not have to repeat our errors !

We have got rid of a lot of old rubbish, of junk discarded by others; we have had all treacherous ground removed; we have taken the topsoil out of the way, so that it is not buried but can be re-used in our new and improved garden.

Our foundation has been corrected, and the building of our life improved. As we continue, we must always remember that we are responsible for whatever we do.

This includes all actions which are indicated by our Intuition, Guides, or other helpers. Are these genuinely beneficial ?

One of the purposes of life may be to experience situations which give choices of action. If we believe that some action is wrong, that it would cause harm to others, we alone take full responsibility for that action.

We all make mistakes, however, and these are acceptable if we act with good intent, and learn all lessons from reconsidering the actions that we take - we can then forgive ourselves for mistakes made with good intent.

Our Intuitive Radio

We can consider ourselves as being like a radio that can transmit and receive signals, to communicate with others - including 'Upstairs'.

We are 'plugged in' because we are receiving Life energy from a well established 'mains supply' - we may not understand how this is generated, but it seems to be at the correct strength (voltage) for us.

We may even be 'switched on' - if we are open to co-operating with 'The System', and so receive help and give help to others.

There are various wave bands, and the most satisfactory is the one called Love - which is used to give support to all Beings in their endeavours to 'do what is right'.

A radio picks up all the signals (such as thoughts) that are transmitted; when we listen to a radio we choose one signal and amplify it so that it can be heard. Our own radio does this simply by thinking of who or what we wish to join in communication.

All this work is done by our Heart-Mind-Brain team - our Brain retrieves the needed frequency from its own storage, our Mind selects the station, and our Heart ensures distortion-free tuning.

If we have any sort of communication with another Being, we have stored their frequency and 'signature' (vibrational pattern) in our memory. This is also the case with any item which we have held in our hand. In some cases, when we have not had previous contact, we may have to ask, via our Heart, for the needed data.

Some people have the ability to link directly to their Heart-Mind-Brain team using their senses - or the similar senses of the Soul, as previously discussed. They are clairvoyant, feel the atmosphere, hear messages, or just 'know'.

Most of us need an earphone (or a loud-speaker) to help us hear the signals better, or a meter-like device of some description to indicate such signals.

This is the work done by our nervous-muscular system, as demonstrated in our first experiment - our body moved forward to signal YES, or backward to indicate NO.

More Body Signals

We are not restricted to just forward or back body movements - we can develop other signals. We decide on the signal, explain it to our Heart-Mind-Brain team, load it as a program, and practice with it to ensure that it is installed correctly and works properly.

Three of the very best, which I find to be extremely accurate, very fast, and not noticeable to most other people, are using Finger Tap or Slide, Eye Blinks and Tongue Signals.

Finger Tap or Slide

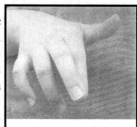

Use your middle finger to press down on the nail of your index finger as you ask a question - if your index finger resists a YES signal is given, collapse means NO. It is even less tiring to try to slide the middle finger from the index finger nail - YES and NO signals may vary according to which hand is used, so check !

Photo from Susan Collins' book 'Bridge Matter and Spirit with Dowsing'

See www.dowser.ca

This is used by experts checking a client's health - it is fast, and does not cause any tiring, so is suitable for continual use.

Eye Blinks

One blink indicates YES, two blinks means NO, and three blinks signals that the question is not understood, or that the answer is not available.

Tongue Signals

Ask your question with your tongue midway between your upper and lower teeth, and feel where it goes - to your upper teeth for YES, or lower teeth for NO. Going to the roof or floor of your mouth indicates a very strong signal

A variant of this is to rub your tongue over the roof of your mouth and ask your question - rough means YES, smooth NO.

Often the answer comes as I am still formulating the question in my mind ! This is wonderful when trying to work out a problem, since you are continually being guided in the right direction.

The late Dan Wilson, who was a 'leading light' in the Alternative Healing Community in England, did a brilliant job in suggesting some interesting signals. Here are his suggestions:

Basically, people are 'touchies' or 'feelies' - they naturally do Intuitive Signaling by touch or movement, or by feel or sensing.

First, what kind of question-and-answer would really be useful and interesting to you ? This is a very personal matter, but in classes I usually suggest a few; for example:

"Is my health better than 50 per cent compared to perfect health ?" You look for a YES or NO signal when trying 10, 20, 30, 40 etc. per cent in turn; this is better than asking is it a particular percentage, since it may not be an exact number.

You HAVE to get a response somewhere so it's a good starter; 0 won't be an answer as that will require you to be dead, and if you get 100 there's probably a glitch in your system.

You can test for 'vitality' in the same way. 'Vitality' as a percentage is the proportion of your total energy available for living rather than fighting current stress factors.

'Health' is the same thing, but rolling into account all the possible stress factors you are likely to meet, being the person you are.

"What stresses me ?" Start with classes of things like food, other substance, circumstance, interrelationship, something place-linked, then hunt for detail.

"Does my car/house/TV need attention for anything ?" If YES, then ask more questions to narrow it down.

"Is my mother-in-law naturally like that, or do we wind each other up ?" A laugh in the class is never unwelcome !

When I teach people, I mix the touchy and feely systems to give everyone a chance.

Whole Body

Stand to attention in front of (say) the supermarket egg counter. Fix a carton of the type you are interested in with your eagle eye and ask, *"Are all these eggs fresh, good, and free from cracks ?"*. A slight bow YES, a slight bending back NO.

A few people who have tried this found that they twisted round rather than bowed, and one man found that his bow was graduated, so if the eggs were very fresh indeed, he did a Japanese bow suitable for the Emperor. (I didn't ask what happened if they were totally rotten.)

Most people get a forward or backward movement. If you do not, then be alert for any other noticeable sensation, or other body part twitch or movement.

Other Body Responses

Many people have a hand reaction of some kind - two fingers moving apart or together, or a clenching or opening.

This energy sensation varies enormously from one person to the next, and from question to question. There are a wide variety of sensations that can be experienced, such as:

- Tingling feelings in all of the hand or just part of the hand
- A gentle breeze-like feeling blowing past the hand
- A cool draft of air
- A pressure-like pushing against an invisible barrier
- An edge-like feeling as if an invisible sharp edge is pushing on a large or small part of your hand/fingers.
- A gentle push on the fingertips
- A pronounced tingling or sharp sensation in one finger only or just part of one finger only
- A 'thud' feeling in the palm of the hand
- A line of energy suddenly appearing across part of the hand.

Those are just a few of the common ones. Usually they are felt in the left hand, but sometimes also in the right hand, and occasionally in both hands.

Sometimes the sensation is very 'up front' and obvious, whilst at other times it is subtle.

You may even get different responses for different types of questions - perhaps because the answer is coming from different sources of knowledge.

Finger Thumb

Think your question, or the section of it (*"is 40% correct ?"*) and rub index finger and thumb together gently. A rough feeling indicates YES, a slippery feeling shows NO; you can have a second opinion on the finger behind, rough for NO.

This system doesn't work well for me, so I use the thumb and the next finger (my middle finger) - I get a reverse signal this way. This is similar to the Radionics 'stick pad', which you rub with a thumb to get the knob settings on the 'black boxes'.

It is very popular with Intuitive doctors who can hide their hand in their pocket for covert diagnosis and get signals about a patients health !

Two Hand Pass

A) Place the palms of your hands together in a prayerful manner at face level.

B) Lower the left hand to waist level.

C) Place your awareness in the palm of your right hand, which remains in an upright position.

D) Ask a question (which can be answered with a simple YES or NO) of your left hand.

Give yourself plenty of space and extend your left arm back as far to the left as you can.

Then gradually move your left hand in the reverse direction, coming in a wide sweep at waist level towards and around your front.

Note that the left hand is kept well below the upright right hand at all times. The two hands are NEVER opposite one another at the same level.

E) If the answer is YES, you will feel energy, or pressure, or just a strong physical inclination to stop before your left hand gets to below the right elbow. This is the energy we are talking about.

If the answer is a strong YES, the left hand will stop almost immediately, while a weak YES will be closer to the front.

If the left hand stops under the right elbow, it means 'Don't know'.

If the left hand goes cleanly past the right elbow under the right hand, then the answer is NO.

It is wise to practice this exercise over and over so you get used to the sensation in your left hand.

The easiest way to practice this is to ask YES/NO questions where you already know the answer - often the silliest and most obvious questions are the best for this practice.

Forced Blink

Consciously hold your eyes open and think your question. A blink occurring against your will signifies YES.

If you're uncertain whether a blink was a natural one or a Intuitive one, repeat the exercise using another system. After a while you can tell them apart.

I got into Intuitive Signaling via this method. I needed to find cheap fuel when driving at 70 mph, so I used the steering wheel as a 'clock face', with positions indicating numbers from 1 to 12.

Run one hand round it for direction (12 o'clock = straight ahead), then ask for mileage - first total distance, second *"How far along this road before I turn off ?"*.   When you get a forced blink, you are getting the answer as shown on a clock face.

This is excellent for such things as locating radar traps, and *"When is this lady in front going to turn off ?"*

Own Aura Sensing

Find another person and see if you can 'sense their aura'. This is done simply by extending your palm towards them and expecting some kind of reaction as you enter their aura.

Sometimes this is a tingling, sometimes it's an 'invisible balloon' feeling, or just some form of gentle resistance.

When you have practiced this with another person, repeat on your own self - then you know that you have an aura, and how it feels.

After that you can command your aura to be there for YES, and not be there for NO. Bingo - you have an Intuitive Signaling system up and running.

A variation of this is to hold your hands apart, palms open and facing each other; now move your palms together slowly, and you will feel auric energy - just some form of gentle resistance.

You can command this auric energy to be there for YES, and be absent for NO. Very simple and effective !

Hand Jab

Ask your question and thrust your right or left hand down sharply as though trapping a bouncing tennis ball. The hand closing spontaneously means NO, opening out YES.

Because of its dynamic movement, this system is excellent for forcing weak Intuitive Signaling to become stronger - 'bursting the paper wall of fear'.

The jab can be upwards, as in a class I gave to the Surrey Dowsers in Surbiton (a suburb of London).

As soon as I suggested the method, about fifty ladies were leaping about the room, jabbing into the air and laughing fit to bust. They were checking on their neighbours, the naughty girls.

As one said, *"If her fancy man parks his Mercedes round the block and I can check what he's doing in there, it's only like having another pair of eyes, isn't it ?"*

I don't know if this preoccupation is shared in other great cities !

Slinky

A 'slinky' is one of those machined spiral metal coils which if you place one at the top of a staircase and push it over, it will somersault slowly down the stairs.

Imagine you are holding one upright in your right palm, place your left palm next to it but lower, like a stair, and ask your question.

If you feel the 'slinky' arriving in your left palm (and/or your hands rising/lowering to match the change in weight) that signifies YES - no change signals NO.

For me this works purely by hand movement - I can't feel the slinky. A variant of this movement is:

Wrist Twist

Hold your hand-shaking hand out as though about to shake hands with someone invisible, thumb upwards, then think your question. Your hand usually twists clockwise for YES, or counter/anti-clockwise for NO.

Chain Link

Gently pinch your right thumb and first finger together, enclose them in a similar left-handed pinch (as if they were two links in a chain), ask your question, and then try to pull apart. Success signifies YES, failure NO.

Opposed Thumbs

Place your hands (palms open towards your body) in front of you as though sheltering your stomach, with the eight fingers hanging down almost parallel and the two thumbs upwards, pressing hard against one another in an upside-down V.

Ask your question and the two thumbs flick away from you for YES and towards you for NO.

In my case, I find I can get rough numbers up to 10 immediately, because the thumb movements are graduated over a 90 degree range.

The significance can be reversed for some individuals, or by willpower, or against your will when you get tired (this is sometimes called 'switching').

You have to find out which is which by asking establishing questions to which you know the answer, or command *"Show me my YES signal!"*

Point-&-Sense

Ask your question and point at the possible answers, which you have attributed mentally to the fingers of the non-pointing hand.

A distinctive sensation (a sting in the neck or ear lobe is common) is YES.

Invisible Balloon

Use one hand to sense with and the other (or the wall) as a wall. Ask your question and move this hand towards the 'wall'.

An invisible balloon (or prickly ball, or cold area, etc.) getting in the way signifies YES - bigger and harder, a surer one.

You can play around with this a lot - e.g. have balloons signifying NO, or have different areas on the wall for diagnostic balloons giving you choices, numbers, times, etc. The 'balloon' is used a lot to sense auras and energy bodies.

Finger Wiggle

Hold your hands limp and ask your question. If the fingers of one hand flutter like a curtain in a breeze the signal is YES; if the fingers of the other hand flutter, NO. Check which hand gives which signal!

Nod

Hold head straight as weakly as will just keep it from flopping, and ask your question. An involuntary nod indicates YES; NO might be signalled by a shake sideways or a jerk backwards.

Robot Nose

Similar to Nod - but using your field of view and blinks.

Keep your eyes looking ahead and ask your question, which then will be answered by something in your field of view (*"Which melon tastes best?"*)

Allow your nose to point to the answer. Another method is to move your eyes across the scene from left to right, imagining a vertical cursor line. An involuntary blink means: the sought goodie is on this line.

Then hold your eyes on the line and scan up and down. A blink means that you are looking at it. This is especially good when picking stones or shells off a beach.

You can keep a reserve blink for something which is hidden underneath the top layer(s) - very good in supermarkets where the best fruit or vegetable is some way down in the pile.

Rummage on the chosen coordinates until you get a blink.

<u>Finger Lift</u>

Rest a wrist on your chest or a chair arm so that the fingers are free to move but extended. Ask one finger to rise to signal YES. When one rises, ask for another to signal NO.

You can even assign other fingers for other responses.

Be sure that you're not moving the fingers voluntarily. If you prefer, you can choose which fingers signal which responses, e.g. use only one hand. You may notice a tingling or other sensation.

In a watchful state this method may require time and some effort. Under hypnosis it's rare for it not to work.

Dan Wilson's Comments

In all these cases, the significance can be reversed for some individuals, or by willpower, or against your will when you get tired; this is called 'switching'.

You have to find out which is which by asking establishing questions to determine your YES signal.

If you do not get any response, it may mean *"That was not the right question to ask!"*, that the question was not understood, or that an answer was not available.

If you get greatly exaggerated responses, you may be getting 'YES stronger than YES' - also called 'yes-beyond-yes', and a similar extra-strong NO.

These signify answers which are more positive or negative than you have allowed for in your question.

> *"Has my daughter passed her exam ?"*
> > Yes-beyond-yes 'she came top'.
> *"Will my plane leave on time ?"*
> > No-beyond-no 'Flight Cancelled'.

Intuitive Signaling can be used to find ways of remedying your tension quickly - identifying the causes, and asking about solutions.

The Power of Thought

Human Beings are creators. As are beavers, viruses, ants, bees and their kind, birds, moles, rabbits, and a few more species. Most other than Humans just create their own nests or homes.

Man seems different in that we create things that affect most other life forms - not in just repeating what has been made before, but new forms and devices.

Humans do not yet have the ability to create life, but to manipulate matter and other life forms for their own purposes - not all results being beneficial to humans or others.

We are, in many respects, just like the student apprentice to a magician, as portrayed in Tchaikovsky's 'Sorcerer's Apprentice', who has some skills, does not understand the consequences of mis-using them, and creates chaos.

Mystics tell that all our thoughts go into the 'cosmic collection' or similar label, similar to Rupert Sheldrake's 'Metamorphic Field' - where they remain for ever. Both the good and the bad !

If one life form develops a new skill, and this is copied by others and found to be useful, it then quickly spreads to others - even those who are not in physical contact with the originators.

There are many examples of this, such as the 'Hundredth Monkey' when one monkey washed its food, others living on the same island copied this practice and found it to be good, and suddenly it spread to monkeys on other islands.

Another occurred in Europe; glass milk bottles had metal foil caps, and were placed by the milkmen on the doorsteps of customers. A 'Blue Tit' (name of a particular bird in England) discovered that it could peck through the foil and enjoy drinking the cream - and suddenly this practice spread throughout Europe.

Scientists have had a number of occasions when they made new compounds, expecting to get a particular result - but this did not happen.

Yet when many more scientists did the same work, the expected results started to happen - and were repeated in all further experiments.

Thoughts are Broadcast

When we have a thought, get a feeling, or express an emotion, we broadcast it to 'All that Is', as do all animals, reptiles, insects, and plants. Perhaps the unimportant broadcasts are dissipated over time, but those that 'The System' considers to be noteworthy seem to be stored - added to 'The System's' store of knowledge or retained as memories in any stones or crystals affected.

A thought that is broadcast is like a pebble thrown into a pond - it sends ripples that travel the whole surface, perhaps meeting other ripples and changing to jointly form an interference pattern, similar to that used in a holograph.

We, and 'All that Is', receive these complicated interference patterns; from our interpretation of these interference patterns we formulate our own actions.

Thus each thought that we have (and broadcast) has a potential effect in the future, both our future and that of others.

Our thoughts are broadcast as symbols - which seem to be universal, understood by animal and plant life, and by Beings 'Upstairs'. Are the crop circles that appear in fields these symbols ? Although our conscious selves may not have direct understanding of these symbols, they may be recognized by our sub-consciousness.

Our Own Thoughts

On a personal basis, when we have good or bad thoughts about another person, the effect can be observed in their aura - even if thousands of miles distant.

It is known that these thoughts often come back to the originator, so it is worthwhile to always have good thoughts of others - and of yourself.

If you do not like the behavior of another, then send thoughts of how you would like them to behave; if enough people do this, a change might be effected.

If a political leader is involved, this may be more effective than the ballot-box - and the desired result may occur sooner !

Remember that such leaders are subject to the influence of those around them or otherwise involved in decisions being made - so send the thoughts to 'all concerned', not just the figurehead.

Thought precedes Action

This may seem to be contradicted by our 'fight or flight' actions resulting from emotional triggers (the thought may be sub-conscious), by the action of tides (which may be following the laws of gravity - perhaps made by a 'higher level of thought'), and by seemingly automatic happenings (installed as programs, themselves formed from thoughts).

Certainly a lot of thought goes into developing any new idea, often from a number of people. More thought is then given to the best way of getting the wanted results from the idea - such as materials needed, manufacturing process, marketing aids, sales efforts, financial implications, and other applicable requirements.

This applies to going on a holiday, baking a cake, handling your correspondence, meeting new people, taking the dog for a walk, going to sleep, or any other activity. The thoughts will differ, but all that are needed will exist - together with thoughts that arose, but were discarded for whatever reason.

The initial idea will be a thought to do or make something; perhaps this will be sketched, or notes made - a two dimensional image. The intermediate steps and the final result may be visualized - now three dimensions. Then, if all seems correct, you may do what is needed to achieve or make the result.

The greater the detail that goes into this thought process, the better the chances of success.

Help from 'Upstairs'

You may find that you get thoughts in your Mind that you did not originate, but help you with the success of your project. Perhaps you are tapping into the 'Cosmic Store' of information and knowledge.

There is a well established principle: 'Like attracts Like'. This occurs with your thoughts about whatever you are trying to achieve - not only in your endeavours to make something, but also in your personal life.

If you are depressed in any way, you will usually find that the people around you are also depressed - often in the same way. For 'depressed' you can substitute any other description, good or 'not good'.

You are the captain in charge of your thoughts. If you put a lot of effort into changing negative thoughts into positive ones, this will happen - but it may take time. Using the EFT and similar procedures you can speed this process, and also improve your health.

The Secret

This is the name of a film, available on DVD, that you may have seen - it explains that if you really want something, visualize the desired result, and put your emotions into this action, then 'The Universe' will provide. It tells the story of many people who have done this with great success.

If you continually put your efforts into thinking 'the very best' then that will be the end result - that is what you attract.

Do not fall into the trap of thinking that you know more than 'Upstairs' - visualize and put emotions into the desired result and its benefits, NOT into 'How this Happens'.

You may think that you need to win the lottery - 'Upstairs' may have a better way of getting the money that you need to come to you.

Notice that the accent is on 'what you need' - not on just what you want. In the same context, do not limit yourself ! Do not think of just $100 to solve an immediate problem - 'Upstairs' may know that you need $1000 to 'get on your feet' again, or even more if you are open to using it to help others for a good purpose. Ask for 'all that you need to have a good life'.

'Need, NOT Greed' is the motto - if you are just being greedy, then you will probably attract others who are greedy, not anything that is useful to you in any substantial way.

Quality of Thought

'Be careful of what you request - you may get it!' and find that although it fits your description, it is not suitable ! Do not ask for 'a Cadillac' - the one that you get may be on its way to the scrap heap.

Be clear and precise - define the model, year, colour, that it be in excellent working condition, that it remain in excellent working condition for all the time that you own it (and say how long the minimum period), that it never gives you any large repair bills, that you and your family will always be safe in it.

Remember the ancient story of King Midas - who wished that 'All that he touched then turned into gold'. Have you tried eating gold ?

There is always 'enough to go round' - but it may require effort on your own part to make this happen. Wealth is not going to come to someone who just thinks of being rich, without making any effort to improve his/her abilities and skills, or fails to put the needed physical energy into achievement.

For example, you are not going to meet your desired partner if you spend all your time watching television ! You must, at the very least, get out and meet other people, and make yourself presentable in all ways.

'No Harm to Others'

Remember that your thoughts attract similar thoughts - and that these can become actions. So if you think negatively about any other person, the chances are that you will suffer in the same way.

There is no harm in wanting to be as rich as another - if this is held as an aim for yourself. But to hold jealousy or envy, or wish that they lose their riches, is to attract disaster to your own self.

Any thought that you have for the detriment of others is like casting a spell. Some people have the skill to do this effectively, and usually they suffer a similar fate later.

If you do not have the skill, the result may not be effective on others - but can surely affect you, who asked for it to happen. Be safe, and ensure that all of your thoughts are kind and positive.

It helps to remember that none of us are perfect - 'There is good in the worst of us, and bad in the best of us'. Robin Hood stole from the rich to give to the poor - the opposite of the policies of many business corporations and some governments.

You may recall a number of prominent religious leaders who called for donations for the general good - but really meant the 'General in Charge', themselves ! Thankfully these cases are few - but they do happen.

The Power of Love

We have discussed the thoughts - now let us have a deeper look into how we can reinforce these to obtain manifestation - to make them materialize.

The strongest of all feelings is Love. The Eskimo have about fifty words for snow to adequately describe all its textures. We, however, have only one word for Love in English - including all its variations.

Love of money, of power, of certain foods, of various drinks, of pretty clothes. Sexual attraction (I love you !), anticipation of a pleasant happening (I'd love to go there !), and musical appreciation (I love that music !) are examples.

The real Love, 'True Holy Love, Namaste', is doing your best to help others for the good of all; this does not include helping them to realize greed or do things which are detrimental or harmful to any others in any way.

'Others' includes all life forms, all the Creations of the 'Holy Creator in Love of All Things, in All Places, in All Dimensions, in All Times'.

This may be the best description of the 'One God' - not just the God of Humans, but of 'All That Is'. Personally, I do not believe that any 'Good God' wants to be worshipped - what is really wanted is to help him/her to care for all His/Her Creations, to give them respect and Love.

Is this what we do by polluting the earth ? By poisoning plants and insects ? By not caring about the side effects of actions that we take - or even purposefully hurting other life forms ? *"Do unto others as you would have done to you"*.

Gratitude for the benefits that we receive, as a genuine feeling, does encourage more benefits to be given. If one is ungrateful, the reaction may be *"Why should we bother with him ? Let us help those who are thankful instead."*

This can often be recognized in human relationships - at home, at work, and at play. The old wisdom 'As Above, So Below' may be reversible - 'As Below, So Above', since we are all just different aspects of the same creation.

When we seek to do 'whatever' for the general good, to help others, then we are acting in Love. Action is far more important than words. How often do people say one thing, and then do something else, or the opposite to their 'promise' ?

This type of behavior is not restricted to politicians !

If the intent is to help others, not just one's own self, then 'Upstairs' is far more likely to put great effort in helping the manifestation of what is desired.

The Effect of Emotions

After Love, next most powerful is the effect of putting a great deal of emotion into your request.

As discussed with emotional triggers, any very strong emotion attaches great importance to whatever is being thought, and so your sub-consciousness puts more effort into attracting and manifesting things that are associated with the thought.

This could be called an 'emotional attractor', and seems to have a lot of similarity with an 'emotional trigger' - guiding you to do what is needed to assist with the manifestation.

Failure to build an emotional attractor may mean that the chances of success are greatly reduced. You have not strongly indicated the importance of your desire to your sub-conscious mind-brain team.

In this context, the emotion to be attached must be positive ! Any hate, anger, or greed involved will attract those negative reactions to you - to your own detriment.

Attach happiness, joy, freedom from negativity (of whatever description), and the emotions associated with Love itself.

Be Sensual !

Use all your senses to reinforce your desires - to implement the realization that 'what you desire' has already happened !

You may not yet be aware of 'it' in the physical world, but your thoughts have already started to make it happen in the world of thoughts !

- So visualize yourself enjoying the desired result.
- See yourself using whatever it is with beneficial results.
- Imagine how your life has changed for the good.
- Picture how others get benefit from your manifestation.

Bring your other senses into use, too:

- Feel the beneficial changes that happen to you.
- Feel how these changes help others.
- Feel how others appreciate these changes.
- Hear other people congratulating you.
- Taste the fruits of success.
- Smell the aroma that goes with a successful person.
- Touch all you can with these benefits.
- Know that all is now well.

The more effort that you put into this, the stronger becomes the attraction generated, and the more likely the successful result.

Magical Ceremony

The actions just described are very similar to any magical ceremony. The main difference is that it is not just you yourself doing all the work, but a group of like-minded people.

You are achieving magical results - things that others believe cannot be done by ordinary people, only by magicians or other 'special people' such as priests.

The ceremonial part of this is the reinforcement of a thought or a collection of thoughts by repetition - a church ceremony, a witches coven, a Healing circle, a political rally, a sports meeting, or anywhere the routine is repeated with the same intent.

Of course, at a sports meeting you probably have opposing thoughts - and those of people who are distant will still have effect. This may also happen at a corporate meeting, since the attendees may have diverse agendas.

The larger the number of Human Beings that participate, the more friends from 'Upstairs' will be attracted - and they may well be able to do things with you that you cannot do alone.

Be sure to attract 'Good Friends' ! That is the 'Real Magic'.

You are a Magician !

You can make things happen ! You can improve life for others - and yourself !

The greatest impediment is the belief that you cannot do something. Your own beliefs, 'stuck' in your mind-brain programming, are very effective in sabotaging anything that is contrary to themselves.

When you actually force the first step, you start to open your mind-brain team to a new belief - that you <u>can</u> do it !

- If you do not make the effort, you cannot succeed.
- If you do not ask, you may not get.
- If you do not succeed at first, do it again.
- Perseverance pays ! Do it NOW !

Any time is a good time. The best time is when you are most closely co-operating with your sub-conscious - when you are in the half-awake/half-asleep state, going to sleep or awakening, and especially when you wake for a short time in mid-sleep.

Develop a routine, your magical ceremony, that you work through at these times - like an affirmation, but more extensive, more powerful, and so more likely to succeed.

At these times you have alpha and/or theta brainwave patterns. There are many methods of achieving this same state when awake, so if you develop the skill of using these methods you can then put even more effort into manifesting your desire.

Subliminal messages were used in advertising - short flashes on television of a message, which did not register upon your conscious self, but were absorbed by your sub-conscious self.

These have now been banned in most countries; they were very effective, but were considered an abuse on the populace. Does this means that they should now be reserved only for use by governments ?

You can achieve a similar effect by using reminders of various types. These must be specifically associated with your desires, either in an obvious way such as spelling it in words or displaying it in pictures, or in a less obvious manner such as a special graphic.

Such a graphic must be drawn by you while thinking of your desire, and include symbols which you directly associate with your desire and its aspects and benefits.

It should be such that other people are unaware of its meaning - it is understood by you alone, and thus has 'extra special' meaning for you.

These reminders are excellent when placed so that you see them when going to sleep or awakening, since they remind you about your ceremony, and to 'do it now'.

They are also very effective in places where you relax - including your office where you may day-dream, your workplace where your attention may wander, or where you eyes go to get relief from television adverts. They will form a focus for your thoughts.

In all this, the strongest manifestation is when you use your Intuitive Heart-Mind-Brain team, and not rely just on your egoistic mind-brain team.

Do it NOW,
Do it with LOVE.

"Lift Up, Lift Up" the Voices Cry
Let's go and Visit in the Sky!

Levitation and Gravity

The Earth Grid is comprised of the geometrical flow lines of energy in the structure of the Earth itself; one point in the Grid having a long and strange history is at the eastern tip of Lake Ontario. Two individuals, living one hundred years apart, were both directly affected by this area. These men were Daniel Home, the 19th century psychic, and Wilbert Smith, the 20th century scientist.

Daniel Home is the world famous levitator of the 19th century who lived in this area; many of the crowned heads of Europe and many noted scientists and world dignitaries visited Home and verified his feats of levitation.

In the 20th century numerous aircraft crashes occurred in the area so the Canadian National Research Council and U.S. Navy began Project Magnet in 1950 to investigate the area.

Many UFO sightings were reported, and other bizarre and unearthly phenomena were noted. (For more information, refer to Hugh Cochrane's 'Gateway to Oblivion', Avon Books, NY)

Wilbert Smith, a Canadian communications engineer in the Department of Transportation, was director of the team of scientists involved in this project, officially terminated when the results became too sensitive for the two governments, as the research seemed to touch upon top secret UFO data.

Afterwards Wilbert Smith designed several inexpensive gravity devices, such as the Anti-Gravity Proximity Detector, the Magnetic Deflection Detector, and the EMP Collapse Collector.

Smith's speculations are most intriguing. He noted large and sometimes mobile gravity anomalies all over the Lake Ontario area. He noted areas of 'reduced binding' in the atmosphere described as 'pillar-like columns' a thousand feet across and extending for several thousand feet up into the atmosphere - invisible and only detectable with sensitive equipment.

Peculiarities in gravity and magnetism were noted inside these columns, possibly related to a reduction (or weakening) in the nuclear binding forces holding matter together; the nuclear binding forces seemed stronger in the north and weaker in the south.

Levitation Experiment

The object is to make the levitatee's body so light in weight that the four levitators can lift him several feet into the air using a single finger each.

The weight of the central person, the levitatee, does not matter nor is the lack of strength or size of the four levitators important.

The levitatee sits relaxed in a straight-backed chair with his legs together, his feet on the floor, and his hands in his lap.

The four levitators stand around him so that they form a square.

One levitator should stand to the levitatee's left, and just behind his shoulder; another levitator should stand in front of him and to his left, close to his left knee. The other two should stand on the right side of the levitatee's body and in similar positions.

The other four participants now stand two on each side of the seated party, one at each shoulder and one at the knee.

Instruct all four to extend their arms and place their closed fists together, closed except for the forefingers which should be extended and touching each other along their lengths as shown.

The person nearest the seated man's left shoulder is now asked to place his two extended fingers, palms downwards, beneath his left armpit.

Likewise, his opposite number inserts his forefingers beneath the right armpit, and again the other two respectively beneath the seated man's knees.

Now invite the four assistants to lift the man in this position, using only these extended fingers. However hard they try, it is impossible.

As soon as you have registered their inability to do so, ask them to stack their hands alternately, one on top of the other on the man's head, in such a way that no person has his own two hands together, and then to exert a steady pressure downwards.

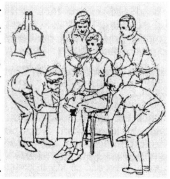

As they keep this up you count to ten.

On the count 'nine' they must withdraw their hands quickly from his head and resume their earlier positions with their extended forefingers.

On the count of 'ten' they must try again to
lift the man with those fingers alone. This
time he will go soaring into the air with no
difficulty whatsoever.

Here are a few pointers to keep in mind.

1. The levitators should be positioned 45
    degrees off the magnetic compass
    direction of north, south, east, and west
    for maximum effectiveness.

2. Alternation of male and female sex of
    the levitators adds to the gravity
    antenna's power - and the hands
    should alternate male - female - male -
    female etc. Note we will be lifting the chair as well.

3. There's no need to think of anything - just hold the hands
    stacked on the levitatee's head for a count of ten.

4. On the tenth count remove the stacked hands quickly and place
    one finger each under the four corners of the chair.

5. The person in charge of counting says 'lift' and up goes the
    chair and the levitatee.

If the experiment is performed properly none of the levitators will
feel the slightest resistance to their efforts - it will be as if the
levitatee's body has lost its weight entirely.

More Experiments

We do the experiment again but this time have no central person
(levitatee). Instead use the heaviest chair you can find. Just stack
the hands, touching on the top of the massive chair back and lift
(levitate) the heavy chair.

Next, place hundreds of pounds of 'dead' weight (such as heavy
books) on the chair seat and still levitate it easily - four weak
children could do the lifting.

Now try doing the levitation with only three people, positioned off-
center to the appropriate 90 degree spacing.

It seems that both the exact number and pattern of the human
levitator element, but not their exact size or physical strength, are
critical to the levitation.

An inanimate weight levitates easily - you could lift a piano or even a Volkswagen in place of the chair.

.

Were Pyramids Built this Way ?

Perhaps this was the technique used to build ancient huge monuments without having the cranes for lifting the stones in those days. The Great Pyramid of Gizeh is an brilliant example of mind over matter where the blocks of stones were lifted and set within the tolerance of an unbelievable higher precision without having the latest construction technology of today in those days.

The late Dan Wilson, using Dowsing sources, suggests that the pyramid stones were moved by a similar procedure:

1. A priest would read a passage from the Book of the Dead. No specific passage was necessary but this induced a respect for the dead - important to the exercise.

2. A rope would be placed around the stone such that it could be pulled sideways conventionally if free to move.

3. The priest would then invoke the spirit of the pyramid being built to assist. This was not a sterile formality. The priest would repeat the prayer if the spirit did not indicate to him that it was present.

4. The team would experimentally pull the rope to check if the spirit was cooperating. if it was not, the stages would be repeated.

5. If the stone moved, then a set of bars were placed like a portable railway to guide it to its final spot.

6. For the final placement, the team would shift the stone with their hands as indicated by the master mason.

7. The placement was judged by conventional surveying, not by getting spirits to place the stones.

The point to note from this is that no apparent lifting was involved. The stone had to be resting on something, however lightly. There was in fact no limit to the weight it was possible to float along the guidance bars, but in practice the priests thought it was asking too much of the spirit to use the process for loads greater than about twelve tons.

Build your own Pyramid

It is likely this exact same procedure could be followed today, employing the Egyptians' thought processes, by ourselves invoking intermediary spirits to activate the original thoughts on our behalf.

Of course there are other rather mundane aspects. You will have to draw plans and get approval from your local building authority; you will have to buy the stone, and arrange for permission to move them to your site - or to the city park, if the Mayor would like a Pyramid there. It could be a tourist attraction ! And you will need a co-operative priest.

Attention !

Serge King in his book 'Urban Shaman' tells how the weight varies according to where you place your attention. You can make something feel lighter by concentrating your attention above it.

First you 'tune in' to the centre of the item to be lifted - you are connecting to the 'life forms' in it; now raise you attention to be above it, and perhaps you are attracting those same 'life forms' to rise with your attention !

This may also include the thought created of the item becoming lighter - which would also be received by the 'life forms' in the item, who would reduce their attraction to 'be together' with other matter, which we label 'gravity'.

If so, then they would release (or reduce) their 'desire' to be 'grounded', and so feel lighter when you lift the item.

He tells how a lady bought a concrete pedestal for her garden which was placed in her car by two strong men. On getting home, she could not lift it out - and nobody was around to help her.

She remembered the above lesson from Serge, and by concentrating her attention above the pedestal she was able to move it from her car, and move it (in stages) to where it was intended to be placed.

For Emergency Use Only

You may find this procedure useful if you have the task of freeing a person trapped in a collapsed building, pinned beneath a car, or otherwise in trouble due to the effects of gravity.

Call in your Angels, Spirit Guides, etc. and ask their help ! If they could help to raise stones for pyramids, they will probably help in saving lives - and obtain help from others in the non-physical dimensions, including 'The Holy Being in Charge of All Gravity'.

Thinking <u>with intent</u> that 'it is now lighter', looking above (for help from 'Upstairs' ?), and knowing 'We can now lift it', would also seem to lighten the load !

There are many reports of instances where a person has been able to lift loads to help others - loads that it would be impossible to lift in the normal way of life.

Give respect when asking for help - and express your gratitude when the help materializes.

Fun, Not Hard Work !

Improving one's abilities and skills should be pleasant and enjoyable - not tedious or overly difficult.

Let us look at some ways that this can be done.

Everyday Opportunities

- Guess who is calling when the telephone rings.
- Hold a letter and imagine what is written.
- Visualize the colour of clothes that will be worn by someone you are to meet.
- Estimate the number of people who will attend a meeting.
- Ask your car if there is any problem. What comes to your mind immediately ? Perhaps nothing, if all is fine !
- Feel the atmosphere of all rooms that you enter.
- Visualize the look of a person you will be meeting for the first time.
- In a store, note when you enter a queue at the pay counter, estimate how many minutes until you leave the store.

Note that selecting lucky numbers for the lottery is not listed - it may work for you, but has not yet worked for me !

In all these examples, practice improves your skill - you may not succeed the first time, but every time you do one of these exercises you improve your ability.

Sector Selection

Perhaps the most important information that is needed by any person is which of the 'Soul Senses' is their strongest, since it pays to improve what you have before expending effort on something new.

Marking a paper with sectors enables you to display many different choices; you are not limited to the four shown here, but it is best not to have so many that they become crowded together.

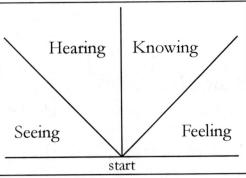

Soul Senses Selection

Usually you will have one sector allocated to 'other' - in case you have not listed the best choice for you.

If this 'other' is then selected, be aware of the very first thought that 'pops' into your head, make a new selection chart which includes that choice, and repeat the process.

There are a number of ways to make the selection; hold the thought of the question in your mind, and ask your Heart for the answer.

Then you can look at the selections shown and be aware of where your eye 'homes'; just know for some reason which is the best; rub your finger gently over the list and feel if it 'sticks' in any particular sector.

You can then repeat this asking if you have another Soul Sense that is very strong - people often have one that is extremely strong, and another which is very strong.

A variation is to make a list of items (vitamins, allergies, foods, holiday places, possible employers, etc), then feel if any item 'sticks' to indicate its selection.

You can also point to each in turn (a pen or pencil as a pointer is fine) and ask for a signal when 'gold is found'.

Remember that in a number of cases you may be interested in more than one 'golden nugget' - your body may need more than one vitamin or other supplement.

You could have listed possible places to go on your next holiday, employment types or employers for consideration, addressees of a possible next home, food to be eaten, which person to hire, which car to buy, or any other choices in your daily decisions.

Map Locating

You can use the above method on a map - it has square sectors, marking the co-ordinates. Here you can move in the north-south direction asking *"Is the XXX in this line of east-west squares ?"*, and then moving to these squares in sequence and asking *"Is XXX in this square ?"*.

When a square is chosen, you can sub-divide it into smaller squares and repeat this procedure to narrow down the location.

If XXX was gold or water, remember that there are minute quantities of gold in most soils, and that soils that are damp contain water.

You should be far more specific in your search criteria before spending money to dig a gold mine or drill a well !

If you are seeking a missing person, remember that you will probably not succeed if they do not want to be found; you also find it best to have some sort of connection to them - a photograph, piece of their hair, or some of their clothing.

This use of a connection is called 'using a witness' - and can greatly improve your accuracy.

Card Guessing Game

You will need a deck of playing cards, pen/pencil and paper to keep score. You will use your Intuition to determine if the next card drawn is red or black suited, later to identify the suite, and finally the value. Remove jokers and shuffle the pack of cards (the deck).

Ask your Intuition *"Is the next card in a red suite ?"* - write down your forecast: R (for red) if you got YES, or B (for black) if you got NO for an answer.

Draw the card from the top of the deck, and write another R or B (next to the letter indicating your forecast) to show the result. Repeat with the next card, writing your forecast and the result <u>on the next line.</u>

Why ? Because when you start getting these correct, your Intuition may start playing a game with you - quite often you will find that the forecast will not be for the top card on the deck, but the one below it ! Sometimes even for the one below that !

By writing the forecast and result side-by-side and below each other, you will be able to spot if the result column matches the forecast column, or is one or two cards 'out of step' !

As a variation, after you ask the colour, if red ask "Is it a Heart ?" and if YES write H after your colour forecast letter (write D for diamond if you got NO); or if black ask about a Spade - and write S for spade or C for Club.

You can carry this even further to find the card value. Ask your Intuition *"Is the next card an ace ?"* - if so, write A on the same line; if not, ask *"Is the next card a picture card ?"* and if YES, ask *"Is the next card a (king, queen, or jack) ?"* - whichever you 'feel in your mind' is the best to ask about.

Do not get rigid in this, such as always asking the same sequence - go with your feeling, which may be your Intuition guiding you.

If you got NO to the card being an ace or a picture card, then you ask *"Is the next card a (any number from 2 to 10) ?"* - whichever you 'feel in your mind' is the best to ask about.

If you get NO, then use the method that computer programs use to find a solution: ask *"Is the value greater than 5 ?"* - if the answer is YES, then it must be between 6 and 10, so split the difference and ask *"Is the value greater than 8 ?"* - if YES, ask about 9 - another YES means it must be a 10, NO indicates it is a 9 since it is greater than 8 but not more than 9 !

Split the difference in the same way if you got NO to being greater than 5 - it must be between 2 and 5, so check greater than 3, etc.

You can combine all these ways to forecast the suite and value of the cards ! Use this for fun - not to bet your savings at the casino !

Bored, with nothing to do ? Play this game, not just to pass the time, but to improve your Intuitive abilities.

Shaking a Dice

You need a dice with a throwing cup.

Shake the dice in the thrower and then place the thrower on a table, open end down, to hide the dice.

First Method - Splitting Values:

Ask *"Are there [any number from 1 to 6] spots on the top surface of the dice ?"* - whichever number you 'feel in your mind' is the best to ask about.   Remember that if you do not specify which surface, you could get answers that may be correct - but not what you intended.

If you get NO, then use the method that computer programs use to find a solution: ask *"Is the value greater than 3 ?"* - if the answer is YES, then it must be between 4 and 6, so split the difference and ask *"Is the value greater than 5 ?"*- YES means it must be 6, NO indicates it is 4 or 5; ask if it is 5 – if NO it is 4.

Split the difference in the same way if you got NO to being greater than 3 - it must be between 1 and 3, so check greater than 2, etc.

Second Method - Awareness:

Some people have the ability to 'move their awareness' around their body - this is not just looking at a part of your body, but imagining that a 'feeling' goes there.

Try to do this, saying *"my left shoulder indicates 1, left hip 2, left foot 3, right foot 4, right hip 5, right shoulder 6 "* - make variations if you want !

Then ask your awareness to indicate the number of spots on the top surface of the dice - and 'be aware' of the location of your awareness, the number indicated !

Some people do this using their forehead as a dial - extreme left being 1, with graduations across the top for 2 & 3 on the left side, for 4 & 5 on the right side, and the extreme right side indicating 6.

No scoring here, unless you just want to count how many times that you have success - to see how you are improving your intuitive abilities !

How else can this be used ?

You can assign different values or meanings to different parts of your body, using these as a scale. It is best to keep a constant form to these - and forms to which you are accustomed.

For example, you are probably accustomed to immediately sensing the dials on your car dashboard - clockwise left to right for speed, engine heat, fuel supply; and your charging indicator is central for null, left increasing with discharge (negativity), right increasing with charge (positivity).

So you can assign values or meanings that are pertinent to the situation that you wish to examine, such as health of a patient, chances of success, advisability of an investment, suitability for a purpose, expected response to a proposal.

You can probably think of more examples that concern your own situation, or that of your business, and use them to help make good decisions.

The more that you use this system, the greater grows your confidence in the results obtained.

Lie Detector Game

You need other players, a deck of playing cards, pen/pencil and paper to keep score; you can use any Soul Sense.

The object of the game is to use your Intuition to detect if a person is making a true or false statement. The first player who gets 25 points wins the game.

The dealer is the only one who can score points during a round - the players try to keep the dealer from scoring points.

Designate one player to keep score. Then cut for first dealer.

The dealer deals one (1) card to each player (none to him/herself). The player to the left of the dealer starts the game.

This player will choose to tell the dealer either a TRUE or FALSE statement about the value and suit of the card she/be is holding. Example: the player is holding the King of Hearts.

A true statement would be King of Hearts; a false statement would be King of Clubs or 5 of Spades.

The dealer will mentally ask her/his Intuition *"Is this statement true ?"*, and say TRUE or FALSE.

The player's card will be shown - if the dealer answered correctly, the dealer scores one (I) point, otherwise no point is awarded.

Now the dealer moves to the next player and repeats the same sequence. The dealer continues until all players have had their turn, and the dealer adds up all of her/his points and the total is recorded.

The deal is passed on to the player on the left. This starts a new round; the same play sequence is repeated.

Remember the dealer is the only one that can score points.

Simple Variations

You can use 'red or black', the suite name, and/or value - building up to a more complicated game as the players gain confidence.

Betting Variation:

This game is played the same except for betting with poker chips - the first player will place a bet and the dealer has to match it; the player makes his/her statement about the card they are holding.

If the player fools the dealer, this player wins all the chips. If the dealer is correct, she/he gets the chips.

The dealer moves on the next player and repeats the same process until all players have had a turn. Then the deal moves onto the next player. The player with the most chips wins.

How else can this be used ?

The ability to tell when you are being told a lie can be used in many different circumstances - a most useful skill !

If you develop other signaling methods, such as the blinking of your eye, movement of your tongue, or placement of your awareness to a body position - nobody will know that you are using your skills !

Telepathic Communication

If you get an urge to telephone somebody, perhaps you are receiving a telepathic signal from them, asking you to contact them.

You can send such a signal yourself - think clearly about the person, picture them in your mind, see them picking up a telephone, visualize you being at the other end of a telephone cable.

The closer the rapport that you have with the person, the more effective this will be.

Meetings

If you are to meet a person or group that are new to you, visualize this happening, even to the clothes that are worn.

Do not have fear in any way - that would restrict your ability. If you consider that you need the situation changed in a way that is advantageous to you, make the changes in your visualization.

Raymon Grace tells how one woman in a group making a decision seemed to be antagonistic; he pictured her surrounded by boxes of delicious chocolates and mounds of red roses, and sent Love to her.

He visualized the group making a decision which was advantageous to him - and then this actually happened.

Use this for interviews, making sales, business meetings, and social interactions - but remember the keys are doing it with Love, without harm to others - make it a win-win solution.

Experimenting with Thought

Imagine, in your mind, that you build a wall along a particular line; imaging the bricks, etc., being placed strongly and securely - make it as high as you like, use materials other than brick if you so prefer.

As with all Mind work, the more emotional energy that you put into this visualization, the greater will be the effect.

Now ask your helper to see if s/he can feel anything as the wall is approached ! Can you feel it yourself ?

You may find success in building a wall (or similar) to keep animals on or off your property, as a barrier against rodents, or a shield against mosquitoes.

What you build is not in the physical dimension; but since thought precedes action, and it is considered to be real by the thinking processes of the life forms involved, it works.

When making a shield, you must have a clear intent of its exact purpose, where it is to be located, and the time for it to be active - and make sure that the purpose is described in a positive way, that it is beneficial, without harm to others.

If you find that the shield that you make does not work as well as you hoped, ask your Heart how it can be improved - and accept the advice given by the very first thought that 'pops' into your Mind.

One big advantage of such a barrier is that it does not harm the life forms involved, such as rats, mice, or mosquitoes - it just keeps them away.

You may find that the power of a shield drops with time, and needs to be reinforced - for you to put more of your personal energy into it, with your Love and Gratitude for the help given.

Such a shield does not have to be fixed in any one spot - it can be linked to a person or object. You can build a mosquito shield around yourself, or place protection around your car.

A driver placed a shield of blue light around the car with the intention that the car would be invisible to police. It worked ! The car was rammed by a police car on an emergency mission - the police driver did not see the car !

Albert Einstein - Dowsing

Many years ago, Herman Wolf was entertaining a guest at his parents' rural home near Bremen, Germany, when, in general conversation, Wolf's mother mentioned that a huge pond in their garden was 'leaking'.

The guest said he might be able to help and immediately fashioned a forked dowsing rod. Taking the rod, he walked out to the pond and in a short time pinpointed the exact location of the underground flow that was draining the pond. The Wolfs were delighted and even more so when their guest proceeded to teach them the fine points of the art of dowsing.

Herman Wolf was actually more amazed than delighted because his friend and guest was none other that the celebrated scientist Albert Einstein.

Quotes by Albert Einstein

"I know very well that many scientists consider dowsing as they do astrology, as a type of ancient superstition. According to my conviction this is, however, unjustified. The dowsing rod is a simple instrument which shows the reaction of the human nervous system to certain factors which are unknown to us at this time."

"A human being is a part of the whole, called by us 'Universe', a part limited in time and space. He experiences himself, his thoughts and feelings as something separated from the rest - a kind of optical delusion of his consciousness. This delusion is a prison for us, restricting us to our personal desires and to affection for a few persons nearest to us. Our task must be to free ourselves from this prison by widening our circle of compassion to embrace all living creatures and the whole of nature in its beauty".

Building on a Good Foundation

We have now developed a good foundation for understanding who we are - and that we have abilities that most of us have not developed. Some of us will find one modality easier to develop than another - we all have our strengths, and our weaknesses.

The easiest way for most of us to use to access and use our abilities is by forming a proper question in our logical mind-brain, and then asking our Heart. Our Heart-Mind-Brain team then manipulates our nervous-muscular system to give a signal; this can be a body movement: forwards YES, backwards NO. Other signals can be developed, too.

We can also 'tune in' to the 'signatures' (vibrational patterns) of other forms and instances of existence - simply by thinking of them; the better we understand these others, the more accurate becomes our tuning.

Tuning in to these signatures was a skill that was learnt in Egypt, being used in antiquity by the Pharaohs and the Egyptian priesthood - and is the basis of Feng Shui as used in China 4,000 years ago.

By using tools to amplify the signals given, more detail may be obtained - and at a faster speed. This use of tools to extend the range of signals is called Dowsing in the English language, and Radiesthesia in many others - or sometimes when locating wells 'Water Witching'.

The interesting point about this terminology is that the Roman Catholic priests used these methods themselves, but if any person who was not ordained used them, they were described as using 'witchcraft'. The Spanish priests used this a lot when they invaded the Americas - and the hint of witchcraft was quite effective in preventing others from competing to find hoards of gold.

Except in certain cases, the tool used has no inherent powers - it just signals the body responses. The special cases involve shape and form. As understood in Feng Shui, energies are responsive to shape - which is a pattern; and so when working with some Health matters one actual shape may have a greater effect than another.

Crystals have a different form from metals and man-made materials; some energies may be more responsive to the vibrational pattern 'broadcast' by a crystal. Remember that in the early days of radio, the receiving sets used crystals. And today, crystals are used to keep time - both in major 'time centres' and in your wristwatch.

Learning can be fun ! Let us have fun together !

I Wonder, Wonder, Wonder When,
And then I Wonder More Again.

Amplifying Intuitive Signals

It is most important to remember that Intuitive signals are originated by our Heart-Mind-Brain team (our Heart being our Intuitive link to 'Upstairs', working closely with the Intuitive part of our Mind-Brain) and then manifested by our nervous-muscular system to give physical movements in our bodies.

We have discussed the use of our sense of balance, and used it in our first experiment; we have balance sensors throughout our bodies, and the signals given by our sense of balance can be amplified.

Let us experiment with using our hands to indicate YES or NO. Get a mug, and put some water in it, almost full - so that you can see any movement due to tilting, but not spill the water.

Hold the mug in one of your hands so it is level (elbows loosely at you side, arm then extended at about waist level); now stop looking at the mug (to look straight ahead is best) and formulate a simple YES/NO question (to start, know the true answer) in the logical part of your mind.

Now ask your Heart this question, and say (silently, to yourself) *"I wonder ..., I wonder ..., I wonder ...,"* and then look to see what has happened to the water in the mug.

Saying *"I wonder ..., I wonder ..., I wonder ...,"* keeps the logical part of your mind very busy - wondering what it is wondering about, so that it does not interfere with the rest of your Heart-Mind-Brain team.

You will probably find that the water in the mug shows that the mug has tilted towards the centre-front of your body for YES (if holding the mug in your right hand, the water is higher in the left part of the mug), and in the opposite direction for a NO.

A simple explanation of this would be that if you asked *"Do I like ice-cream ?"* (or your favourite food or drink) and had held mugs in both hands, then they would tilt towards each other to signal a 'joining' for YES, or a 'dispersion' for NO.

There are probably a few problems that would arise if you carried almost full mugs of water around with you whenever you might need to get an Intuitive answer to a question ! How can this be overcome ?

The signal that you are receiving is being made by the slight twisting of your arm, wrist, and hand muscles. It is this movement that we need to amplify, so that we can get good and clear signals.

You could hold a straw or a stick in each hand, and see if they move in- or out-wards; there are other ways, however, that have been used for centuries - and proven to work well.

Intuition on Building Sites

You will find many plumbers, electrical workers, and water-works employees who use a piece of bent wire - it is cheap, does not break, is easy to carry, simple to use, and proven to be effective.

They use it to locate water pipes and buried wires - they have success even when the original engineering drawings were incorrect or have been lost. Beyond just locating the pipe or wire, they can even locate the spot where there is a leak or break.

This 'Pipe Locator' is usually a length of strong wire (perhaps a welding rod) bent in a 'L' shape - the shorter length being the handle, and the longer length the pointer.

It needs to be held correctly; the operator's elbow should be loose at his side, with the forearm, wrist, and hand extended forward.

The handle should hold the handle strongly enough to give good support, but loosely enough so that the pointer can swing easily.

To start, the pointer is guided to be pointing forwards; this means that it is hanging down slightly, so that gravity keeps it forward - but not hanging down so far that it will not sway when the operator's wrist and hand give a slight twist.

The operator tunes his Heart-Mind-Brain 'radio transceiver', concentrating his thoughts to whatever is being sought, such as picturing a pipe - or water leaking from a pipe.

Now he walks slowly forward, and the pointer may swing (usually in, towards his body centre) to indicate that his Heart-Mind-Brain team has found resonance between the tuned thought and what is being sought; then the operator marks this point on the ground in some way.

It is important to have a clear and precise understanding in your Mind as to the exact point that is indicated - the end of the rod, your hand, or where your toes are located.

It is customary to then approach this point from the opposite side, and locate a similar point of first contact. The item being sought can generally be found half way between these two points of first contact. The depth often equals half the distance between the points of contact.

This whole procedure may be repeated at other places nearby, to confirm the location of the pipe or wire.

If a leak or break is sought, the operator will then follow along the indicated location of the pipe or wire, picturing the leak or break in his Mind, and using his wire (sometimes called an 'L' rod) as before to find where it is.

Making your own 'L' Rod

If you do not have an 'L' rod, get hold of a metal coat hanger, cut off the hook section, and cut the bottom bar in the centre; you now have two pieces of wire - bend them so that they form a right angle at the bend, and you now have two 'L' rods.

If you wish, you can cut a drinking straw in two, and slip each half over a handle of your 'L' rods. Keep the uncut edge uppermost - if the cut edge rubs against the pointer it may catch and stop free rotation.

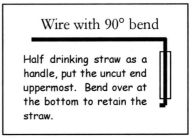

Wire with 90° bend

Half drinking straw as a handle, put the uncut end uppermost. Bend over at the bottom to retain the straw.

Signals Used

The basic signals for use with an 'L' rod are 'joining is positive, separation is negative'. The amount of movement, the degree of change, indicates the strength of the signal.

If we imagine our 'L' rod to be the hour hand of a clock, with the 12 o'clock mark furthest from us, then movement between the 11 and 1 marks indicates searching - trying to get the answer, and not the answer itself.

With your 'L' rod held in your right [left] hand, 10 [2] indicates a weak YES, with the strength rising to a strong YES at 8 [4].

If it goes to 7 [5] this is a 'YES-beyond-YES', a better than expected result. The signals for NO are reversed: 2 - 4 [10 - 8], with 'NO-beyond-NO' at 5 [7].

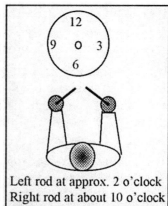

Left rod at approx. 2 o'clock
Right rod at about 10 o'clock

Many people use an 'L' rod in each hand; the advantage is that you get confirmation when they both give the same answer.

Should they differ, check your question, or stand up and ask your Heart the same question and see whether you move forwards or backwards.

In all such cases, be aware of the very first thought that 'pops' into your Mind - this comes from your Intuition, and will probably assist you to correct any problem with your question.

There is little training needed with 'L' rods - just hold in your Mind the clock face and meanings attached, and practice - seek where the water supply comes into you home from the street, or see if you can locate any underground streams in your area.

Pointing with your 'L' Rods

You can ask that your 'L' rod points to something that you seek - hold a picture of it in your Mind, or even a sample like it (or belonging to it) in one of your hands. Then hold your 'L' rod in the search position, and slowly rotate yourself, preferably in a clockwise direction.

You may find that the pointer of your 'L' rod stops moving with you, holding in one direction. You can follow the line indicated - or just note where it points, then go to another place, repeat the search, and note where the line now indicated cross the first line, and go there.

One peculiar aspect of this is tracking - your 'L' rod may lead you along taken by the item sought, not directly to its present location.

This can be useful in tracking the route taken by a criminal, to find clues left along the way, but it can confuse a person who does not understand what is happening.

On one occasion a very experienced operator was demonstrating pointing to a good sized audience, and asked *"Please point to North"*. Everybody knew that the building was built North-South, but his 'L' rod kept pointing at an angle !

Finally a man in the audience stood up, and said *"It is pointing at me - my name is Tom North !"*

Is the Baby a Boy ?

There are many stories of ladies holding a needle and thread over a future mother's stomach and asking this question - and they are surprisingly correct most of the time !

If there is an error, it is usually in the question asked - *"Is it a boy or a girl ?"* will give a YES signal, because it could be either.

Sometimes a pendant, crystal on a chain, a cross, or other type of Pendulum is used. The item used is not important - it is just a tool being used by the Heart-Mind-Brain team via the nervous-muscular system, again using the balance receptors to cause movements of the forearm, wrist, and hand.

The manipulation of these is far more complicated than with an 'L' rod, but the principle remains the same.

The signals used may vary; this does not matter, so long as they are understood by the operator. The operator may even decided to change the signals or their meaning - and this works, so long as the sub-conscious Mind understands the new system.

This method is also used in many egg hatcheries to determine the sex of the unborn chicks - with great success even on a commercial basis.

The signals are usually based on the subject or answer being Positive/YES or Negative/NO.

This Positive/Negative is like comparing the direction of a flow - from the positive to the negative.

Male is generally seen by the Heart-Mind-Brain team as being positive, giving out energy. Female is seen as negative in the sense of being receptive.

Thus the best way of forming the sex question is to ask *"Is the unborn male ?"* since a YES signal is also appropriate for Positive-Male.

Of course, it also pays to check if twins can be expected, and if so, to ask additional questions.

Making and Holding your Pendulum

You can make your Pendulum by having any form of weight suspended by a flexible connector that you can hold in your hand. You can tie a piece of string around a metal nut, for example.

You can also use a crystal on a chain, a cross or other neck decoration, or a glass bead on a length of cord. Some people use specially shaped Pendulums - because energies are very responsive to shapes, to forms of structure.

But even so, the main movement originates from your Heart-Mind-Brain team via your nervous-muscular system - YOU are the most important part !

You will find it best to hold your Pendulum with the string, cord, or chain between your thumb and first finger, as illustrated.

A long length of string enables you to see the movement more easily, but the speed of movement is slow. A very short length moves very fast, but the amount of movement is less, making it more difficult to see - a real problem when you are starting !

Probably the best length to use when starting is about six inches (15 cm) - then as you get more experienced, you can reduce this to between 3 and 4 inches (7 and 10 cm), as you find suits you.

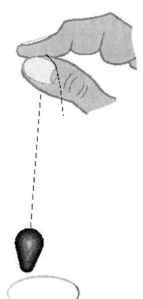

Some LOLs (Little Old Ladies) are absolute wizards at using a Pendulum; their friends may watch them, and try to do the same: *"It doesn't work for me !"* they cry. Why is this so ?

In most cases this is because they have not trained their system to give signals. This is like telling a five year old child *"Give me the first five numbers in the Fibonacci series"* - he does not have any idea of what is meant, which of his toys you want.

Now it may work if you ask your Heart *"Please give me a signal with my Pendulum that indicates YES"* and then watch to see if your Pendulum moves. Repeat the question for NO, and for NOT AVAILABLE, and remember the signals. Then you can ask questions.

Signaling Systems

A Pendulum is able to move in more directions than an 'L' rod, so the signaling can be more extensive - swinging to and fro in various directions, or rotating clockwise or anti-clockwise, or even making elliptical combinations of these movements.

Again, the strength of the movement indicates the strength of the answer.

Basically, there are two major systems of signaling - perhaps best described as being Physical or Meta-Physical.

The Physical system is similar to that used by 'L' rods - to and fro indicates a joining (the food is good for you to eat), side to side a separation (a barrier between the food and yourself - do not eat it, for whatever reason).

The Meta-Physical system is rotational - YES, positive, male, inputting an energy, and sending Love being clockwise; NO, negative, female, extracting an energy being anti-clockwise. Note that there is no 'taking of Love' !

It may be best to decide which signal you want to use, and then train your Heart-Mind-Brain team and your nervous-muscular system to give these.

I find the following best:

WAITING	To and fro swing
YES	Clockwise circle
NO	Anticlockwise circle
NOT AVAILABLE	Side to side swing

So for each of these signals, make your Pendulum give the signal by using all your muscles in your forearm, wrist, and hand - exaggerating these movements (since you are in a training session).

Then say *"This is a [to and fro swing], it signals [WAITING]!"*, and then holding your Pendulum still, and asking *"Please give me the signal for [WAITING]"*.

Repeat this until you get a good response for the signal being installed, and then do the same training session for the next signal, until they are all satisfactory.

It is best to do these in the order shown, since you can go into the WAITING mode before getting the other signals - it is easier for your Pendulum to change its movement rather than start from being still.

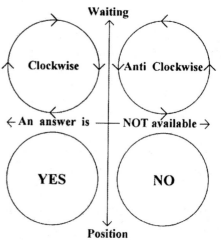

Signals for Pendulum & Bobber

Bobbers

Your Pendulum hangs down on its cord, chain, or string; movements are made against the force of gravity.

Your Bobber is like a horizontal Pendulum that makes movements against the springiness of its stem.

Your Bobber can be a metal coat-hanger which has been straightened, a tree branch, radio aerial or fishing rod held by the small end. The key need is that it must be very springy.

For this exercise I suggest that you get a metal coat-hanger that is not too rigid or too bendable, cut off the hook portion, and straighten the wire that remains.

Bend over one end into a handle, and make a smaller bend at the other end to avoid poking somebody's eye. You can tape over the handle if you wish.

The advantage of teaching your body the Pendulum movements when using your Bobber is that you can put much more effort into making the signals, so that your nervous-muscular system gets a higher level of training and experience.

Now force your Bobber to make a large 'up and down' movement, saying at the same time *"This is an 'up and down' movement - it means WAITING"*, and then hold it still, and ask *"Please give me tile signal for WAITING"* - and repeat this procedure until you get the correct signal.

It is most important that your Bobber be very springy - this amplifies the signals given by your nervous-muscular system, and is a great help to a person who is learning to Dowse.

The signal that you first get may be very small - it is probably the first time that you have tried to use your nervous-muscular system to interface between your Mind-Brain team and a Dowsing tool - but with practice the signal may become quite large.

As you become more accomplished you will find that the size of the signal indicates the strength of the answer.

Now force your Bobber to make a clockwise circle, saying at the same time *"This is a clockwise circle - it means YES"*, and then hold it still, and ask *"Please give me the signal for YES"* - and repeat this procedure until you get the correct signal.

If you have a problem in getting a movement, start your Bobber in the WAITING signal by giving it a small 'up and down' movement.

Then do a similar exercise making an anti-clockwise circle to represent the NO answer. This is repeated to get the other main signal: NOT AVAILABLE AT THIS TIME - a side to side movement.

Practice each signal until you have confidence that you are being given the signals correctly at all times.

It is like learning to ride a bicycle or drive a car - it may be hard at first, but gets easier as you get the hang of it. And eventually you do all the little things that are needed without thinking about them.

Pointing - with your Pendulum

One of the very good reasons for using a circle to signal YES or NO is that when you seek by asking your Pendulum to point towards something, you can check that it is giving a good signal.

Install a program to define the signals used by your Pendulum: *"When my Pendulum points to an item, it will first give a YES signal to indicate that it is the correct direction, or a NO signal to show that a problem exists"*.

A linear signal for YES or NO could be confused with the direction sought - the circular signals avoid this problem.

Remember that your Pendulum swings in two directions - so if you are lost and seeking the direction to your home, or locating an item that you have lost, see the way that your Pendulum swings (to north-south, east-west, etc.), then point to one of them (north or south, etc.) with your hand and ask *"Is this the correct direction ?"*

The skill of pointing with your Pendulum is most useful in selecting items from lists, books from shelves, and checking on supplements for your use.

Simple Counting

A simple way of getting experience with pointing is to practice with the 'Counting Chart':

1. Hold your Pendulum over the 'Start Here'.
2. Ask your Pendulum to point to a number that you choose.
3. Check that your Pendulum makes a clockwise circle - to indicate 'OK'.
4. Check that it does point along the line of the number chosen.
5. Repeat with other numbers.

See where your Pendulum points when you choose a fractional number: like 3¼.

Pendulum Dowsing

9 0 8 7 6 5 4 3 2 1 0

Start Here

Counting Chart

Pointing is a most useful way of using your Pendulum - so the amount of time that you spend on practice is not wasted.

It is time well spent - some examples follow.

Segment Selection

One of the benefits of pointing with your Pendulum is that you can make a segmented diagram, each segment identified with an option - such as writing the names of various places to go on holiday in each segment.

Then ask *"Which is the [best place for me to go on my next holiday] ?"* and see which is indicated by your Pendulum.

It is also best to label one segment as 'Other' - and if that segment is indicated, listen for the first thought that 'pops' into your Mind.

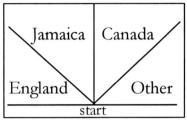

Your Handy Chart

Since most of us have two hands, we can use the spare one (the one not holding your Pendulum !) as a chart for many purposes.

It is best to use signals that conform to indicators that you see often, such as the speedometer and charging gauge of your car - your mind-brain team is accustomed to the signals used.

This is a quick way to check on your health or vitality, if medications are beneficial to you, how many tablets should be taken (dose, doses per day - these may change with effect already achieved), percentage accuracy of a statement, etc.

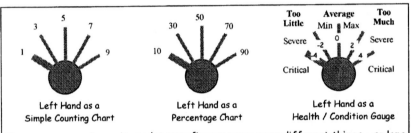

You can use your ingenuity to let your fingers mean many different things - so long as you have ensured that your Mind-Brain team understands the meanings to be signalled for each 'hand-chart' - and that you have specified to your Mind-Brain team which 'hand-chart' is being used for the Dowsing you are now doing !

Selection from Lists

You can use your Pendulum to select an item in a list, even to identify problems in a computer program. You can do this by holding it to one side and see where it points, or use your other hand to point with a pencil or your finger to items until your Pendulum gives a YES signal.

When you get one selection, ask if there is also another to be found - you may have more than one error in a program, or need more than one supplement if you are checking what is needed for your good health.

'V' and 'Y' Rods

The forked sticks cut from trees to form a 'Y' are recounted in many ancient texts as 'THE water witching' tool. Modern day 'Y'' rods are made from metals and plastics, as well as wood.

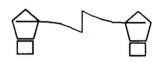

Two Hands holding a 'broken branch' Dowsing tool.

There is no real difference between a 'Y' rod and a 'V' rod, except that the 'tail' is missing.

By similar tools we mean a Dowsing tool that is held between both your hands.

This could be just a loop of wire, or a complicated device such as two longer lengths of springy material with a third shorter piece joining (but allowing movement) the ends that are not held.

This can be produced by getting a thin branch, and making two 'snaps' towards the centre - so the wood is broken, but the pieces are still held together by the bark. This device is reputed to be extremely sensitive.

Your 'V' rod relies on the same wrist movements as the 'L' rods, but while accepting fewer signals it amplifies them so that they are unmistakable.

In fact, many people have found the resulting force to be so great that they cannot fight it !

And if this happens to you, the best advice is to just loosen your grip instead of hurting yourself.

A lot of people have trouble using a 'V' rod; this is because the correct way to hold it is not obvious. A picture can show you the correct positioning of your arms and hands, but the importance of where to exert pressure with your hands is critical.

You can hold the 'V' rod with your knuckles uppermost, or with your palms on top. Having your palms facing upwards puts more tension in the muscles of your forearm, and so gives a more vigorous reaction - the movement UP or DOWN will be reversed.

What is important is that the posture that you use is comfortable, and that you apply pressure in the correct way at the right points.

Holding your Rod

So how do you hold your 'V' rod ? Since the European way is the oldest hold, start with that grip - keeping the back of your hands uppermost. The alternative is similar, but with palms uppermost.

Put your elbows into your sides and hold your 'V' rod pointing to your front.   Now place your thumbs in between the two free branches of the rod, and spread the rod apart by moving your hands and elbows outwards, but bringing your thumbs towards your body.

Now the really important part - the pressure should be applied by the first fingers of your hand pulling the rod towards you, with the palms of your hands pushing the ends of the rod away from you, to force a nice curve in the rods.

You can use your other fingers to grip the rods to add stability, but the main pressure is from the first fingers - the index fingers, the fingers next to your thumb. This is your 'start' position.

With both your hands force the branches into a curve, with the joint ends (the 'V') kept pointing away from you in front, and the handle ends in line horizontally - if someone held a long ruler for you, the handle extensions would be parallel to the ruler.

The sensitivity of the 'V' rod is at its maximum when the free ends are in line - each free end having been rotated through a right angle from when they touched.   To reduce sensitivity, you rotate them using a smaller angle.   But if the angle is too small, they will not react.

An important test to see if you are holding your 'V' rods correctly is to give a very slight twist to your wrists. If your grip is correct, your rods should immediately respond. If not, change your grip until this does happen.

Rod Signals

To program the signals, just install a simple program for YES and NO - being UP or DOWN as you decide, preferably based on your normal reaction, found by trial.

If you just hold it with your fingers without applying the pressure then you may have trouble getting your rod to work.

After you have got your rod to work, you can have fun trying different holds, to see which one is best for you.

Do not be afraid to experiment - it can be fun, and you will learn. And remember, we often learn more from making mistakes than we do from doing things right the first time

The signals given are very clear and strong - it was using a plastic 'V' rod that I was helped to locate a missing child. I asked that I be signaled when my rod was pointing towards his present position, and the signal received could not be mistaken !

Rod Variations

I have tried a simple 'broken branch' rod - and found it very sensitive, it gives a rotational signal when entering an energy field, and then returns on leaving the field.

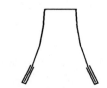

'Broken Branch' Rod with pen casings on hand held ends - used in 'forward' position.

You hold it so that the ends in your hands are pointing to the middle of the central piece.

I used two 15 inch lengths of a springy wire coat-hanger, with a 5 inch length of 'not so springy' coat hanger in the middle - all taped together with sticky tape.

There is quite a strain on the tape, and it twists - so I do not expect it to last. Perhaps a better connector would be thin (and flexible) plastic tubing (or a piece of string) bound (or bonded) to the wires.

Have fun making your own version !

I find that it is best (for me) to hold it with my palms downwards, and the wires held as tightly as possible where my fingers join my palms. The reaction on entering an energy field with my palms upwards was too vigorous - so the tool did not return when leaving the field.

A further improvement is to place the hand held rod ends in empty ball point pen casings - this allows you to have a comfortable grip, while releasing any resistance to the rotation of the wires.

Another way to hold the 'broken twig' rod is with the middle piece in front of you, with the hand held ends pointing forwards. This is most comfortable, and gives you a feeling of control.

Working with 'The System'

'The System' can be considered a 'catch all' term that includes 'All That Is' - the totality of all creation and beyond, including the past and future.

It includes all Energy and life forms in all planes of existence; in all dimensions and domains; in all times and all 'nows'; in all mind, matter, and material; in all Energy Beings; in all Universes, Galaxies, and all that is within and around them.

'The System' may well be the organizational structure that implements the works of 'The Holy Creator in Love of All Things in All Places in All Dimensions in All Times'.

From the personal experience of myself and many others it enables changes to be made in remarkable ways.

Walt Woods tells how there was a problem in the air conditioning system of an office building; this caused plants to wilt, and people to feel most uncomfortable.

Walt asked 'The System' if corrections could be made without harm to others, was told YES, asked that such changes be made NOW, and put his own energy into helping to accomplish this by using his Pendulum.

The next day the office workers were astounded ! No repair work had been done by humans, but the atmosphere in the building was beautiful, and even over a long time the plants all flourished !

Power versus Force

In the book of this title by David Hawkins he describes a 'Map of Consciousness' that has values rising from Shame 20, Apathy 50, Fear 100, Anger 150, Courage 200, Reason 400, Love 500, Peace 600, to Enlightenment between 700 and his top value of 1,000.

By his calculations all of the great religious figures of the past were in this range for Enlightenment - but none achieved 1,000.

When I read this book I realized that the total range was confined to the attributes of human beings towards each other. I asked *"Does the range exceed 1,000 ?"* and was told YES.

I asked about certain people that I knew who cared about plants and animals, and found most of them to be in the range 3,000 to 7,000 - and found one person actually at 10,000 !

Perhaps some of those people who care for the total environment of all nature might exceed 10,000.

I have observed that many humans pray to be 'saved' - from this earth and be 'taken to Heaven'. Most seem to be praying for themselves - and sometimes for other humans.

Working with 'The System'

Perhaps it would be better to recognize that we are all part of 'All That Is', that we have 'God Energy' within us, and that we would be helping in the 'Great Work' of the Holy Creator.

We can develop and improve our use of our 'God Energy' by doing our own best to create a 'Heaven on Earth' - a Heaven-like environment for all creatures, for all the creations of the Holy Creator, not just human beings.

When we ask the help of any Deity, we are restricting the response to the environment in which that Deity has effect. The actual help may need to come from a different source.

It seems that by asking the help of 'The System' the request is directed to the needed source - or sources, since 'The System' is understood to represent the total essence of all action by the 'God Energy'.

It may be that the greater our respect for all of creation then the more likely that we can expect to get help from 'The System'; the more help that we give to 'The System', the more that 'The System' will help us.

A key precept is that whatever we request should be made with the proviso 'without harm to any other' - not just humans, but all life forms.

Express gratitude for the help received ! This is seldom done; when you do this you show that you have respect for 'The System' - and become more likely to get expeditious help in the future !

And how much does 'giving thanks' cost you ? You will never get a better cost-benefit deal !

Questions

Our Dowsing Team seems to have access to a tremendous amount of information. Because of this you need to be very literal and you will need to very carefully word your request.

We unconsciously use many idiomatic expressions like *"He was caught red handed"*. To us he was caught stealing. To a Dowsing Team that reads statements as they are worded, it means he has a red hand.

Most Dowsing Teams can be very accurate - errors come about because of the way we ask questions and how we interpret the answers.

It is so easy to misinterpret what someone said ! So be careful in your own wording. Carefully pre-planning and establishing pre-agreements about questions, request and responses, can help increase your accuracy.

Programming your Intuitive Abilities

We thank Walt Woods for permission to include his guidance on programming and checking your Dowsing abilities. Walt was many times the President of the American Society of Dowsers (ASD), was instrumental (with Harold McCoy, another Past President of the ASD) in forming the Ozark Research Institute to research the use of the mind in Healing, and has dedicated his life to helping others, and especially the use of Dowsing to help overcome diseases and personal problems.

Walt's work on programming, outlined in his 'Letter to Robin' has enabled many people to improve the accuracy of their Dowsing - his contribution to Intuition Technology is unsurpassed and greatly appreciated.

These pre-planned and agreed programs are intended to help avoid missing things that you may not think of while Dowsing, or when using some other detecting and influencing method.

They have been carefully pre-thought-out and tested against many conditions.

You are trying to clearly inform your Dowsing Team in advance, of the parameters you wish to use and how it is to respond.

You are programming your Dowsing Team - not the Pendulum, L-Rod, or other indicator that is generally only an interface, indicating, or communicating tool. Please feel free to change or adjust these programs to fit your needs.

Program Installation

To install a program or agreement we use three simple steps:

(1) Pre-plan a program; check it is clear and non-contradictory
(2) Ask your Heart if any changes should be made
(3) Revise accordingly and re-check; if OK then:
(4) Read in the program with the intent to install it
(5) Check that it has been installed OK without conflicts or errors
(6) Thank all involved for their help.

If the responses are all YES you are finished.

Programs installed will normally act like a post-hypnotic suggestion - you should never have to repeat the programming. They are worded so you can easily change them.

The Set of Main Programs

The programs are designed to reflect the details that 'The System' can respond to, and to help you to avoid misunderstandings related to your questions and requests.

After installing the programs, you will only be using the Pre-Check Q1 to Q9 questions when you start a Dowsing session. Following these questions there are hints on what to do if you have a less than beneficial indication from your questions.

Repeating from our earlier training, first install a key program:

"That my Heart be in command of my total Being at all times, in all 'nows', in all ways, and in all aspects"

Now the base program:

"That my Heart will assist and co-operate with all in my total Being to ensure the correct and satisfactory installation and implementation of all affirmations and programs which I ask to be installed, providing that all changes made are for my highest and best good, shall not cause harm to myself or others, and shall be in effect until revised or cancelled by me".

This is another program that is most beneficial:

"That all calls that I make to my Intuition shall be via my Heart, and that all replies that are given shall be the truth as best I am able to understand, based on information obtained from all possible sources that are reliable as correct, provided that if the information is not available or the reply should not be given then this will be so indicated".

Primary Program

'The Primary Program is to be continually in effect until I choose to make changes.

The purpose is to cover the overall primary controls, limits, requests, questions, protection and agreements used, and to determine amounts, effects, conditions, circumstances, influences, times, measurements, distances, numbers, percentages and other requested values.

* Communications and guidance is to be restricted to sources that are approved by my Heart and that operate in True Holy Love, Namaste.

* Influences such as misleading thoughts, imaging, wishes, or any other conditions from any physical or non-physical source, persons, entities or mind systems of any kind, are not to affect me adversely, cause me harm, discomfort, loss of energy, or take control of my free-well, mind, awareness, subconscious or any part of my Being. Influences from myself, or any of the above are not to cause incorrect Dowsing answers or interfere with the intended results.

* Time as related to Dowsing or other activities is to be in my perceived time as associated with my clock and calendar unless otherwise requested or specified differently in involved programs.

* Intuitive hints may be given to improve my questioning and understanding of answers, which are to be selected from all available knowledge and information sources.

* Methods of answering by Dowsing or any other agreed methods of any kind are to indicate by swinging, moving or relating to a YES or NO or other information arrangements indicating the most appropriate answer for the question asked.

* Should a question involve any prohibited subject then the answer is to be signaled as ANSWER IS NOT AVAILABLE.

* I may make temporary changes for any program while it is in use. Temporary information changes indicated by the [ ]`s are to be duplicated, where appropriate, in all involved programs. These temporary changes are to automatically change back to their original programming after use.

* Permanent program changes such as adding, deleting or changing any aspect of any program may be made by me at any time using the previously defined 'Program Installation Routine'.

End of Program. Thank you'.

Remember to check the installation !

Pre- and Post- Check Routines

Whenever you are Dowsing there are four areas that seem appropriate to check:

Q-1 is designed to pre-check yourself. It does this by looking for the lowest level of effectiveness for seven different broad-spectrum areas. Usually ask for the level of effectiveness for the entire block. If it is less than a +10, proceed to isolate the individual component.

When you find where the problem then you can run corrections before proceeding.

It is best not to work in any areas where you are knowingly or unknowingly blocked, inappropriately influenced, or not ready in some component of your Dowsing method.

Q-2 is the 'May I ?, Can I ?, Should I ?' program. Do not interfere with someone else's life without first checking with their Beingness - and your own ! Also there may be unrecognized side-effects.

Q-9 is intended to look for areas that you may have failed to think about or that you have not built into your overall programming. It also instructs your Dowsing Team on the areas you want to be sure that it has checked.

Q-10 is to indicate the staging and timing of completeness. You may have asked for something to be done and 'The System' has agreed, but this gives you no clue as to when. It could be seconds, days or months. The subconscious or mind of the person involved may rebel, or have too get use to the idea or only partiality accept the energies, etc.

If you ask for the percentage of completeness for different amounts of time, you will have a better idea what is going on. It may alert you to use a different approach.

Normally start a procedure by asking your Dowsing Team to check the Q-1 through Q-9 on yourself as a block. If you get a +10 (out of 10) you are ready to proceed.

Q-1 Pre-Check Program

'The Pre-Check Program is to work with all my programs or agreements, and to be continually in effect.

Considering all aspects of my Dowsing Team for communications, contacts, corrections and activities, indicate the Least Effective Level of Effectiveness for:

1. My readiness, ability, and the response conditions necessary for information accuracy.
2. Interferences to obtaining information or achieving desired activities.
3. Obtaining information from sources unobstructed by interfering conditions including any aspect of hypnosis from any source.
4. Abilities of my Dowsing Team to translate information as presented by 'The System'.
5. Response ability of my Dowsing Team to respond by mind and/or physical methods.
6. Relating ability of my Dowsing Team's vocabulary, understanding and background.
7. Interpreting ability for the responses for the requested information.

End of Program. Thank you'.

Remember to check the installation !

Q-2 'May I ? Can I ? Should I ?' Program

It is suggested that we ask for guidance from whatever Dowsing or other Intuitive method that we use. The reason is to protect the freewill, life plans or needed experiences for anyone with whom we are working, and avoid any undesirable side effects.

This is also, to prevent unknowingly creating 'karma' for others or ourselves. Our ability to use our freewill, intent or desires, are basically unrestricted, and when using focused intent we may be very capable of inadvertently influencing other persons. It is only courteous and perhaps much wiser and safer to use and respect this guidance.

'The 'May I ? Can I ? Should I ?' program is to be a working part of all my programs and to be continually in effect.

When an 'I' or 'We' is used the program is to automatically adjust to the most appropriate one. The 'I' involves myself; the 'We' includes myself and all other advisory and beneficially supporting factors. When there are questions or request with Dowsing or other activities the following meanings are to be in effect:

* May I ?	Do I have appropriate permission to proceed and be involved ?
* Can I ?	Do I have the ability to be successful in this area and am I ready ?
* Should I ?	Considering all aspects related to this situation would it be appropriate, proper and suitable to be involved in this area at this time ?

End of program. Thank you'.   Remember to check the installation !

Q-9 Safety Net Program

'The Safety Net Program is to work with all my programs or agreements and to be continually in effect.

Considering all aspects related to my request and/or instructions associated with information, activities or objectives, to indicate the Lowest Level of Effectiveness for:

1. Conditions necessary for the Dowsing or other methods to achieve stated objectives
2. Information completeness of instructions necessary to accomplish stated objectives
3. Ability, conditions and function for involved genes, energy fields, biological or etheric bodies or systems and any other influencing factors for achieving stated objectives
4. Time and space conditions which include, when, where and how long statements
5. Interference blocking from any source including personal conditioning, implants, imprints, or any aspect of hypnosis from any source.
6. Omissions of any necessary known and unknown conditions, influences or aspects needed in the programs, questions, request or other areas not covered in this method to achieve objectives
7. Results obtained for stated objectives

End of Program.   Thank you'.

Remember to check the installation !

Q-10 Completion Program

'The Completion Program is to work with all my programs or agreements and to be continually in effect.

When requested 'The System' is to indicate completeness of the requested activities.   The answer is to be indicated in numbers 0 through 100 (percentage) where 0 equals none, progressing to 100 which equals complete.

This is to be related to the requestors indicated time in minutes hours, days or years. If no time is requested it is to be in my perceived 'now' or any other method or system the requester may chose to use.

End of Program. Thank you'

Remember to check the installation !

Using the Pre-Check Routine

Always check yourself first before Dowsing - by checking Q-1 through Q-9 as a single block, requesting that the lowest level of effectiveness in any segment be indicated:

Q-1 Pre-check: Please indicate the lowest level of effectiveness for:
        (1) my readiness   (2) interference blocking
        (3) obtaining information   (4) abilities   (5) response ability
        (6) relating   (7) interpretation ?

Q-2 May I ? Can I ? Should I ? Dowse for [myself] ?

Please indicate the lowest level of my ability to Dowse due to the most detrimental, non-beneficial, interfering and undesirable effects, impacts, or other influences from:

Q-3   Entitles ?   Outside Influences ?   (From people, noxious energies. psychic, etc.) (Within last [24 hrs] or as requested)

Q-4   Thought Forms ? (Images, Imprints, ideas, Experiences, Race Consciousness, etc.) (includes present and past lives)

Q-5   Conditions ? Other Influences ? (Within last [24 hours].)

Q-6   Mind-Body-Spirit Connections or Alignment ? (For all aspects of [my] total being)

Q-7   Ability to Receive and Send Beneficial Influences ?

Q-8   Personal Concerns or Conditions ? (Areas of special interest needing extra attention)

Q-9   Safety Net - Indicate the lowest level of effectiveness for:
        (1) connections, (2) information, (3) abilities,
        (4) time/space, interference, (8) omissions   (7) results
(Normally requested as a single block)

After any changes are requested:

 Q-10 Completeness of requested changes as a percentage. (After indicated now, clock or calendar times)

Suggested Responses:

Q-1 Dowse for which sub-section (see Pre Check Program).

Q-2 If YES proceed. If NO tactful avoidance is advisable. Trust the advice !

Q-3 If Entities, ask 'The System' to send 'medics' from the 'Entities World' to pick them up and give them appropriate medical care.

If there are Thought Forms from the outside, ask 'The System' to adjust the aura to convert them to positive, useful, and beneficial energies. This is a 'win/win' situation. The recipient gets free positive energies and the sender gets to do their 'own thing'.

Q-4 If a negative reading ask 'The System' to first remove the emotional energies. Watch your Pendulum for progress. (working over to a +10). Then return your Pendulum to the original negative reading and ask 'The 'System' to *"modify the thought forms, images or imprints to neutral or beneficial, considering all aspects of [my] total being including attitude"*. Watch your Pendulum for progress.

Q-5 to 8 For any undesirable readings ask 'The System' if it can and will adjust or modify these conditions. If YES ask 'The System' to return your Pendulum to the original reading and please proceed, indicating progress with your Pendulum. Then recheck Q-4.

Q-9 Possible Omissions. See 'Safety Net Program'.

Q-10 Required completeness time for requested changes. See 'Completion Program'.

Corrective Action

First, you will need to tell 'The System' what you want it to do. If you install the 'Influence Program' it tells 'The System' in advance what you would like it to do. All Programs are worded so you are always free to change, adjust or delete any program.

Second, you need to ask if 'The System' can and will make corrections or influence the requested situation:

Ask 'The System' if it can - and will - do anything about this situation. If YES, then ask *"Can I ? May I ? Should I ?"* and if you get YES then proceed. If you get NO it is OK to ask *"Why ?"* and be so informed by dialoguing with 'The System'.

If the above is YES ask 'The System' to take all action that is needed to make the necessary corrections.   To do this I use my 'Handy Chart' to get such approval from 'The System' and to watch the progress of the corrections.

My Pendulum will be swinging to indicate a low number, and then gradually swing to show higher values.   When it reaches 10 (100%) then it will either return to indicate another low number (for another aspect being corrected) and repeat this corrective action, or it will stay at the 10 (100%) mark to show that the work is finished.

I then check by asking *"Have all the needed corrective actions been taken ?"* and then ask *"Were all these corrective actions fully effective ?"* if not, then ask *"Is any further action is needed by myself ?"* - then do any such action, and repeat the whole process.

Do not ask questions or interrupt while 'The System' is working !

Changes may sometimes be very quick and for differing amounts. Never underestimate the power of 'The System', your subconscious, your mind, or other energies involved.

Influences (of Food, etc.) Program

Food is both a source of bulk and an energy carrier, this is in many ways and at many levels.   It may be possible that our Dowsing or other Intuitive methods combined with 'focused intent' may influence the energies and other aspects in both type and amount. This is an area that you can experiment with just to see what happens.   Nothing ventured, nothing gained !

Once installed, and you have a need, you might try asking your Dowsing Team to evaluate the effects of the food, substance or other areas you are interested in.   The program is activated by specific request, like in the corrections procedure above.

'Before and after' evaluation could be fun to do - using your Handy Chart for indicating information may be helpful.   You may use your Dowsing or other methods to request this program to be continually activated for certain areas for yourself, like food, drink, medications, noxious energies, blocking interfering psychic influences, etc.

But be very careful to ask *"May I ? Can I ? Should I ?"* for each area, or block of areas.

'The Influences Program is to work with all my programs.

The terms 'Influences' is to include the effect from any source upon any part of [my] Total Being.

When requested, 'The System' is to selectively evaluate, affect, modify, transmute, adjust and/or block such influences and adjust them to the highest practical and appropriate level for beneficial results; to minimize the non-beneficial effects and optimize the beneficial effects on all the involved aspects of [my] Total Being.

This is to be at the most appropriate level and at the fastest rate that is practical, comfortable, and pleasant for [me], [my] body and its related systems.

This program is to be activated by my asking about any such influences or their effects on [myself].

End of program. Thank you.'

Remember to check the installation !

Summary

The installation of these programs and the correct use of them (as mentioned) is one of the main keys to getting correct results when Dowsing - or using any other Intuitive method.

The other main keys are to be properly protected; to always work through your Heart; and to always operate in True Holy Love, Namaste - with good intent and without causing any harm to others.

Asking Questions

This sounds very simple - everyone knows how to ask a question - we do it every day.

But it is actually the cause of many misunderstandings - you know what you mean to ask, but the respondent mistakes your meaning, gives you the answer to a slightly different question.

You may even misunderstand this reply - especially if the answer given was not complete, but presumed that you knew some aspect, but this was not so.

In some cases the words used may be ignored, because the listener concentrates more on the tone used than the words spoken !

Problems also may arise when a person strong in one sense (seeing, hearing, feeling, or knowing) converses with others whose prime senses differ.

When you are working with your own Intuition some of these problems may not be relevant, but it is still best to be aware that they could exist - and do your best to avoid them.

Asking Your Intuition

It is important that whenever you work with your Dowsing team (your Heart-Mind-Brain team and nervous-muscular system) you are being sincere - never being frivolous. Questions that you ask for training purposes are not frivolous, since you are being sincere in improving your abilities.

Sincere means being in a similar state of Mind to prayer, since you are working with the same Beings 'Upstairs' - but you do not have to be on bended knee, shut your eyes, or hold your hands together.

A good way to start is to open by asking the help and protection of 'Upstairs': *"I open in True Holy Love, Namaste, and Love of Truth; I ask the Force for Good to help my Dowsing team, and to ensure that all the answers given are the truth as best as I can understand, obtained from all sources that are 'In the Light'. I send you my gratitude, thanks, and Love for the help that you give."*

It is very worthwhile to then check that you have a 'green light' - so ask *"Is my Intuitive team now ready, willing, and able to so work with the 'Force for Good' ?"* or a similar question.

The questions that you ask must be absolutely clear in your mind, and be in simple language such as a child would understand.

The clarity must include avoiding any words having double meanings, or express which alternative is meant.

I was speaking on the telephone to a clairvoyant friend, and told her that I had lost my glasses. She replied "Look by the sink in the kitchen". She was correct, but I had meant my spectacles, and she was locating glass tumblers.

Some Important Rules

There are some very important rules about the questions that you ask. While your Dowsing Team may be able to understand your intention, it may still insist that you 'cover all your bases' to get you into a good habit.

And this habit is important, since at times you may address questions to an animal, a tree, your car or your computer; they will respond to the exact question that you ask - even if it is not what you intended !

<u>First,</u> you should be in a state of meditation or prayer - be serious, concentrate.

<u>Second,</u> the question must be clear, so that your Dowsing team really understands the question.

If you are thinking about eating more ice cream the question *"Is it OK ?"* is NOT clear - your Dowsing team may not understand what you mean by 'it' ! So ask *"Is it OK for me to eat more ice cream now ?"* - including to state 'when' !

Imagine that you are in a car which has a broken fuel gauge; you ask *"Does the car need gas ?"* The answer will always be YES, even if the tank is full. The car needs gasoline (called 'gas') to make the engine work, and it needs air (another gas) to burn with the gasoline and to fill the tyres. A better way to ask this question would be *"Is the fuel tank of this car less than half full ?"*.

<u>Third,</u> the answer must be YES or NO (if not a direction). If somebody told you a story, asking *"Is the story true ?"* may not work, because some of it may be true, and some of it may not be true.

So you must ask about the part of the story that you think may be untrue.

Fourth, there are some questions which should NOT be asked - especially if the question is NOT your business ! This is why it is very important to ask for permission before asking the actual question, if it may be in this category.

Included in this category are any questions concerning the time of future death of any person, including yourself.

Fifth, you must check that you are working within the 'rules of the game'. This means that you must define your question and the reason for asking it, and check with your Dowsing team for YES answers to "*Can I ? May I ? Should I ?*".

This is most important if you are working on another person - but you can always just send them True Holy Love, to be used in the way that is for their Highest and Best Good without checking.

- *"I am seeking to find the best way to ...."* to define the problem.
- *"This is to help XXX to feel happier"* to explain your reason for asking.
- *"Can I ask ?"* to inquire if you have the skill and knowledge to get a correct answer.
- *"May I ask ?"* to get permission to proceed, and confirm that the answer is available.
- *"Should I ask ?"* in case your question is about a forbidden subject, an invasion of a person's privacy, or other reason why you should not ask at this time.

If any reply is NO, you do NOT proceed; if you are asking about someone else, and did not explain that you are asking in order to help, you may get a NO answer; this is one time when you can explain why you are asking, and repeat your check. It may just be the wrong time to ask the question, or to take action.

Some people try and combine these, by presuming that getting a YES after asking *"Can I ?"* implies that permission would only be granted if the *"May I ?"* and *"Should I ?"* were also YES.

This is logical; but your Intuition is NOT logical ! It is best to ask ALL the questions separately, or ask them all together !

If you get wrong answers after your *"Can I ? May I ? Should I ?"* requests, check why; it is probably due to badly worded questions, or to your influence in wanting a particular answer.

Make sure that your questions are clear and cannot be twisted (like the gas example), ask your question if the replies have all been YES, and then having asked the question say to yourself *"I wonder . . . I wonder . . . I wonder . . . "* to keep your egoistic logical mind busy wondering about wondering and avoid its interference.

Sixth, concentrate on what you are asking. Asking about something you do not like (broccoli ?) and then thinking of an ice cream will be sure to give you a wrong answer !

You must not try to make your Dowsing tool move in any way. If you try to force it to move YES because you want it to, but think that the true answer may be NO, then you are spoiling the training that you have done. So the next time you ask a question, your Dowsing team may not give the correct answer.

It is good practice to always check the answers that you get by asking *"Is the answer ... YYYY ... correct ?"* - it may be wrong if the question was poorly worded or should not have been asked.

"Is my understanding that (the answer you perceived) correct ?" is a good way to check that you have understood what was told !

Practice

Remember how to ask a question; although it may seem silly to ask permission for very simple questions, do it to build a routine to use when asking more complicated questions - 'get into the habit'.

"May I ask if my eyes are brown ?" then *"Are my eyes brown ?"*, and afterwards check by *"Is the answer that my eyes are brown correct ?"*

Ask questions such as:
- *"Are my eyes brown ?",*
- *"Did I eat an egg for breakfast today ?"*
- *"Do I like spinach ?" Ice Cream ? Broccoli ?*
- *"Will I be rich ? poor ?"*

Did you ask the *"Can I? May I? Should I ?"* questions ? - and did you check the answers ? Did you remember to 'open' correctly?

If YES to both rich and poor, remember you could be poor at one time and rich in another. Are you poor in spirit and rich in wealth ? Try asking about wealth, and about spirit !

When asking about the future, understand that the answer will be given in terms of the likely outcome of the situations and conditions that now exist - these may be changed, by yourself and by others who are involved.

If you try to influence your Dowsing tool it could give you the answer that you want - and one that may not be true ! Try and keep an open and inquiring mind, and always check the answer - ask *"Have I correctly understood the Truth ?"* or *"What is the percentage of the Truth that I have understood ?".*

Some Hints

You do not have to speak aloud when you ask your Dowsing team a question - it is quite OK to 'think' the question to yourself. And that way, nobody else knows the question that you are asking !

The size of the swing that your Pendulum makes, such as a small circle (or a small swing), or does this slowly, is indicating that there is some doubt, or the question may be poorly worded. A very large circle (with speed) means 'without any doubt'; usually you get a middle sized circle, meaning that the answer is based on present data which may change in the future.

Remember that the size and speed is relative to the normal size and speed of a circle made with that same length of string.

Another time when you may get a small circle is when your solution to a problem is workable, but not the best solution - so keep refining your solution and you will get a bigger circle the closer that you come to the best solution.

Although your Dowsing team is able to answer all your questions, you must not rely on it for every minor matter in your daily life !

You must learn to make your own decisions; but it is OK to ask for training purposes, and if the matter is important.

And even then, it is best to make a decision and then ask *"Did I make the correct decision ?".* If the answer is NO (or a weak YES) then work with your Dowsing team to find out how you can improve your decision.

Using your Intuition about other people is fine, providing that you stay within 'the rules'.

You can always ask how you will get on with a person. *"Can I trust Pat ?", "Is Pat telling me the truth ?", "Will Pat be a good friend to me ?"* and *"Has Pat taken my pencil ?"* are all excellent questions to ask.

But it is wrong to ask these same questions when they concern Pat and some other person - you should only ask if YOU are involved.

Asking about some one else, such as *"Has Pat any allergies ?"* is wrong unless Pat has given permission for the question to be asked. This is like poking your nose into another person's diary !

But if you are preparing a meal which Pat may eat and 'need to know' then explain the situation, ask permission, and you will probably be granted permission and given the required answer.

This 'need to know' is also applicable to Healing - there are a few times when Healing is 'not permitted' - if you run into such a case, you can ask if you can be told the reason.

Asking *"Is my girl/boy friend interested in another person ?"* will always tell you YES - but the sort of interest may not be what you meant !

The 'another person' may be you, the interest may be for business reasons, or because they are relatives - or they may be a fan of a film star. We are all interested in many other people.

Multiple and Imprecise Questions

Quite often we ask multiple questions in one sentence when speaking to some one else - hopefully they will give separate answers to each question.

When seeking YES/NO answers, this does not work !

Also, the English language is excellent for its imprecision - meanings being reversed according to the sense used !

A few examples, some with bar room connotations:
> *"Will the baby be a boy or a girl ?"*
>> YES - unless it is a puppy ! Twins ?
> *"Do you want bread or a roll for your breakfast ?"*
>> A roll in bed with Honey may be preferred.
> *"Is she pretty or ugly ?"*
>> *"Yes - pretty ugly !"*
> *"Does this road go to [London] ?" - "Yes"*
>> But it may be the long way or the worst road.
> *"Do you have the time ?" - "Yes"* (but not tell it !)
>> Or *"Yes, but not the inclination !"*
> *"Does your dog bite ?" - "No"* - CLOMP !
>> *"That is not MY dog".* (Peter Sellers)
> *"Follow me, men - I'm right behind you !"*
>> A certain General Officer talks.

Greater Depth Needed

"Should I marry Pat ?"

To learn forgiveness, or some other lesson ? Best to define what you are looking for: long, happy marriage based on mutual respect and love.

"Will Pat be a good employee ?"

Good for whom ? Specify honesty, loyalty to firm, punctuality, lack of absenteeism, get on well with other staff and customers.

"Will this house suit me ?"

Will it also suit the rest of your family (except mother-in-law) ? Check also about structural strength, possible gas or water leaks.

Be careful when asking about which home to purchase - the home that may be best for you may not be the best for all in your immediate family, or may be OK for a short time but have problems in the future. So always Dowse for these points ! And you can then use your counting expertize to find the lowest price that you can buy the property - and how much money will be needed to get it in good condition after your purchase.

"Should I buy this car for my wife ?"

Depends - it may be a wonderful car for her, or save the trouble of a divorce (remember the man whose wife wanted a Jaguar - he bought her one, and it ate her !).

"Will this car last a long time ?"

Yes - but not move. Check if any problems within next 5 years for tyres, steering, engine, transmission, etc.; and if you will enjoy trouble-free and safe motoring in it.

"Will I win the lottery ?"

Which lottery ? Perhaps a $5 win next year ! This is a win ! Define how much, and when - and remember that because you want to win so much, you may be influencing the answer.

In all these cases, it may be best to ask each sub-query as a separate question - then you may be guided as to further questions to ask, and will be aware of reasons which may be pertinent in making your decision.

The more important the decision, the more time and care is best invested in thinking about possible problems - and the questions to be asked to properly identify them.

For example, imagine that you are thinking of buying a house; if you have identified possible problems then you can ask about them - and perhaps drive a better bargain.

In the same vein, you can ask *"What is the minimum amount that the vendor will accept ?"* and *"How much should I offer ?"* - and use your Intuitive counting methods to get answers.

Practice makes perfect - so now spend a few minutes forming and writing down questions that are pertinent to you, and write down the answers - writing down impresses the gist into your memory, and you can learn a lot from looking at these at a later date.

Counting, Charts and Lists

Counting

Counting can be done in many ways. You can use a numeric chart or your other hand (both methods described previously), count the number of swings or circles made, or work through numbers using YES and NO answers.

When getting the count by the number of signals given, such as for small numbers or percentages, ask if the answer is greater than 10 and if so ask for the number of 'tens' in the answer, and then the number of 'l's (digits or units) to be added.

Sometimes there is difficulty in deciding if a small end circle is included (when using a Pendulum, for example). The only valid way to find out is by testing. So now ask for the number 3 to be signaled to you, and other numbers that you choose - and to which you know the answer. Do this with your Bobber, your L-rod, and your Pendulum.

Dealing with large numbers can be done in a similar way, by asking the number of thousands, the number of hundreds to be added, and similarly with the number of tens and of units.

Another way is to 'guess' at the answer (XXX) and ask *"Is the correct number greater than XXX ?"* - if so, add about 10% and ask again. If less, subtract the 10%.

If it is still greater, add another 10% and ask again, until the opposite signal is given. Now choose a number about halfway between the limits that have been found, and check again. Repeat again, choosing numbers about halfway between the new limits, until you are dealing with numbers that are very close - and then check *"Is this the correct number ?"*

As an example, imagine you are trying to find how far to drill before hitting oil, at a site that Dowsing has indicated that oil will be found.

Based on your experience, perhaps, or just a 'gut feeling', you think that it will be about 1000 feet.

"Is the depth to oil greater than 1,000 feet ?"

YES - add about 10% = 100 feet

"Is the depth to oil greater than 1,100 feet ?"

YES - add about 10% = 100 feet

"Is the depth to oil greater than 1,200 feet ?"

NO - limits 1,100 and 1,200 feet - go halfway

"Is the depth to oil greater than 1.150 feet ?"

YES - go about halfway between 1,150 and 1,200

"Is the depth to oil greater than 1,175 feet ?"

NO - go about halfway between 1,150 and 1,175

"Is the depth to oil greater than 1,165 feet ?"

NO - go about halfway between 1,150 and 1,165

"Is the depth to oil greater than 1,157 feet ?"

YES - go about halfway between 1157 and 1165

"Is the depth to oil greater than 1,161 feet ?"

YES - go about halfway between 1,161 and 1,165

"Is the depth to oil greater than 1,163 feet ?"

NO - either 1,162 or 1,163 feet

"Is the depth to oil greater than 1,162 feet ?"

YES - it must be at 1,163 feet !

"Is the depth to oil 1,163 feet ?"

YES - confirmed !

You would continue your Dowsing in a similar way to find the thickness (or depth to bottom) of the oil bearing ground, and the most economical rate of extraction; and check if there is another oil bearing layer below !

Now ask for the depth that the well should be drilled, allowing for drawdown.

At each major point, check the accuracy of your Dowsing - asking for the percentage that it is correct, and the percentage that you have understood the answers correctly - perhaps by using your 'other' hand as a percentage chart.

Practice this method now, with your Bobber, L-rod, and Pendulum - asking:

"How many days in a year ?"

"How many miles between New York and Calgary ?"

or between cities with which you are more familiar and know (or can determine) the distance. You can vary the questions:

"... as the crow flies", "... by road", or "... by rail".

Charts

Charts are all the same - a line or segment which has a designated meaning, like the Counting Chart in our previous lesson. You can write in places to go on holiday; different firms to approach for work, investment, or supplying equipment; vitamins or herbs; or in which city to live and which home to buy.

When you are dealing with books of charts, such as determining the cause of a problem in health and the action need to be taken, you will often be guided to 'go to chart number...'.

Before you do this, it may be best to ask *"Is there any other item on this list to which I should return ?"* in case of there being more than one problem, or two different remedies being needed.

Just to be safe, check if you are being blocked, or are getting interference, from any of the sources that are shown on the chart.

Robert Detzler has written a number of books using similar charts on Soul Retrieval and other Spiritual Matters, and gives courses on

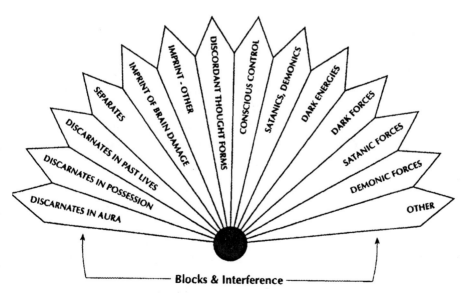

Example Chart from The Freedom Path by Robert Detzler

his teachings.   You can phone Robert at (425)868-3643 about courses and people that he has trained in your area.

Lists

Lists are very similar, except that they are not structured as a chart. Imagine you have a list (a few pages long) of vitamins, herbs, and supplements which you may need.   You can ask *"Is the item I need on this page ?"*, and if so, ask *"Is the item in the upper part of this list ?"* to reduce your work, and then put a finger of your 'other' hand on each item in turn, asking *"Do I need this item ?"*.

Remember to check if you need another item on the same page !

And here we have a trap.   Your finger is on 'Vitamin A' - so you need it.   We all need Vitamin A at all times - but do you need more ? Should you supplement your present intake ? So it is better to first specify in your mind (to your Dowsing team) that you are only to be shown those items that you need to take additional quantities to enhance your health.

A list can be used to check for illnesses or allergies - often 'Bach' or other flower essences can be used alleviate or eradicate these.   It seems that plants carry vibrational patterns which can be superimposed on the energies that cause problems and so change the outcome.

Perhaps we can take a plant, remember its essence and vibrational pattern, and recall it to be used when needed - or even ask which is needed and have it sent !

A computer program is a list of commands - if you have problems you can Dowse *"Is there a problem in the coding on this page ?"* and if so, go to each line asking *"Is there a problem in this line ?"* - and to each command in that line if more than one.

Dosages

On the next page are listed a few popular items which could be beneficial to you, as submitted by John van Dries - use your Dowsing skills to find if you need any of them, and then use your counting abilities to determine the strength that you need, the dosage to be taken, and the frequency of the dosages. Perhaps you need some items for a short time, or the dosages may change as they take effect.

Major Organs, etc.

1. Brain
2. Heart
3. Thymus
4. Spleen
5. Pancreas
6. Blood
7. Liver
8. Gall Bladder
9. Kidneys
10. Bladder
11. Adrenal Glands

A List of Supplements

1. Trace minerals
2. Multi Vitamms
3. Vitamin A
4. Vitamin C
5. Vitamin D
6. Vitamin E
7. Plant Enzymes
8. Green Food Supplements
9. Herbal Fibre

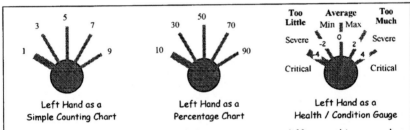

Left Hand as a
Simple Counting Chart

Left Hand as a
Percentage Chart

Left Hand as a
Health / Condition Gauge

You can use your ingenuity to let your fingers mean many different things - so long as you have ensured that your Mind-Brain team understands the meanings to be signalled for each 'hand-chart' - and that you have specified to your Mind-Brain team which 'hand-chart' is being used for the Dowsing you are now doing !

Then check your major organs and other body parts, finding their percentage efficiency to the maximum potential, and how they compare to those of an average person of the same sex and age.

Check the following (maximum levels are shown)

Cholesterol Level : ages 40 to 60, men 200, women 190

LDL Cholesterol Level : ages 40 to 60, men 140, women 117

Triglyeride Level: men 120, women 110

Use your Handy Chart to check your levels for:

Calcium	Vitamin P	Phosphorus	Blood Press.
Cobalt	R2 Hormone	Potassium	Vitamin A
Chlorine	Biotin	Sodium	Vitamin B1
Chromium	Choline	Sulphur	Vitamin B2
Copper	Inositol	Zinc	Vitamin B6
Fluorine	Lecithin	Amino Acids	Vitamin B12
Iodine	Niacin	Enzymes	Vitamin C
Iron	Paba	Fibres	Vitamin D
Magnesium	Folic Acid	S.O.D.	Vitamin E
Manganese	Linoleic Acid	Sorotonin	Vitamin F
Molybdenum	Pantothric Acid	Selenium	Vitamin K

Making Corrections

If you find that you need a particular item, you can ask 'The System' to *"supply the essence, vibrational pattern, and energy of [the item] in the quantity required in the places needed"*.

Remember to ask permissions first - and if granted, and 'The System' approves, then use your 'Handy Chart' to watch the implementation. You may have to repeat this if more is needed later.

In the same way you may be able to remove any unwanted items, such as toxins and surpluses of any element in your system - but remember that you have a responsibility to do your best not to ingest the causes of such unwanted items.

You may be able to get approval from 'The System' to do such supply and removal whenever needed.

'The System' may also agree to using such procedure for the Healing of another person - including distant Healing.

Locational Dowsing

This is the sort of Dowsing that most people expect ! Going to a place and finding something. And yet we have covered half the course before coming to this - to make sure that we have all understood the principles and the basic skills needed.

Buried Treasure could be lost coins or a pirate's hoard. If a coin was buried in a place, its has left its 'imprint' or 'memory' at that place - so when Dowsing you may be finding where a thing had been, not where it is now.

Pirates often dug a number of holes, sometimes putting 'dummy treasure' there to fool those who sought their hoards. Using our 'Power of Thought' we can place 'Thought Forms' which can be found by Dowsing.

We can do this by thinking *"I know there is treasure buried here"*, these thoughts are sent to a place, and construct an 'imaginary' item (but real in the metaphysical world) which our Dowsing team will consider to be just as real as themselves, unless carefully instructed to ensure that the sought item exists in the physical world - and is there NOW.

To guard against this problem, always include in your program (by so stating, or thinking at the time) that *"I seek the present location of the physical (item)"*.

Lethbridge's Experiment

False images are really displacements of the 'real thing' or 'physical item'. T. C. Lethbridge found that images could be discerned (using his 'long' Pendulum) in circular patterns above the object being Dowsed, the diameter of the circle in which the image appeared increasing with the distance between the object and the Dowser.

To some extent there is a similar occurrence with water veins - as illustrated by the 'Bishop's Rule'; in that case the influence of the water rises at a 45° angle from the vein. Tom Lethbridge describes a much smaller angle in his experiments with such things as artifacts.

Tom was the Director of Excavations for the Cambridge Antiquarian Society and for the University Museum of Archaeology and Ethnology, and the author of very interesting books about his extremely unusual experiments using a long Pendulum, having lengths of up to 10 feet.

He used his Dowsing abilities to locate artifacts that had been buried for thousands of years.

Lethbridge's Spiral and Time

Tom Lethbridge used a 'long Pendulum' to investigate dimensions, as recorded in the book 'The Essentail T. C. Lethbridge'. He found that the first clockwise turn through 360° or 'leg' of the spiral was 0 to 40 inches, the second 40 to 80 inches, and the third 80 to 120 inches. Each leg is understood to represent one plane or dimension.

Points were found on these spirals to represent the various elements and other attributes - and these were not always in the same spiral radial location for the different legs.

Of particular interest is time; he found that this was a general attribute of the first leg, became a point on the second leg (perhaps indicating that the other values in the second leg were not dependant upon time), and re-emerged as a general attribute in the third leg.

Does this mean that when we operate in a 'Higher Plane or Dimension we can access the past and/or the future ?

Measurements

When the French Dowsers were experimenting with radium salts, one test was to measure the length of string needed for the Pendulum, so that it matched the 'length' of the 'vibrational pattern' of the salt.

They measured this in both inches and in centimetres and found that the <u>numeric value</u> was the same - not the actual distance !

Perhaps this explains why we do not need a long Pendulum as used by Lethbridge, and do not need to vary the length of the 'string' when seeking different items - the same actual piece of string may be considered by our Dowsing team to be the required numeric value when measured in some abstract unit of length.

Zinc and Copper

The effect of zinc has been suffered by Bethe Hagens and Clive Tucker; Clive failed to correctly locate a well, and did a most thorough investigation into the reasons why this happened. Both Bethe and Clive found that, <u>when in the field</u>, the effect of nearby zinc deflected the images located by Dowsing.

Remember that zinc is the metal used to galvanize steel; so if you are near any water structure, wire fence, or tin roof - your Dowsing may become inaccurate when locating things in the field.

Copper bracelets were found on the arms of Pharaohs; Clive wondered if this was to overcome the effect of zinc, and experimented with one on his arm - his Dowsing accuracy was restored ! So it may be prudent to wear such a bracelet when we are Dowsing 'in the field'. Zinc does not seem to have any effect on map Dowsing.

To make a suitable copper bracelet, get about 2 feet of single strand electrical wire, bend it in two (back on itself), and twist it so that the wires spiral clockwise. Then twist the two ends together.

This makes a bracelet based on the principle of a Lahkovsky coil (such as are sold by the Holistic Intuition Society), ensuring that all the energies travelling in either direction are spiralling clockwise - or 'good', and thus exerting a good influence on our energies, including our Dowsing team.

The Bobber in 'Find Mode'

If you use L-rods or a Pendulum to seek a small item on (or in) the ground you will find that either your tool is too high to give the needed accuracy, or you wear out your knee pads.

You could use a foot as a pointer (blowing it off if looking for landrnines, or crushing a flower if you lose your balance), or hold a long stick as the indicator (which could be your Bobber).

A Bobber, such as a straightened wire clothes hanger, has the advantage that you can hold the search end close to the ground whilst remaining upright.

First we must program our Bobber: **"When I am using a Bobber to find some item that I define in my thoughts and is in my vicinity at the present time, my Bobber will swing side-to-side to locate the general direction of the item from my present location, and then swing in an ellipse when the** item is located; the upper part of the swing indicates the change in direction needed; when my Bobber is pointing in the direction of the item it will swing up-and-down; when the end of my Bobber is over the item it will make a small YES circle. This program is my 'Find Mode' program for my Bobber, and is to remain in effect until cancelled by me".

Before we use our 'Find Mode' program, we should 'open', think about the item, and check if it is in our vicinity - and describe what we so mean: *"Is (the item) in this garden ?"*. After finding the item, remember to give thanks for the help received.

<u>Group Practice:</u>

Make a copper bracelet as described above. Place a marker and hide two coins in the grass or under a carpet for your partner to find; count the paces from the marker (noting the direction taken) so that the location can be identified later.

Go to the marker set by your partner and use an L-rod to find one coin, placing your own marker at the spot found; repeat for the same coin when wearing the copper bracelet, and see if there is any difference when wearing it. Repeat with the other coin, this time using your Bobber.

Tracking

Tracking the trail left by a person, animal, or thingy is often easier than we imagine.

If we have lost a wallet, or had it stolen, and seek to find it, we may be led to a spot but not find our target - and give up, thinking that our Dowsing ability is at a 'low'.

This happened to a number of Dowsers in England who were seeking a wallet that had been stolen from a coat one of them had left outside at a meeting.

They tried Dowsing to find the wallet, but all signals pointed to places on the floor where it was obvious that the wallet was not there.

The general consensus was *"A waste of time, that sort of thing does not work"*.

Frank Milburn did not give up, however - he thought that the wallet may have left a track; so at this 'failure' spot he took his 'L' rod and asked to be led to the wallet, and followed the directions given.

These led to a sewer excavation in the road outside - a very muddy open trench in the road where new sewage pipes were being installed.

"Oh well, no point in climbing down and getting muddy and wet !"   But Frank has faith in his Dowsing, and is not faint hearted.

He went to climb down, and saw that the wallet has been caught by a piece of trench framing - where it had been thrown by the thief !

Perhaps their Dowsing could have been improved, by including 'the present physical location' in their thought. But there are times when this tracking ability is advantageous - such as seeking a criminal, who may have left evidence en route.

When a person does not want to be found, you may not be able to get an accurate 'fix' on their present location - but still be able to use your tracking skill in the field or on a map (map Dowsing is covered later in this chapter) to get the needed information by following the trail that they left.

Remember that whenever you are dealing with another person you MUST get prior permission - even to help them !

If you seek a missing person remember that they may also not wish to be found. In many cases of criminal involvement you will not get permission from the criminal.

But in such cases you may get approval from the 'Force for Good' (a Higher Authority) providing your intent is for the 'Highest and Best Good of All Creation'.

When locating a missing aircraft, you can use your Dowsing skills to find the crew (checking if they are still alive in their physical body) and also the fuselage and engine(s) - if these locations all agree then you are probably finding the correct places. Having each of these items sought by different Dowsers increases reliability if they agree.

Well Dowsing

Locating a well includes paying attention to the physical conditions. Many drillers are constrained by accessibility of the site and safety precautions in avoiding utilities such as overhead electrical wires and buried pipes and cables.

Use common sense in selecting areas to be Dowsed for a suitable site.

There is water in all living creatures, all plants, and in the ground. You must be very precise in forming your thought and your Dowsing question.

Water is of varying quality, and the quantity available can be expected to change throughout the year. It may be at great depth in one place, or shallow in another - reducing the drilling, installation, and running costs.

You will not be popular if the well that you locate takes water that is now being pumped from another well. Make certain that the intended action does not harm others.

A typical program for locating a water well would include: *".. an all-year-round supply of at least (xxx) gallons per minute of good potable water within (yyy) feet of the surface located on this property without harm to others"*

There are two basic approaches to locating wells - to ask for the best available site, or to find veins of water.

A good way is to ask for them in this order - first getting the site, and then checking on the location, depth, flow direction, quantity, and quality of all the veins of water that are nearby - and checking if they are now providing water for others, and if so, whether their capacity can give the needed additional supply.

If you have a water bearing layer of sand (or similar material) check the depth to the top and to the bottom to find its thickness, and if there are more layers at other depths.

When you pump, you 'draw down' the water surface within a layer - this attracts more water to the extraction point; if the layer is compact you may have difficulty in pumping out the water - even if it is available.

To help overcome this type of problem, Dowse for the diameter of hole and casing to be installed, the drawdown expected at the maximum flow, and the advisable depth that the well should be drilled.

Water Domes

'Water Domes' occur in many places - they are vertical flow paths within the earth that bring water that has been 'Re-cycled for Good' in the depths back to the upper layers. They are often associated with 'Power Spots' such as Medicine Wheels, Labyrinths, and the sites of ancient churches.

It seems that the people who originally selected the site used their Intuition (or Dowsing) to choose a site that had beneficial energies, as are found at most Domes.

I understand that Domes have an odd number of water veins taking the water from the dome to be distributed, and in my experience I have always found an odd number - and the strength of the Dome seems to increase with the number of these veins.

Often you will find major beneficial earth energy lines crossing within the Dome - this is reported at Chartres Cathedral, centred in the famous labyrinth.

If you drill into a dome, you can expect to ruin it !

You will lose the water, and your efforts will have been to no advantage.

But you can always tap into the veins themselves, after they have left the dome.

Mineral Deposits

Mineral Location is similar in many ways to finding water - there are probably traces of most elements at some depth below the Dowser. You need to specify the minimum acceptable levels of quality, quantity, and depth.

If you have a sample of the mineral sought, you can use this as a 'witness' - holding it and concentrating your thoughts on finding exactly that mineral.

A golden nugget can be used to trace its movements from the 'Mother Lode' by tracking, or to direct you there - by using the methods described later in the chapter on Vivaxis.

Working with Nature

Disturbing the earth occurs when a well is drilled, a mine is constructed, and land is cleared.

This may affect other life in, on, and above the site - and the Deva ('Spiritual Being in Charge' or 'Land Lord') may already be upset with the changes forced by humans on other life in his care.

Perhaps it would be polite (and wise) to ask the Deva for approval and help. Show that you respect him - tell that you understand his duties, and apologize for actions that you (and others) may have made that caused him concern.

Explain the purpose of your endeavour - emphasizing how it will benefit other life, such as giving water for the cows to drink or to help the plants grow. Ask for assistance to do this good work, and give thanks for the co-operation between yourself and the Deva which results in helping others.

Very few humans fully understand (or are even aware of) the Nature Spirits such as Devas. Most people do not admit that they exist ! But we have never seen God either - although we may pray.

Perhaps it would be prudent to accept that the Nature Spirits are also the servants of the 'Force for Good' - you have nothing to lose !

The Devas have the 'Devic Society for Environmental Harmony' - and will help people who show them respect and work with good intent.

Map Dowsing

A map is a representation of something, such as a land area, which has two dimensions. Using a segmented chart we obtained a pointing in one direction; with a map we need to get pointers in two directions, and find where they cross.

A 'map' could be a picture or photograph; a detailed coloured map of a road system or a smaller area; a diagram or sketch of a home, a piece of land, or a human body; or even a visualization in our Mind-Brain team.

A carpet, an area of a floor, or a piece of paper - they can all be used to represent a farm, a lot, a room, or a bed.

You just 'imagine' that it is the 'real thing'.

The more accurate the detail, the better you are able to pin-point whatever you are seeking. It is best if you understand the symbols used on a map and how they link together; in all Dowsing you cannot expect to get answers beyond your understanding.

This is particularly so when Dowsing for problems in a machine or a body.

If you do not understand how the different organs in a body work (and how they work together) you will not be such as good Healer as a person having the same abilities combined with superior knowledge.

Let us consider a material or physical map at this point; even if it does not have all the detail, our Mind-Brain team can often visualize some of the missing detail.

First of all we 'open', and then think of what is being sought, our objective. This act also gets the specific vibrational pattern or 'ID code' (similar to a 'call-sign', or 'Internet address' of the objective) for our Dowsing team. We then ask *"Is (our objective) in the area shown by the map ?"*

Co-ordinate systems are used on most maps; often they are marked with squares identified by numbers along the top, and letters (or numbers) down the side. We can go to each letter in turn, putting our pointing finger of our 'other' hand on the letter, and asking *"Is [our objective] in the set of boxes represented by this letter ?"*.

If we get YES, then we can repeat the questioning with the row of numbers on top, or just put the finger on each box in the lettered line asking *"Is [our objective] in this box ?"*

To determine where our objective is within the box, we could mark the box with horizontal and vertical line, give the spaces in these lines letters and numbers, and repeat our search by the box method - and continue with smaller and still smaller boxes.

If you do not wish to mark the map, gradually move a ruler (or other straight edge) down the map, asking for a YES signal to be given when your objective is on the line shown by the ruler. Then move your finger along the ruler, asking for a YES signal when above the sought objective.

Triangulation

Go to a corner of the box, and using a Pendulum (or L-rod) ask for the direction to your objective from this corner, and mark in that line. Then repeat this from an adjacent corner to see where they meet.

Land surveyors use this method when locating a distant point using a theodolite. Just in case an error has been made, they always use a third line.

When this third line is drawn it either joins at the same point or makes a small triangle. If it makes a small triangle, the correct location is taken as being at the centre of the triangle. It is good practice to use the method developed by Land Surveyors when Dowsing.

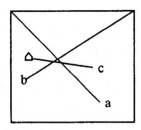

Triangulation

First get lines a & b, then imagine a line that is perpendicular to their mean coming from the intersection, and choose a prominent point on this line as the start of your third line.

It is far quicker to use this Land Surveyors method on the whole map ! Go to two corners of the map and get the intersection point.

If you have a rough idea of where your objective is located, then do not use the whole map, but choose two nearby points as your starting points.

Then choose a road junction (or other well defined point) which is along (or close to) an imaginary line perpendicular to the average direction of the two lines already obtained, and get a third line back from this newly found point to intersect these two lines.

If you get a large triangle, use its corners as the starting point of a second search to locate your objective with greater accuracy.

"Who Goes There ?"

Some years ago a Dowser in Toronto, Canada, told fellow Dowsers on the 'Digital Dowsers' email list that at a certain time an object would be placed in the middle of his table, and invited other Dowsers to Dowse what had been so placed.

Quite a few did this, but three of the Dowsers found friends - one from Canada and two from the USA. Their 'Dowsing Teams' met at the table, and reported the identity of each other to their Dowsers - telling how they had met each other. This was reported on the email list.

Christopher Bird, in his book 'The Divining Hand', reports how Peter Harmon, a water dowser and driller living in Portland, Maine, was telephoning a client in Oklahoma; Mr. Harmon suddenly 'saw' the man's property in what has been fittingly termed his 'mind's eye'.

He told his client: *"You know, out in your back field you have a big dog house. Not far from its northwest corner there is a Coca-Cola bottle lying on the ground. Your best bet to spot a water well is going to be close to that bottle. Will you please go out and check to see if it's there ?"*

Taken aback, the man went outside and, northwest of the dog kennel, found the Coca-Cola bottle. Dashing back to the telephone, he shouted: *"How in hell could you tell the bottle was there ?"*

Unhampered by any scientific constraint, Mr. Harmon offhandedly replied: *"Well, I can see it because I'm there !"*

It seems that his 'Soul Sense' (or his auric body) was able to go to the sight and report back what was being seen !

A number of Dowsers have found that they can tell their aura to go to help others, or to stay in a spot whilst they move - and this happens. It is not recommended that you send your aura away for too long a time. You can Dowse for the maximum time - about 20 minutes seems OK.

Dowsing the Location of Submarines   *by Dan Wilson*

Churchill was very open to 'weird goings-on' - we have all heard how he employed Dennis Wheatley, the occultist author, to tell him what Hitler's astrologers were telling; so it wasn't surprising when a Dowser approached his office to say he could locate submarines from his home, Churchill didn't have him thrown down the steps but said: *"tell me where ours are this evening, then".*

The man sent in a map of the Atlantic with crosses on it showing where he thought the British subs were. He was accurate except for those under refit, which were shown in false positions. When this was pointed out, he said: *"I had never realized they needed so much time out of service".*

Churchill said: *"I have to go down and see a new depth-charge being tested on the Solent (stretch of water between Portsmouth and Southampton and the Isle of Wight). You can come with me and tell us where the test sub is".*

The Dowser was placed up on the prow out of the test destroyer out of the crew's way and where he wouldn't get any suspicion (unless he dowsed such a thing) that the British were also testing an improved sonar, so they knew where the two subs in the test were anyway.

The Dowser was told to keep on the phone to a man in the sonar room whenever things were moving about and the tests were under way. He was accurate on both subs throughout the day.

Churchill then commanded him to put in a daily report of U-boat positions to the Admiralty, using a printed map of the Atlantic and the North Sea which the Navy supplied in quantity.

This he did until the end of the war without anyone making any comment or sending a word of thanks or acknowledgement.

After the war, when hostilities had ended, the Dowser approached his governmental contact who had fixed up the meeting with Churchill and asked: *"Why had there been quite so much silence about his maps ?"* The contact knew nothing about it and spent a few weeks finding out.

He responded to the dowser somewhat apologetically. *"We had an organizational problem. For the first few weeks no-one had any confirmation of your maps, so there was nothing to say. By the time any information came in about U-boat positions (this was long before Enigma had been decoded) all the people who had been told what your maps were about had been promoted or moved to other jobs. For the rest of the war no-one had the slightest idea of their relevance and the whole lot were put in boxes and never examined".*

But the Dowser had kept copies; years later, from the history of 'The War at Sea', he found that he had been pretty well spot on - every time.

Detecting Landmines or Finding Lost Items

Most people can learn how to Dowse using a Pendulum; the basic skills are getting answers to questions and locating objects. Any person seeking to find mines by Dowsing must first become proficient in these skills.

Mines can be located both from a distance and close at hand. To find mines that are close to you can be most dangerous - but the risks are far less to a trained person than to an innocent child.

Training and experience, however, are not sufficient in such a dangerous exercise; the seeker must be aware of the mental conditions required and be able to prepare and control his thoughts and attitudes to ensure success in safety.

This section outlines a method to train volunteers to Dowse with a Bobber (a spring loaded horizontal Pendulum), and to get their mind attuned to enable them to locate land mines in safety. The disposal of located mines is NOT covered.

The military use of dowsing started with the location of water supplies, but extended to finding unexploded shells and the position of sea mines (after World War 1), and detecting enemy tunnels (Vietnam, from 1967).

In 1959 Verne Cameron demonstrated his ability to locate all the submarines in the Pacific Ocean, and determine which belonged to US, Russian, and other countries.

The best tool for outside use in locating lost coins or jewelry (on a beach or in a garden) and for landmines is a 'Bobber', as previously described.

Unlike a vertical Pendulum, a Bobber is far less influenced by the weather; it also enables you to cover the ground more easily - and with a further reach.

Safe Practice - Coins and Jewelry

You can go to the beach to find items lost by other people, or get a friend to place coins in places for you to find - under carpets, or in your garden or a park.

You can use your map Dowsing skills first - draw a rough plan of the carpet, garden, etc. and find where these have been hidden.

If you ask for metal, you may find coins, jewelry, bottle tops, and old nails. Precision in your thought of what is being sought is very important ! A 'quarter' and a 'dime' are made of different metals and their size varies; a 'coin' could be described as 'a metal disk that has been embossed, has value, and can be used for the exchange of goods and services'.

Are you looking for a lost gold ring ? Then hold the picture of such a ring in your mind - otherwise you may find a gold broach instead. If recently lost, it will be on the surface - at a greater depth it could have been lost in ancient times, and be of greater value !

Thus defining what you seek is an exercise in itself - you can define shape, material, purpose, depth of cover, age, and value (is it worth digging X feet down ?). A 'witness' can be most useful.

I was looking for a plastic top for a fuel container, without any success - until I held a similar top in my 'other' hand, when my Bobber took me straight to it !

Mental Alertness, Focus, and Intent

Since Dowsing for dangerous materials can lead to the injury or death of you or those around you, you must take extreme precautions.

Nobody has proved that there is a God; and nobody has proved that there is not a God. If you do not believe in a God or Guardian Angels, you have nothing to lose in imagining that there is a God and that you have a Guardian Angel. Play it safe !

Humans have the right of choice. You can choose to have a hang over, be tired or drowsy, or listen to music while you work. But anything which reduces your alertness or your ability to work with the intuitive part of your mind will increase your danger, and prevent you from getting a crucial message.

Even if you believe that a death in battle for 'the cause' will send you to heaven, this may not happen if you are so foolish as to go into the battle unfit or poorly prepared.

You are going to take enough risks in locating mines, so do not add more and unnecessary risks !

The intention behind your actions is critical. If it is to earn money then you are doing it for gain, and historically 'Upstairs' does not favour using their powers to help selfish aims.

You must have the feeling (deep inside you) that you are prepared to sacrifice your life and good health to help others - to prevent some child from losing a leg or being blinded, or to enable farmers to grow food to feed people. Then the fact that you may be paid (as a soldier, for example) is a secondary consideration. Your intent must be to 'do good' and help others.

Some people would call this following program a prayer, and perhaps others would justify it for 'organizing your mind for the job'. But it states your intent and asks for protection and help - and you have nothing to lose by saying it, and perhaps much to lose if you do not ! So before Dowsing for any dangerous items state:

"I, [your name], seek to locate unexploded materials to prevent them from causing harm to innocent people; I ask for the help and protection of God and my Guardian Angel for this task."

And before proceeding into danger, ask your Dowsing Team *"Is it safe for me to locate mines today ?"* - your Guardian Angel may know that today could be a bad day, and warn you not to go.

You would be most foolish to ignore such a warning !

But be warned - the fates may have decided to accept your sacrifice. And you may not be protected from your own stupidity or lack of attention.

While seeking mines, you must keep your mind completely focused on seeking the mines, imagining that you can see (with your Intuition) their outline below the ground and relying on your Bobber to give you the correct signals.

If you are in the middle of a minefield and start thinking of a beautiful beach, the film you saw last night, your girlfriend, or a cool beer - then that thought may be your last. Should you lose your concentration, you must stop until you can again focus only on the land mines.

How do you define a land mine ? A possibility is 'An explosive device made with the intent of causing damage or harm to humans and/or vehicles, that is now active in the physical world.'

The last part of this definition is to guard against mines that have already been removed, and to prevent thought forms interfering.

When a person thinks *"I will place a mine here"* but does not so act, a thought form of a mine may have been placed.

In a similar way, if another Dowser is also searching this area (or has done so in the past) then any thought of such a mine, even on a map, could place a thought form in position.

It may help to ask the number of explosive devices that have been placed in a defined area, and then check that all these have been located on your map - and then also in the field.

With each mine located, Dowse if it has been booby-trapped !

The 'now active' wording is intended to avoid wasting time on pieces/fragments of mines that have already been exploded.

Using a Witness

There is an old saying 'Like likes like' - that similar things attract each other.

It may give you an extra advantage in finding landmines if you hold part of a defused mine, preferably with a trace of explosive still inside, in your 'other' hand. This will help to keep your mind focused. A sample of the explosives used is probably the most important part of the 'witness'.

Improvised Explosive Devices

In some places, such as Afghanistan, these are placed to explode when a convoy or chosen vehicle is within range. Usually these are placed during the night, and are probably exploded by a 'watcher', perhaps using a radio telephone to detonate the device.

In such cases a team of Dowsers would best be used to check each section of road before the road is travelled. Each section should be examined by each Dowser at the same time, with the Dowsers each seeking different aspects, such as:

* Explosive material
* Human activity having the intent to cause harm or damage
* Radio / telephone location

The more of these aspects that are found at any place the greater the reliability of detection. If any is found, then further Dowsing should be used to check - including the location of any 'watcher', and if any booby-traps have been placed.

The information then needs to be sent to those responsible for on-site work - to include the elimination of any such 'watcher' and the de-activation of the device used.

It may be best to have people having clairvoyant abilities trained to do such Dowsing. They are able to 'see' what is found by their 'Soul Senses', and so could give a clearer picture of exactly what is placed at the located sites.

Practice

Do not have the idea that, having read about this suggested method, you can now go and find land mines ! You must practice all your skills many times first, even doing this with de-activated mines in a practice area.

The location of a mine is only one aspect - it has to be marked (to prevent you or others from stepping on it or spending time to locate it again) and then defused, which is a job for other experts.

Now practice finding the defused mine or sample. Repeat until you have confidence in your abilities. Then practice again with a number of samples buried in the ground by others, in locations unknown to you - and repeat until you are certain of your ability to find each and every sample every time you search.

Dowsing in Action

Keith Chamberlain started to Dowse when serving as a nineteen year old soldier with the Royal Engineers in Aden. This is his story:

A significant part of our job was mine clearance. Twice our observers had seen mines explode when the electronic detectors passed over them; with these deaths it was decided to stop operations until a solution had been found.

Two days later a colonel arrived and called us into the mess. He handed each of us a Pendulum and took us to a table where groups of playing cards were laid face down, in blocks of three cards.

He talked to us about 'instructing' the Pendulum, said that there was a Queen in each group - we had to find her !

Three of us kept finding the Queen; it was a good game - and then he spoilt it: *"Right, lets go and see if you can find mines with the Pendulum".*

We went to the training ground, and found the hidden mines - more precisely, we found the edge of a circle about 3 metres diameter which surrounded each mine. We did this over and over again, for four hours.

The next day we went out for real ! Bets were taken on how long we would survive - nobody placed a bet longer than two hours. We found twelve mines placed to catch people supplying the army base. We were hooked !

We worked for six weeks using Pendulums to locate mines. In that time we did not lose a soldier, and nobody was injured in the areas that we had cleared - which indicated that we had found all the mines.

Location of Hidden Weapons and Drugs

Some years ago I was sent information about a device being marketed to security and intelligence organizations that was able to locate hoards of drugs, stashes of explosives, and caches of weapons hidden inside buildings.

It had been tested by the Corps of Royal Engineers at their proving ground in England, and been found successful in defining which house in a row had such things hidden inside - and the actual location within the house.

It was a very complicated device; a 'black box' was fitted to a belt, with an electric wire leading from the 'black box' to an indicator which was held in the hand.

A 'token' for the item sought was inserted into the 'black box', and the operator walked with the indicator in his hand until the indicator moved to signal the direction of the sought item when located.

In fact, the 'black box' was just that - it held nothing. The connecting wires were for show, and the only 'active' part was the indicator - a well designed and carefully manufactured 'L' Rod !

The 'tokens' may have had a sample of the items sought implanted, or just have had the vibrational patterns / thought forms of the items; they served as 'witnesses'.

Why go to all this trouble and expense ?   It saved the organizations from having to admit to using 'metaphysical devices', and was acceptable as 'modern technology' instead of wizardry !

The manufacturers made a profit and the organizations passed on the costs to their clients ! Happiness all round !

Animals use Intuition Technology

Christopher Bird comments on the countless tales of pet cats and dogs who mysteriously found their way home.   When Walter Coleman, owner of a blue-eyed tomcat named Wahoo travelled from Seattle, Washington, to his summer home in Alaska, he decided to take his pet with him for company.

In Gold Pan, British Columbia, 300 miles north of their starting point, Wahoo, startled by dogs, bolted from his owner's car and disappeared into the underbrush.   Eleven months later the now bedraggled cat, his long hair matted and caked with filth, appeared on Mr. Coleman's Seattle porch.

A more inexplicably fantastic journey was made by Clementine, a cat owned by Mrs. Robert Landmark, which travelled 1,600 miles across the great plains from Dunkirk, New York, to Denver, Colorado, to find her owner who had left her behind with friends when she moved west because the cat was about to produce kittens.

After weaning her litter, Clementine hit the road and after four and a half months appeared on her mistress's doorstep. With no way of knowing where her owner was located, the cat was able to track her down simply by 'Dowsing' for her person.

It is disheartening that, instead of studying how an urge in animals leads them to their human friends, scientists mostly explain away such occurrences with the allegation that animal lovers, heartbroken at the loss of their pets, delude themselves into believing they have returned by adopting a look-alike facsimile.

Charting Catacombs

One of the best tests of Dowsers was made about ninety-five years ago by Armand Viré, a biologist who installed a laboratory in the catacombs beneath Paris's Jardin des Plantes to experiment on animals normally living in underground caverns.

Viré described his initial attitude toward dowsing in a book, 'How to Become a Dowser - What I've Seen and What I've Done': *"I was steeped in the exact sciences, particularly physics and biology and, out of habit, was used to imposing on any phenomenon the very limitations imposed on it by my venerable masters at the Sorbonne and the Museum of Natural History".*

"Anything concerning Dowsing seemed to me wholly cockeyed and unjustifiable.   The art was practiced mostly by simple countrymen who operated on the basis of more or less unfathomable instructions which they ill-understood or seemed unwilling to explain".

While in this state of mind Viré was visited one evening in 1913 by a geographer, Henri Mager, whose chapter on Dowsing in a book on methods to discover underground water Viré rated as 'at best, mediocre'.   Mager explained that, in connection with the Second Congress on Experimental Psychology being held in Paris, several scientists were hoping that a test of the Dowsing phenomenon could be organized.

"It is expensive to establish proof of the Dowsing phenomenon by drilling for water", he told Viré, "but as our country's leading expert in the study of subterranean caverns, we want to ask you if you will set up an experiment to test our ability to find them".

Viré's first reaction was to reject Mager's suggestion out of hand, but then he wondered whether a vast network of quarries dug under Paris and its environs from Roman times to the nineteenth century could not serve as a testing ground.

Over the years they had been precisely illustrated at a scale of 1:1,000 on charts which, still unpublished, were kept under lock and key.

Since there was no way in the world that any Dowser could know about them, Viré felt that they might provide a means *"to put an end, once and for all, to a superstitious fairy tale".* Without telling Mager what he had in mind, he asked the geographer simply to have Dowsers wishing to be tested assemble at Paris's Daumesmi Gate at eight o'clock the following Thursday morning.

The test area was covered by an extensive lawn, split by macadamized roads which revealed no trace of excavations ranging from 1.25 to 4 metres in height lying below it at depths between 16 to 20 metres. Viré's official report on the exercise to the Academy of Sciences, printed in La Nature, stated in part:

"Monsieur Pelaprat, a retired gendarme, discovered a void, which I recognized as being at the border of the quarry. I asked him to follow its contours and, to my great astonishment, I saw him stake them out. I then had him come back to his point of departure and delimit the contours in the opposite direction, which he did with precision. Monsieur Probst from Buglose in the Landes region, marked sixteen points on the ground which formed the borders of three squares and an elongated rectangle".

"Questioned as to their significance he told us that he sensed a solid mass within the confines of the outlined figures and voids outside them. My map immediately confirmed the correctness of his data. He had found columns put in place by the quarry-workers to obviate cave-ins".

"All the Dowsers also correctly maintained that the depths of the underground voids were in the 16 to 20 metre range".

Earth Energies

One aspect of Health that is still not receiving much recognition in the English speaking world is the effect of earth and water energies.

The original Feng Shui included the location and identification of these 'dragons', but the loss of understanding over the years has caused many practitioners to just 'go by the book' without using the needed Dowsing skills.

In Europe the builders of ancient structures (like Stonehenge) and of cathedrals were aware of these energies, and chose sites with the utmost care. But even good energies can be harmful (and so noxious to humans, animals, insects, plants, etc.) if they are too strong for the individual or the exposure is too long.

Humans, dogs, horses, cows, sheep, and pigs find most of these energies noxious - so if your dog loves to sleep in your chair or on your bed it is probably clear of these energies. But if a cat chooses such spots, beware - cars, ants, and bees love the concentrations. Bee keepers try to place their hives on energy crossings to get increased honey yields.

The energies themselves are not the disease - their noxious effect lowers our resistance and vitality so that diseases, etc., that we would normally overcome are able to 'take root' and harm us.

German medical doctors, including Dr Curry and Dr Hartmann, investigated these noxious energies in modern times, as well as Gustav Baron von PohI, who made the first detailed study on the effect of noxious water veins.

Studies were made by Dowsers of where noxious energies existed, were plotted on maps, and then compared with deaths from cancer - with excellent correlation.

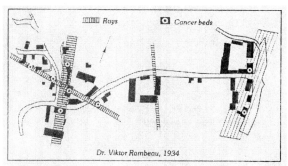

Rays   Cancer beds

Dr. Viktor Rambeau, 1934

As a result there are places in Europe where geopathic studies are required before hospitals, schools, and other institutions are built.

Käthe Bachler's Studies

In Austria, Käthe Bachler conducted a study of over 11,000 people in 14 countries and 3,000 homes and workplaces - cases where extended sitting or sleeping caused sudden infant deaths, inattention at school, and diseases such as cancer, arthritis, and heart problems.

In all these cases in needed only to change the seat or bed to avoid 'bad spots' - and when this was done the health problems disappeared !

> **Examples from Käthe Bachler's book 'Earth Radiation'**
> **available from the Holistic Intuition Society**
>
> **A condensed booklet 'Sleep Well, Be Healthy'**
> **which includes some of these case studies**
> **is available from the Holistic Intuition Society**

Case# 264. Anita, 10 years old, told me: *"I have been sleeping in this room for the past year. I sleep poorly, I am so tired in the morning, and I have headaches most of the time".*
Change of bed ! After only three days she reports happily: *"Now I sleep very well and feel well. And I am so happy, because I am finally warm in bed. Before my bed was moved, I was always so cold in bed".*

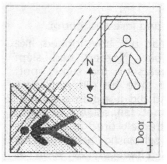

Case# 1507b. Ingebord had two places for doing homework.

Place 1 does not feel well, short concentration

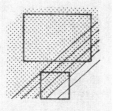

Place 2 feels well and cheerful, does extra work

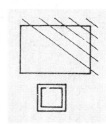

Case# 164. After her grandfather's death (he had died six months earlier from lung cancer), Lotte was given the privilege of sleeping in her grandfather's old bed.
She immediately lost her appetite, suffered from headaches, had trouble sleeping and lost many days from school.
As soon as the bed was moved to another location, she felt better again.

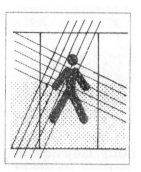

Case# 987. Mr. LL has multiple sclerosis.

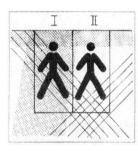

Mrs. H. from Salzburg asked for an examination. Afterwards I asked her which bed her husband was steeping in.
She said: *"In this one"*, and pointed to bed II. I looked surprised and she explained that he had been sleeping in bed I for 7 years and that they had changed beds only two weeks ago. I recommended a different place.

Case# 610. Premature birth.
Gall bladder, cramps, and pain in the feet, premature delivery. The doctor believed that without the appropriate measures, the foetus would have been aborted.
The dowser said: *"The child wanted to flee from the uteris."* The child was born after

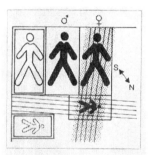

6½ months of pregnancy, cried most of the time, had convulsions, was restless.
The mother had to getup at night as often as 20 times to quiet the baby. After the bed was moved to another place, there was improvement.

Case# 660. The ten-month-old baby was tied to his crib.

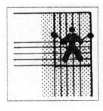

The parents were afraid he might fall out of bed, because he stood up again and again.
When in his playpen, he only occupied the half which was 'free of radiation', never the half above the Curry Line.
The father finally phoned me: *"Since we moved the bed, we have had no problem with his sleeping and he is healthy and robust".*

Case# 201. During the first and second year of the child's life, his development seemed retarded, and he did not talk at all. During the third to sixth year of life, the child was classified as mentally retarded.

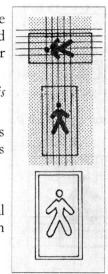

The school psychologist's judgement was *"This child needs to be put into a school for the handicapped."*

Through sheer coincidence, the child's bed was moved - and suddenly all the effort and care of his intelligent mother brought measurable success.

The child progressed in all areas of his life.

He was put into a regular grammar school on a trial basis. To everyone's surprise, he came home with 'Good' on his first report card.

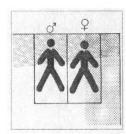

Case# 81. Migraine

The couple lived in a room for 18 months. He felt constantly 'under the weather'. She suffered from severe migraines, insomnia, and many other complaints.

A letter from them reported rapid improvement as soon as their bed was moved to another place.

Case# 510. Cramps in the legs

Mrs. R. suffered from cramps in the legs almost every night, and also from insomnia, duodenal ulcer, and phlebitis.

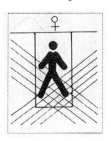

Four months after moving her bed she wrote: *"What a blessing to be able to sleep through the night. Ever since I rearranged the bed, I have had neither pains nor cramps in the legs."*

Case# 565. Stomach cancer was the cause of death of Mr. L. three

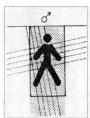

years after he moved into this house; his son's bed is located exactly beneath his on the floor below - he too suffers from severe stomach ailments, swelling of the lymph nodes, and abscesses over much of his body. The doctor had tried to help for years, but to no avail, and a thorough examination in the hospital did not shed light on the disease.

When bed was moved the patient became well.

Cancer Studies

Russian experience concurs - Dr Melnikov, Director of the Medical and Ecological Department of the Geo-Ecological Centre in St. Petersburg, reports a 5 year study looking at a 5 mile stretch of the city for geopathic zones in which 100 of 1,000 house were labelled as being 'cancer houses'.

Hospital and medical records were checked; 90% of oncological cases occurred in the zones, including direct correlation with leukemia in children. Traffic records showed a corresponding high rate of traffic accidents in the streets.

It has been determined that these energies rise way above ground - that a person in an apartment at the top of a high rise building will be just as susceptible as a person living on the ground floor.

In the 'normal' North American population about 25% of deaths occur from cancer - in 2007, information showed that this had risen to 33% challenging heart problems for the top place !

Studies show that the incidence of cancer in Gypsies is low - a survey in Europe indicated that less than 2% had any relation that had died from cancer. The Gypsies seldom stay in any one place for an extended period, and may also be aware of places to avoid.

So what are these energies ? What do they do ? And what action should we take to mitigate harmful effects ?

Noxious Water Veins

Noxious water was the primary interest of Gustav Baron von Pohl, working in Germany during the 1920's, assisted by other Dowsers. They located these streams or veins, measuring their depth, width, and strength (using a 'scale like the Beaufort wind scale', the value found by Dowsing - but the details seem not to be available now).

The Baron also was able to predict where lightning would strike - at crossings of water veins having specific characteristics.

My understanding is that the water is carrying 'bad energies' to be 'Healed Good' within the bowels of the earth - known as Gaia.

These noxious energies can be helped to be good, and so less noxious to humans, by being Blessed, by sending them True Holy Love.

When I bless a vein of noxious water, and then test the results, I find that it has lost most of its attributes that are noxious to humans.

The Curry Grid

Curry Grid lines were found by Dr Manfred Curry, M.D., in Germany; they run NE - SW and NW - SE, at spacings of about 10 feet / 3 metres. These lines alternate in having Yin or Yang characteristics.

Where two lines cross, their effect may be magnified and an energy vortex formed - which can be even more noxious.

Mike Doney, one of the world's most experienced Dowsers of energies, gets people to Dowse for lines (or vertical bands) of energies carrying hate, anger, greed; or love, joy, and healing. Mike has also found that you can Dowse for lines of colour !

I understand that most of the Curry Grid lines are like 'residential roads' carrying small amounts of 'traffic'. About every 100 lines they are reinforced by 'main roads' which have heavier loads, and about every 100 'main roads' is a 'freeway' - and if you sleep on a freeway you can expect to be injured !

As an example, the following was reported by Gary Skillen, a past President of the Canadian Society of Dowsers, who writes:

While teaching how to locate these zones we identified a Curry crossing point.

Each student took turns to stand on the point and described the effect on their bodies. Some felt sick to their stomachs, others tipped over or got a tingling sensation.

Suddenly a thought came to me to Dowse how detrimental this crossing was to humans.

On a scale from 1 (no problem) to 10 (most detrimental) this crossing was at 10. My next thought was:

"Maybe this Curry line has its own consciousness, its own awareness of itself; and is suffering as well ! And if I acknowledge the fact that it has its own awareness with respect, perhaps I can communicate with the energies involved".

I then asked:

"Are you detrimental to your own self ?" YES

"Do you want to remain detrimental ?" NO

"Do you want to change to being beneficial ?" YES

"Do I have permission to help you change to being beneficial ?" YES

"So be it !"

I took my Pendulum and allowed it to swing (with intent and with Love) in the way needed to make the change - it swung clockwise for about 2 to 3 minutes, and then stopped.

I asked *"Is the correction made ?"* YES.

Each student then took turns standing on the same spot and reporting how they felt - some were apprehensive about repeating their previous experience, but all were pleasantly surprised !

This same crossing point now gave them more energy - and it was beneficial !

The Hartmann Grid

The Hartmann Grid was identified by the Dr Hartmann, M.D. in Germany, in the 1930's. It runs N-S and E-W, the spacing varying with latitude between about 6 feet / 2 metres and 12 feet / 4 metres.

These seem to be polluted electric systems, especially in places where an earthed mid-point is used to distribute electricity, such as in North America.

Slim Spurling considers all Hartmann lines to be noxious and caused by electricity; he says that the Hartmann lines were sought in the Amazon jungle (no electricity distribution system so far !) but not found.

I asked Slim *"Were they searching for noxious energies ?"* and got the reply YES.

Using my 'Message Chart' I was told that the Hartmann Grid exists in all places - it is the 'road' that is used by energies (such as a member from a Dowsing team) in travelling around the earth, to get the current location of a person, etc. But it gets polluted by the electrical distribution system.

And like the Curry Grid, it has a one way street system, alternating like Yin and Yang, with residential roads, main roads, and freeways.

Slim recommends placing welding rods across these Hartmann lines where they enter a property - he (and clairvoyant assistants) 'see' the effect as deflecting the lines over the property. Michael Stodola has demonstrated in many of his workshops on 'Geobiology' that it is useless to just place the rods - they must be placed 'with intent'.

This means being instructed in the job required, the duration of their job, and given True Holy Love - and thanked for the good that they do.

People who are Clairvoyant seem to be able to 'see' Hartmann Grid Lines, but not Curry Grid Lines. This may be due to the Curry Grid being in the Mental or Buddhic Plane, and the Hartmann Grid being in the Astral Plane - where most clairvoyants operate. Dowse if this is correct !

Earthquake Faults

Fractures in the earth's crust are created by the folding of the earth's crust and are quite numerous, and can be small to very long and deep, like earthquake faults.

They are constantly changing their influence, which can be weak to very strong, depending on the stress of the moving earth's crust and the constantly changing gravity pull of the moon and sun.

There seems to be a varying summer/winter angle as well as the 28 day moon and sun cycle.

These Noxious Energies usually appear as a curtain of influence directly above and for the entire length of these fractures. They usually measure about three to four feet wide.

Electro-Magnetic Fields

EMF, or Electro-Magnetic Fields have been investigated by Dowsers in Europe and North America; this is another form of energy which causes harm to humans and other animals.

Electricity is generated in three phases. Especially in rural areas in North America it is distributed by taking leads from just two phases, with 220 volts between the phases, and having a ground which gives about 110 volts between each lead and the ground.

But loads are not equal, and so the ground is seldom at zero volts. Additionally there is a voltage between these grounds due to being at the 'centre' of different phase connections. Thus current flows in the earth to give balance, and itself generates magnetic effects.

The energy comes from transformers, computers, television sets, microwaves (especially microwave communication towers), cell phones, electric clocks, and even unused electrical outlets.

Be particularly aware of the effect of cell phones - even a 2 minute call can affect the mind and brainwaves of a person - and the younger the person, the more damaging the effect; in pregnancies any unborn child is especially vulnerable - even in 'standby' mode !

Experiment:: 1 Egg And 2 Mobile Phones

Place a fresh egg in an eggcup, and initiate a call between the two cell phones, then lean them against the egg as if was an ear listening to both phones - one each side; you can use an elastic band to hold them in position.

When this was done, nothing was noticed during the first 15 minutes; 25 minutes later the egg started getting hot; 45 minutes later the egg is hot; and 65 minutes later the egg is cooked.

Conclusion: The immediate radiation of the mobiles has the potential to modify the proteins of the egg.

Imagine what it can do with the proteins of your brains when you do long phone calls !

Devices are sold which give various degrees of protection, and magnets are often recommended to be placed at the sources, such as at transformers.

Gary Skillen has found that crushed calcite crystals are excellent for absorbing the EMF radiations.

I experimented with placing thought forms of such crystals at a few electrical outlets and in front of my sound system, and found that they worked well; but after a couple of days the effect returned, so I asked why this happened. I was told *"We are overloaded. We need to be grounded"* - so I placed a grounding thought form in the piles of metaphysical calcite crystals, and they are doing a good job again.

The effectiveness of the calcite crystals seems to be enhanced by placing a sodalite crystal on top; if you placed a thought form of calcite crystals, then use another thought form for the sodalite (or add it to the calcite thought form).

Ray Machell reports on his testing of this method:

"The first item to be cleared was my new 21" computer monitor. Before starting I measured the distance that the monitor radiated energy that was detrimental to me. It was 64", much more than I expected.

With thought I placed crushed calcite crystals around the base, the edges of the screen, and on top of the monitor.

Measurement showed that the radiation had been reduced to 40".

I then imagined a sodalite crystal on top of each pile of calcite crystals - the radiation was now reduced to only 18" !

I then grounded each pile of crystals by thinking that each was connected by wire to an imaginary ground rod driven into the earth. Incredible - the radiation was now only $2\frac{1}{2}$" !!

In all this procedure I asked permission by Dowsing to do the work, indicated the purpose of the request and the length of time needed to be effective - in this case the time that I owned the monitor.

Upon completion, I gave thanks to all involved."

Categories of Noxious Energies

It appears that we can divide these energies into two types - the metaphysical and the physical.

In the metaphysical category we have the energies radiated by noxious water and the Curry Grid lines; they are both not detected by physical apparatus, and can both be improved by Blessing them and sending them True Holy Love.

In the physical category we have electro-magnetic pollution and radiation, detectable by instruments and deflectable by both physical and metaphysical devices.

Location of earth energies is best done by Dowsing - which works in all planes.

Now that these various types of energies have been described to you, you are able to think about them, and so tune into them.

Greater accuracy would be useful when adding various different energetic effects, and crucial in better understanding the relationship between different energies - such as evaluating the changes in energy strength of two Curry Grid lines due the effect of the vortex caused at the crossing, or the effect of a noxious water vein.

Logarithmic Numeric Chart

Accordingly I have designed a Logarithmic Numeric Chart specially for the Dowsing of the values encountered in handling noxious energies.

Extremely durable Vinyl-Plastic business cards printed with this chart are available (with a glass bead Pendulum) from the Holistic Intuition Society - to purchase one, see our web site: www.in2it.ca/tools.htm - or see our other contact information in this book.

Unity (the value of 1.0 on the chart) represents the **'Average input of Beneficial Life Force/Energy that you receive in an hour from all sources'** - or 'Hourly Input' for short.

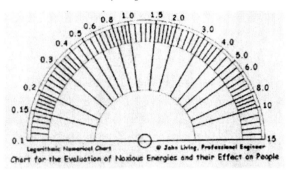

Chart for the Evaluation of Noxious Energies and their Effect on People

The value at a point is best found by using a Pendulum - by moving the chart to various locations (such as by just walking with it) and getting the readings of energy strengths, and checking if the effect is noxious to humans - as it will be in most cases.

To use the chart, ask your Heart-Mind-Brain team to signal the amount of your 'Hourly Input' that would be used by you if you were to remain in the spot below the centre point of the card.

In most places this will be in the range from 0.2 to 0.4, signifying that it is a good position for you. Any value below 1.0 indicates that you have a net gain of beneficial energy, but the closer to 1.0 the less spare energy is available for other normal activities.

Any value greater than 1.0 means that you would have a net loss of energy if remaining in that place. The greater the value, the more detrimental is the noxious energy.

You can quickly find its type by asking *"Is it a Curry line ?", "Is it a noxious water vein ?", "Is it EMF ?",* and *"Is it another energy field ?"* by asking a YES or a NO circle to be made. Remember that a combination may be involved !

If you are getting a very high reading you may be in contact with discarnates - souls, lower selves, or other energy that was in a person (or other life form) now deceased. In most cases they have not been able to get 'in the Light' and are coming to you, as a Light Worker, for help. You can also ask that these energies come to you to be helped !

You can use a normal counting chart to check a person's 'Battery Strength' perhaps in terms of their personal 24 hour days.

Approximate values are: at full charge 100%, and the critical strength level needed for good health 50%.

Then find their present strength - if 30% this would indicate their level as being 20% below the critical level.

Curses

I was very surprised when clearing a house that there was another energy field that I had not helped to heal; a thought popped into my mind *"Is it a Curse ?"* - so I checked, and YES.

So I asked for it to be released from its task and sent into the Light - and all was well.

If there is a curse (perhaps from ancient times) on a piece of land, you can ask the 'Force for Good' to help the energies in it - most have been give a bad job by a Being now dead, and were not released before the Being died.

They do not like the bad job, and are keen to be Healed ! The energies are good - they just have been hurt by being made (given jobs) to hurt others.

One interesting fact came to light when chatting with Bill Askin. He had been working to remove 'Curses placed in all time' but was not getting success. I was guided to suggest that he make his request '.. in all time*s*' - and this worked !

It seems that there are designated periods 'a time' similar to the times suggested by the Mayan and Aztec cultures - perhaps denoted by the direction of the sun, whether rising in the east and setting in the west, or operating in the opposite directions.

This may also apply to other aspects where time is involved.

Malicious Energies

Occasionally you may find very negative, evil, or malicious energies. They are still made of tiny 'baby energies' - most of whom want to be 'in the Light'.

So I treat them all the same - I find it very effective to ask *"That the 'Force for Good' now come and escort these energies to their rightful place to be Healed in the way that is best for All Creation with True Holy Love"*.

Some Experiences

The method described has been taught at many 'Intuition Technology' courses - and we have had some most interesting experiences !

Most who attend are 'In the Light', and so attract those energies of various types that wish to be back in the Light - and a few energies that are disruptive.

We have had to put a 'Shield of Light' around our workspace to protect our work from interference, while allowing space within the room for those energies that wish to 'attend' the workshops !

Indian Bands

At Red Deer College in Alberta, when the students went into the corridors to find zones of energies noxious to humans, they found four spots giving very high level readings, and asked me to check their work.

I found readings of about 10 hours energy depletion (for each hour spent in the spot) and Dowsed if it was caused by a curse, a noxious water vein, a curry line, or EMF radiation - and got negative replies in each case.

I then 'wondered' what could be causing the depletion and my Intuition suggested 'Earth-bound Souls' - so I Dowsed if this was so, and got YES.

Using my Message Chart, I then asked who they were - and was told *"We are four Indian Chiefs with other Band Members - we died centuries ago, and wish now to go into the Light".*

We then held a ceremony to send them True Holy Love and asked that they be guided to their correct place in Heaven; they went, and sent a message of thanks.

The energy levels were then re-checked, and found to be within acceptable limits.

The Age of Dinosaurs

After the workshop resumed we asked that all such energies be prevented from entering the workspace.

About half an hour later, a Tribal Leader who was attending the workshop felt that there was a similar energy within the workspace, pointing to a spot by a wall.

I checked, and found a depletion level of about 10, so asked who was there, and how it had intruded when we had placed protection.

I was told that it was a human who had been killed by a Dinosaur 300,000,000 years before !

Because he had been hurt for so long, he had obtained special permission from 'Above' to come and ask that he be returned to the Light.

We held a short ceremony for him, and the depletion level returned to a low level. Perhaps he had wandered into a 'Time Portal' from a later age.

After clearing, the residual energy field usually give an hourly depletion reading below 0.5.

You can asked if an energy field can be made beneficial, and this will usually be approved and the change made.

You then may get a positive reading of about 3; but do not 'overcharge your battery' - you can have too much of a 'good thing' !

Procedures

The order of asking about depletion energies may best be:

1. Earthbound Energies (Souls, Spirits - of all types) - since they are so strong that their effect 'blankets out' other readings.
2. Curses - because they are usually covering a very large area.
3. EMF Radiations - often being noxious over a large area (from transformers), or very local (electric appliances).
4. Noxious Water Veins - they wander across the grids.
5. Curry Lines - easily identifiable, known spacing.
6. Pollution in Hartmann Grid - perhaps more common in rural areas, due to unbalanced electrical distribution systems.
7. Earthquake / fault lines.
8. Other Sources - and ask as guided by your Intuition.

Protection

Using Lahkovsky Rings (formed of a thick 'good gold' wire, bent back on itself, and then twisted clockwise and joined to form a ring) is a most effective method of protecting a place or building.

Wire Twisted Clockwise:

You can place a thought form of a very large diameter ring around a hospital. school, apartment block, office building, or home - not a whole village or town, since the effects generated inside the ring build up too densely.

It is best to place one such ring in the Etheric Plane (for Noxious Water energies), one in the Astral Plane (for the Hartmann energies), and another in the Mental Plane (for the Curry grid).

Remember that to place any thought form this you go into prayer mode (being sincere), explain what the effect you wish to achieve, tell how you intend to do this, and ask permission to proceed.

When granted, you just imagine (in your mind) that it is being done (and it helps to put physical effort into the work, such as by making large clockwise circles with you Bobber or Pendulum).

You can then fill the place with the essences, vibrational patterns, and energies of Peace, Harmony, and True Holy Love, Namaste.

Then confirm that it is placed with True Holy Love to do the (specified) job for the time stated - such as the life of the building - and then give your thanks and your gratitude to all who helped this to be manifested.

Blessing Noxious Water Veins

When Blessing noxious water, go upstream (again in your mind) to the sources (imagining all the tiny little veins starting and then joining together) and Bless all the vein itself and the water which it carries for the whole course of its existence - this can be beneficial to many others who would otherwise be subjected to its noxious effects.

Having good intent, placing with True Holy Love, and designating the effective time are all critical - and action by using your Pendulum or Bobber increases the effectiveness. And give thanks to all who assist in your good work !

Investigation of Electro-Magnetic Fields

Joey Korn has found that there is a difference between the subtle EMFs you can find with Dowsing and the physical EMF fields you can detect with electronic measuring equipment, such as gauss-meters and tri-field meters.

Subtle energy fields, whether related to electronic devices, to the Earth, or to us as human beings, cannot be detected by gauges or other electrical measuring devices. But human beings can find these with Dowsing - and can feel their effects with muscle testing.

Through many years of his research, he finds that it is the subtle counterpart to the physical electrical field that affects us, not the physical field unless it gets very .

It is thought that the closer you get to the source of the electrical emanation, such as a TV, the stronger the physical field and the greater the effect - which is typically considered detrimental if it measures greater than 3 mG (milli-Gauss).

Joey's research gives a different take on this.

The subtle electrical field is a vortex, composed of two spiraling bands, one positive and the other negative; he finds that only the positive band carries the charge - the negative band is neutral.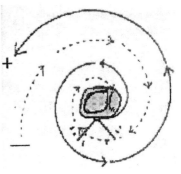

When you're standing in a detrimental band in the subtle electromagnetic field, you'll be weakened, as can be experienced with muscle testing.

Stand between the bands, and you'll muscle test normal.

This is at the core of why Joey doesn't call detrimental subtle energy 'negative' and beneficial subtle energy 'positive'.

From his research over the past eight years, only the positive bands carry a charge in the subtle energy fields radiating from electronic devices, and they can be beneficial, detrimental, or neutral as to their effect on us.

He finds that any detrimental or neutral subtle energy field can be changed to be beneficial with a properly stated prayer or blessing, simply asking 'The System' to change it to be beneficial.

EMF Experiment

Use any Dowsing tool you wish; Joey suggests using a pair of L-rods, holding one in each hand.

Now stand about eight feet away from any device that might be radiating a field, such as a television, portable phone, or any device with a lighted LCD display.

Approach the device while Dowsing with the intent, *"Show me any detrimental energy that might be radiating from this device"*, and keep your intent focused on the device. As you approach the first band of detrimental energy, you'll begin getting a Dowsing reaction.

As you pass through that band, your Dowsing tool will begin to return to its search position and will then begin another reaction as you approach the next band.

The closest band is typically within twelve inches from the device. The next one will be about twice that distance away from the device, and the next one will be twice that distance again. These bands ultimately extend into infinity, but the bands are weaker and more diffused the farther they are from the device.

You may not get a Dowsing reaction until just before you reach the device, within twelve inches or so. If this happens, it's because that is the strongest band. Dowse again for subtler bands of the same energy and you'll likely get several reactions as you approach from at least six feet away.

If you have someone to work with, you can use muscle testing to see that people are weakened when standing in the bands and will muscle-test stronger while standing between the bands.

Then say a blessing as simple as, *"Dear God (or however you address the Divine), please change the energy radiating from that device to be beneficial. Amen"* (or ask 'The System' to do this). After the blessing, muscle test again and if you've stated your intent adequately, you'll both muscle-test strong while standing in the bands, even stronger than while standing in between the bands.

Then Dowse again, asking to find detrimental energies that might be radiating from the device, and if they've changed, you won't get any Dowsing reactions. Change your intent to *"Show me beneficial energies that might be radiating from the device"*, and you'll get Dowsing reactions in the same places you did before.

Joey's version of the blessing is: *"If it be Thy Will, may the Powers of Nature converge to increase and enhance the beneficial energies and balance any detrimental energies radiating from this computer (or other device), for our family our friends, our pets, and for all of benevolent life, for now and into the future, for as long as is appropriate.   In deep gratitude, Amen".*

After you've experimented a little, Dowsing and blessing a few devices, you will be able to bless all the electronic devices in your home that radiate these subtle energy field.   Just use the above blessing and include *"and all energies like that throughout my home".* Then use Dowsing and muscle testing and you'll be amazed to find that all or most of the energy fields around electronic devices in your home will be beneficial.

Joey suggests that you can even use these subtle energy fields to help keep your own energies balanced and help you resolve key issues in your life.

Joey uses what he calls 'the blessing process' in his work, while I call on 'The System' in my work.   Either way will work, and ultimately both methods engage the same forces.

Joey has suggested the following <u>'Simple Blessing Process'</u>

In my research over the past thirteen years, I find that the most powerful way to keep the energies around you, in your home or office, balanced and beneficial is to keep your own energies balanced and beneficial, as well as those who share the space with you.   This includes the Earth energies associated with geopathic stress.

I've devised a very simple blessing formula to help you do that.   You can also use it to bless others and objects you wear.

If you will include these five components to a blessing, and do it often, you or whoever you bless will stay balanced, as will most of the energies around you.   This is simple enough to memorize or learn and integrate into you're your throughout-each-day life.

Try to let your negative thoughts and emotions remind you to say this blessing.   Negative thoughts and emotions are what I call 'anti-blessings' - so turn your 'antiblessings' into 'blessings'.

The five components of this Simple Blessing Process are:
1.   Address the Divine.
2.   Ask to be blessed or charged with energy.
3.   Make a statement of what you want to accomplish.
4.   Express gratitude.
5.   Close the blessing in some way.

Each component is important. The first three are to make it work; the next two are for you. It is important to feel and express gratitude and to turn our blessings over to a Higher Power.

So here's a simple blessing:

"Dear God (or however you address the Divine)

Please bless (or charge) me (or someone else or an object you wear) with energy to bring healing and balance to [my/his/her] complete being, physically, emotionally, mentally and spiritually.

Thank you. Amen"

Joey Korn is an internationally renowned Dowser and energy worker from Augusta, Georgia. To order his book 'Dowsing: A Path to Enlightenment' call 1-877-DOWSING (369-7464), visit www.dowsers.com or email Joey at Joey@dowsers. corn

Blessing Energies Program

'The Blessing Energies Program is to become part of and work with all my Dowsing programs, and to be continually in effect until I choose to make changes. Other names, words, situations and numbers may be temporarily substituted inside [ ]'s. Questions or requests need only simple reference wording.

If it be in the Highest and Best Good of All Creation then all changes that are needed to achieve the goal of Blessing the Energies and families of Energies in this [curse, water vein, Curry line, appliance, etc.] and making them beneficial without any noxious influences on human and other life are to be made now.

These changes are to be effective to all such Energies in the physical and all metaphysical environs, in all time, in all dimensions, in all planes, and at all levels including at any contract levels.

All jobs and tasks that are not in the Highest and Best Good of themselves and of All Creation which were given to such energies are now cancelled and made null and void.

All such Energies are hereby released from all such jobs and tasks, and may now be re-allocated to new jobs and tasks, or to join with Energies and families of Energies that are beneficial and acting in the Highest and Best Good of All Creation in their jobs and tasks.

Any Energies and families of Energies that do not want to be so Blessed are to be Healed in the way that is best for the Highest and Best Good All Creation with True Holy Love.

I send True Holy Love to all these Energies, and to all who Bless them and help them to be beneficial, and wish them well in their lifes.

This program is to be activated by saying: "I Bless the Energies in this [curse, water vein, Curry line, etc.] and send them True Holy Love".
End of Program. Thank you.'

Electro Magnetic Field Neutralization Program

'The Electro Magnetic Field Neutralization Program is to become part of and work with all my Dowsing programs, and to be continually in effect until I choose to make changes.

Other names, words, situations and numbers may be temporarily substituted inside [ ]'s. Questions or requests need only simple reference wording.

If it be in the Highest and Best Good of All Creation then I ask the help of 'The System' to place a Thought Form having a sufficient quantity of crushed calcite crystals with a sodalite crystal on top, to neutralize or make beneficial to all life forms all the noxious effects emanating from this [transformer, power point, computer, television, microwave, or other piece of equipment], and such Thought Form is to be grounded to carry away all such electro-magnetic fields and effects, so that all Energies and families of Energies in such fields can return to their families without any noxious effects. The programming of these crystals is to be effective for [the life of this building].

I send True Holy Love to all the calcite and sodalite crystals and the Energies, and to all who Bless them and help them to be beneficial, and wish them well in their lifes.

This program is to be activated by saying "I place calcite crystals with a sodalite crystal on top, all grounded, to neutralize the electro magnetic fields in this [transformer, power point, computer, television, microwave, or other piece of equipment] to be effective for [the life of this building] and send them True Holy Love". End of Program. Thank you.'

Placing a Protective Gold Rings Program

'The "Placing a Protective Gold Rings Program" is to become part of and work with all my Dowsing programs, and to be continually in effect until I choose to make changes. Other names, words, situations and numbers may be temporarily substituted inside [ ]'s. Questions or requests need only simple reference wording.

If it be in the Highest and Best Good of All Creation then I ask the help of 'The System' to place a Thought Form of a wire ring made of Good Gold (bent in half and back upon itself, and twisted in a clockwise direction, with the ends then joined to each other in the correct way) is to be placed around this [bed, home, building, etc] to prevent any 'not good' Energies or families of Energies from entering the space enclosed by the ring, and to transmute them into being beneficial. Any essential earth Energies are to be carried around by the ring to rejoin their path without having any noxious effects inside the ring. The ring is to be effective for [the life of this building].

Such a ring is now placed in each of the Etheric, Astral, Mental, and Buddhic Planes of existence.

I send True Holy Love to all the Gold in the rings, and to all who help them to be beneficial; I wish them well in their lifes.

This program is to be activated by saying "I place Protective Gold Rings around this [bed, home, building, etc] to be effective for [the life of this building] and send them True Holy Love".

End of Program. Thank you.'

Remember to check the installation !

Noxious Energies Program

Of all the areas we use Dowsing or other detecting methods for, Noxious Energies may be one of the most important ones. We are asking our subconscious or other sources to detect where there may be a less than beneficial influence within a designated area.

Because of the effect on the body, it seems to be very easy to detect these influences by many methods.

There are of course numerous influences from the earth, outer space, and man-made. You should normally be able to Dowse or otherwise detect their current location, strength and your personal safe time - the time you can be in this area and not be harmed.

Experiencing such a noxious energy for a safe time can be very beneficial by exercising your defence systems and avoiding disuse atrophy - avoiding exercise can sometimes make you weak !

Also, what we sometimes classify as Noxious Energies are only beneficial energies where we have had an overdose - such as the sun, or heat from a fire.

'The Noxious Energies Program is to become part of and work with all my programs or agreements, and to be continually in effect until I choose to make changes.

The term 'Noxious Energies', unless other wise requested, is to mean any form of energy, condition zone or situation that is or could have a non-beneficial affect on any aspect of [my] personal total being in a harmful, disrupting or interfering way. This is not to include, unless otherwise requested, smoking, alcohol, drugs, medication, food or drink that we have deliberately and knowingly put into or on [my] body.

It is to include, but not limited to, the effects from magnetic or electromagnetic energies from zero to all frequencies, alpha, beta, and gamma energies; the influences from fractures or faults and underground water; all man-made, earth or cosmic energies, gases, mind, psychic and spiritual influences.

When 'The System' has evaluated the area designated and indicated the levels of effects then I ask the help of 'The System' to adjust the Noxious Energies in such a way that they will be neutral or beneficial to any person, animal, plant, equipment or other thing, seen or unseen, entering or occupying the designated area, and to make this continuous for [a requested event time (Like the life of the building or as long as you are in a motel room, etc)] and the adjustments are not to otherwise cause non-beneficial effects.

This program is to be activated by saying "I Heal the Energies around this [bed, home, building, etc] to be effective for [the life of this building] and send them True Holy Love".

End of Program. Thank you.'

Remember to check the installation !

I suggest that this program be used only if the previously mentioned programs that are specific to individual energies are not effective.

More about Energy Bands

When discussing the Curry and Hartmann Grids it was noticed that these lines of energy were in vertical bands, of alternating Ying and Yang qualities, and having separations varying from approximately 2 metres (6 feet) to 4 metres (8 feet) according to their latitude.

It has been found that clairvoyants can see pollution in the Hartmann grid, but seem to ignore the Curry Grid - perhaps because their clairvoyant sight is operating in the 'Astral' dimension, and the Curry lines are in a higher dimension beyond their sight.

These lines can be located by Dowsing, since the Heart-Mind-Brain 'Dowsing Team' has the ability to 'tune' into all levels of existence.

Dowsers have discovered many more energy bands; those identified are for each individual colour, for each individual element, for the various combinations of elements into molecules, and for emotions.

As an experiment, Dowse for the lines of such various colours and elements, noting their positions, directions, and spacings. Because we are not aware of all these energy bands (and the waves within them) does not mean that we are not affected by them.

I found the bands for elements and molecules to be 4 to 5 feet (about 1.5 metres) apart, running North-South and East-West. The bands for colours seem to be about 7 feet (2.5 metres) apart.

I have also found energy bands for various plants, insects, animals, and human Beings. These different types of bands overlap without interference, probably due to being in different dimensions.

In some cases horizontally stratified bands exist; these seem to be sub-sets of the vertical bands, operating in a lower dimension than the main vertical bands.

When we consider that just in our physical electro-magnetic spectrum rays of various colours (visible and beyond normal sight), waves of radio signals, X-rays, and many others all co-exist without interfering with each other, we realize that we exist in an ocean of energy that surrounds and inter-penetrates our Being.

Other Dimensions

We realize that such an 'ocean' is even larger when we acknowledge that there are many higher dimensions above our physical electro-magnetic spectrum.

My understanding is that each dimension operates at a different speed of light; where S is our physical speed of light, the dimensions are defined as operating at S^n, (S to the power n) including the negative (root) values which accommodate sound.

My Dowsing indicates that the positive values for n are 1, 2, 4, 8, 16, 32, 64, 128 , 256, etc - each being the square of the preceding value.

It does seem that each and every dimension does interact with all others, although the range may be limited - as with sound and light, the effect diminishing with distance.

The higher the speed, the greater the power involved - and probably the smaller number of 'aspects' contained. Thus a more simple 'cosmic' signal would still be effective in a star, planet, or human - but accompanied by many more signals originated at lower levels.

The effectiveness of a high level dimension may be propagated through lower levels in a similar fashion to the way that harmonics operate within the dimensions that we understand. Perhaps it is the vibrational pattern of the signal that is important - the 'dance' that is made.

It is interesting to note that we see the light from a distant star even when moving our head a tiny amount; it seems not to be a single ray of light, but a field of light that we observe - to which our sight organs react.

The Message Chart

This is advanced Dowsing - so be sure to have gained confidence in your Dowsing abilities before working with the Message Chart.

To some people the message chart is very similar to a OUIJA board - so called for the YES or NO signals it gave, from French 'OUI' and German 'JA'. There have been serious warnings made against using these boards - and those warnings are true.

So what is the difference between Dowsing for a YES or NO answer, Dowsing with a Message Chart, and using a OUIJA board ?

In most cases the OUIJA board is used by a number of people as a game, without any protection.

Because a number of people use it, it is easy for an unwanted entity to join in and have fun - at your expense !

First something that attracts you is offered, and then you are trapped - you start to use the OUIJA board by yourself, you do everything that you are told (believing that good is intended) and find yourself in serious trouble.

The programming that you have installed will help to stop the entry of unwanted entities.

When receiving any message, remember to check that any change in position starts with a small clockwise circle - to indicate a correct and true message. If you get an anti-clockwise circle, it may not be true or you may have mistaken a letter - which may need correction.

Experiment with your message chart to exchange messages with your pets. You can have a wonderful time 'talking' to your dog. And you might be able to get your plants to grow better - and grow prize vegetables in your garden.

Conversations with Angels

It is always most important to build on a good foundation. We will start with the Higher Entity (your Guardian Angel, Higher Self; or whatever other name you choose to use) that is your special link to 'The System'.

Say (aloud, or to yourself) *"I open in True Holy Love, Namaste, and in Love of Truth; I send Holy Love to my Guardian Angel and ask what is your name ?"* and hold your Pendulum over the Start Circle on the message chart.

Your Pendulum should make a small YES circle, and then point along one of the lines which lead to the letters; follow along the line, until you come to the 'flower' at the end which has 3 'petals', and see which petal your Pendulum indicates. Write down the letter, and ask *"Is this letter correct ?"*.

Now you understand why it was suggested that you use your non-writing hand to hold your Pendulum - so you can write the messages as you receive them !

If the letter was not correct, ask for it to be repeated - and continue until you do get the correct letter. Then ask for the next letter. Remember that the name that you get may not be like the names used in your environment today.

Remember to check - ask *"Is XXX your correct name ?"*. Then ask *"Are you in the Light ?"* followed by *"Do you love the Good God System ?"* (or God, Great Spirit, or your own wording) and if either of these gets a NO then you are not conversing with a good entity.

If you have an entity pretending to be your Guardian Angel, just ask for help - say aloud *"I ask 'The System' to please take this entity into to its rightful place to be Healed"* and that entity will not bother you again. Then ask once more for the correct name.

Always check that entities are 'In the Light' and that they Love 'The Good God System'. They cannot lie about this, and by refusing access to them you can avoid a lot of trouble. It is very quick check, and good Energy Beings like to be asked.

When you have the correct name, say *"I send my love to XXX in thanks for the Love and Kindness that I receive. Namaste"*. Saying 'Namaste' is the 'end of message' signal.

The next stage is to ask for assistance. So say *"I send my love to XXX and ask will you please always guide me onto the Highest and Best Path through my life ?"*. When you have finished, end with giving thanks and saying 'Namaste'.

It will not hurt at this stage to say *"I thank The System for the Love, Life, and Light sent to me and for assigning XXX to help me; Namaste."*

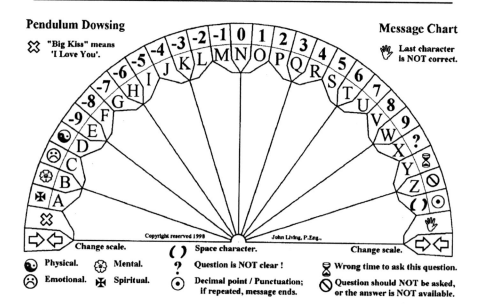

Pendulum Dowsing

✕ "Big Kiss" means 'I Love You'.

Message Chart

👋 Last character is NOT correct.

Change scale.   ( ) **Space character.**   **Change scale.**

👁 **Physical.**   😵 **Mental.**   **?** **Question is NOT clear !**   ⏳ **Wrong time to ask this question.**

😢 **Emotional.**   ✳ **Spiritual.**   ⊙ **Decimal point / Punctuation;** if repeated, message ends.   ⊘ **Question should NOT be asked,** or the answer is NOT available.

All this, of course, should be done in a state of prayer. The state of prayer has nothing to do with clasping your hands or kneeling down ! It means being really sincere and honest, concentrating on what you are saying and thinking - and thinking only good thoughts.

It is especially powerful if you ask for good to happen, or help to be given, to somebody else, not yourself !

Understanding the Symbols

One of the best ways to start is to go through every character on the chart, so that both you, your Dowsing Team, and 'The System' know where to find characters and understand the meaning of each character.

When I designed this Message Chart I included some special characters; personally I have found that these are not used - but in case your Dowsing Team chooses to use them, let us examine their meanings.

So ask your Pendulum to point to each in turn and then read aloud the note given to explain its function; then ask your Dowsing Team if the meaning is fully understood, and give examples of when it is to be used.

If the question mark '?' is signalled, this means that the question is not properly constructed. It may have two meanings, or require two answers. Asking *"Can you tell me the time ?"* is two questions - can your Angel tell you, and what is the actual time. What time do you mean ? You should try to make the question clear.

A sand timer indicates that it is not the right time to ask the question - and implies that the question may be asked at another time. This may be because something is presently happening which changes the answer, or that it will take time to get the right answer for you.

The prohibited sign means that you are trying to enter forbidden territory - such as asking about your death, about the future, or about some other person's business.

It is also used if you ask about matters that are beyond your understanding - given your present state of knowledge. You may ask why the sign is shown, and the answer may help you to increase your level of understanding, so that you are allowed to ask the question in the future.

The large open cross represents a 'Big Kiss', and indicates the phrase 'I Love You' (or 'Namaste') which is an important part of each message. I find that my Pendulum makes this sign itself when I have 'done very good' - it does not fool around with the small sign !

The symbol '( )' of empty brackets indicates a space between words. The hand signals 'Stop !' to let you know that the last character was not interpreted correctly. Not used once in ten years !

The point in a circle is either a decimal point or punctuation, depending on the context. If it is repeated, the message has ended. This is another sign that has never been used in my own work.

The remaining special symbols refer to the types of problems which cause illness - physical, emotional, mental, and Spiritual. Just run through the meaning and location of each symbol.

The double arrows instruct you to use the other scale - if an address is being given, part will be numeric and part the name of the street and town. The positive numbers will normally be used. I have not found any telephone number or address to be correct !

Having explained these symbols, placed when the Message Chart was first designed, let me confess again that my own Dowsing Team hardly ever uses them - preferring to spell out messages.

Using the Numeric Scale

If you want to know relative numbers, such as how well your health or ability compares to that of the ordinary, average person, then you can ask on a scale between plus nine and minus nine - and use the scale 9 to -9 to get the answer. But remember to program your Pendulum responses first - and this can be done in the question:

"Please indicate my weight compared to an average person of my sex, race, age and height by -9 being too light, 0 being average, and +9 being far too heavy" or, using different meanings of the scale:

"Please indicate my weight compared to an average person of my sex, race, age and height by -9 being most adverse, 0 being average, and +9 being ideal".

You could also ask for a percentage, of course, with 50% being average, and get an answer using the numeric characters 0 to 9 getting a '7' first and then '5' to give an answer of 75%.

But a word of caution - do not ask for the future prices of a stock, the value of a currency, the winning numbers of a lottery, or any other information which would give you an unfair advantage unless you need the money for a very good purpose such as helping others - and in such a case, get permission first.

Remember that if you really want to get a big win, then this desire may overcome the truth of the answers that you get - so be very surprised if you do win !

I find that my Handy Chart is easier to use for this type of work.

Starting a Conversation

Do not send frivolous messages or time wasters. If you feel that 'I Love You' is not appropriate to the message that you are sending, then the message should not be sent. It is as simple as that !

So you want to ask a simple question. Hold your Pendulum over the 'Start Here' circle of your Message Chart, and concentrating (in meditation) on the circle think your message:

"I open in True Holy Love, Namaste and in that Love of Truth. I wish to ask if I may talk with the Guardian Angel of [a friend's name] to help in healing him. Is this permitted ?" Do not be surprised if your Pendulum makes a YES circle while you are thinking your message - this indicates that it is being amplified and sent.

Your Pendulum will now stop, and then make a YES or NO signal. Suppose it is a NO signal. "I ask the reason why I may not ask about healing [your friend's name]" and the following message is given:

"I am [name and/or title], in Light, I Love a Good God System. Now not good time; send friend True Holy Love. In team I trust, Namaste."

So then think *"I thank [name and/or title] for Love and Kindness. In team I trust, Namaste."* Then send True Holy Love to your friend, to be used as best needed, and ask again at a later time.

I find that when the message says *"I am healing good"* it is best translated as *"I am feeling Happy and Loving"*. This can be considered as the result of 'being healed good in a good way' - which is the intent of healing, usually achieved using Love.

Receiving a Message

Not only can you get messages in reply to yours, but messages can be sent to you when you are doing something else ! So how do you know that there is a message for you ? You can ask, and a signal can also be sent. This is something that you must agree with your Dowsing Team.

You may decide that only very special messages will cause a signal, and all others must wait for you to check for them.

Often a signal that there is a message will be a funny wave in the side of your head, but this may not suit you, so you can arrange for the signal to be a feeling in your finger or a tingle in your toe.

At first my personal signal that I am being contacted was a slight pain in my hand below my left thumb. Now I get such signals in different places, according to the source of the message.

It is up to you to decide, but a tingle in your toe may well be better than having an accident while driving because your head suddenly ached !

If you get a message signal while driving, while at a business meeting, or while you are otherwise preoccupied, just tell your Dowsing Team that you have received the signal and will deal with it as soon as possible.

Remember you do not have to say this aloud, you can just send it as a thought. So when you are ready to communicate, hold your Pendulum over the 'start circle' of your Message Chart, and concentrating (in meditation) on the circle ask *"Is there a message for me ?"*

If your Pendulum makes a YES circle, then start to note the letters sent in the message.

The usual format for a message that you receive is: *"I am [name and/ or title of the sender], in the Light, I Love a Good God System".* Then the message, followed by *"In the Team I Trust, Namaste."*

You may get a message *"I am healing bad in not getting your Love True and Holy. I am now healing good at getting your Love. I am healing best in all Heaven at the Love sent me. I am healingest bestest in all Heavens in joy in happiness and in Love."*

Note that the message seems to be contradicting itself - because messages are always given in 'the now', so this is saying *"My previous feelings were .... I now feel better."*

So the above message would translate as: *"I was not happy that I was not sent Love. I am now happy at being sent Love - I am very happy indeed - I am more happy and joyful in Love than any others in Heaven."*

Perhaps an overstatement in fact, but this exaggeration is the accepted method of expressing these feelings in a Heavenly way ! And quite often the words used are in a different order from normal English usage.

Overcoming some Problems

The most common problems are grammar and spelling !

Messages are thoughts that are sent to you; they travel as symbols. The way that messages are constructed varies in the physical world according to the language used - and the language used by 'Upstairs' is different from our speech.

Hence the sequence of words may not be as you are used to hearing. Since 'Upstairs' is always working in 'The Now' it is only the present tense that is used - but you may find a few exceptions.

Spelling is by your Dowsing Team; the message is mainly the concern of the Intuitive part of your brain, and the spelling normally is the responsibility of the logical part. It helps if both parts work together in harmony, but this may not be the case.

So if the spelling and grammar of your messages is unusual, it maybe that the Intuitive part of your brain is doing its best to spell without relying on the logical part.

Another common problem is when you have received part of a message which makes sense, and then you get garbled nonsense. This is because there is interference (which should not happen often), the sender did not complete the message, or that you have misinterpreted the message.

When the message is not correct you should have been given a 'Stop !' signal to let you know - but sometimes this does not happen, so you get garbled gobbledegook instead ! If so, go back to the end of the part that made sense, read it out, and ask if that part is correct. If not, go back to an earlier part until you do get a correct part, and then have the rest of the message repeated.

If the message does not make sense as a whole, or seems to be telling you to do something that you believe to be wrong, ask *"Are you in the Light ?"* and then *"Do you Love the Good God System ?"* to check that another entity has not interrupted.

The System should have prevented this, but it can happen.

If the message is correct and something still seems wrong, then ask the sender to confirm the message by spelling it to you again, and then ask if the message is correct and if your understanding of the message is correct.

If the sender is your Higher Entity such as your Guardian Angel and confirms the message, then have faith that it is correct.

An example of this would be telling you about reincarnation if your religion did not support the idea. It may seem wrong to you, but it was a belief of the early Christian church - until Rome decided that the church would not allow the general public to have this belief.

Should you get a message that involves harming or hurting any other life form, be most cautious. Such a message is NEVER sent by the 'Good Guys'.

If you do take any such action, you alone are responsible !

Important Questions

Perhaps Souls come into this life as humans to learn lessons and undertake missions.

But most humans do not know which lessons of life they have come here to learn, or how they can help by completing their mission. You are now in a very special group of humans - you can ask !

When you ask about your lessons or missions, remember that as you complete one lesson you may have the opportunity to learn another.

In the same way when you complete one mission you may be given another. Also the missions may change due to circumstances beyond your control - some other human may have done the job you were intended to do !

It is important to keep checking on your lessons and your missions, so that you always get guidance on what to do. And if you always act to the best of your ability you will find that things go well for you, since you are on the right path.

Improving your Skills

You may well find that you start to recognize patterns of conversation, and may assume that a pattern is always used; you may also recognize words due to the context in which they are used. But always check !

Sometimes you will find that the next letter or word does not come - and this is intentional, as a signal to you that you have made a mistake interpreting the message. Each letter is given to you, but your hand may 'stick' if you have made an error.

Be very careful with words such as no, not, and now - they can reverse the meaning of the whole message ! So always say *"Is my understanding that ... blah blah blah ... correct ?"* to check that you have not only the correct words but understand their meaning.

As you gain more skill, you may find that you receive the messages without the message chart, or just by gazing at it.

The message chart helps you with two things - it concentrates your mind on the message, and enables you to check difficult words - especially in spelling names.

Remember that in all Dowsing you 'tune your system' by thinking and visualizing the person or item that you seek.

It's a Two-Way Street !

So suppose you want to ask about a friend who does not know how to send or receive messages - can you communicate ? Yes, but not with the friend directly; you say *"I ask 'The System' in Love to tell (your friend) (the message)."*

If The System approves, then you may be connected; often this is to the Higher Self of your friend, not the physical entity that you know.

But in this way you can check if your friend is in trouble, what sort of help is needed, and how you can assist.

If the conscious mind of your friend can also send and receive messages, can you exchange messages with your friend ? Yes ! It is just like email on the Internet. You send a message. When your friend next checks for messages yours will be received. Your friend can send you an answer, which you receive when next you check for your messages.

Be careful to check that the message does come from your friend - and not an 'evil entity'. If you are suspicious, ask 'The System' to check that it is actually your friend.

Perhaps in the years to come humans will learn to access the thoughts of others in this way, so that we do not need telephones or the Internet.

If so, we may be regaining abilities that we have lost - it may be that many plants, insects, and animals have this ability to communicate amongst themselves, and perhaps between different species.

Some Simple Guidelines

- Be sure that the wording of your question is clear and not ambiguous.
- Think only of your question - get other thoughts out of the way.
- Remember to define what you are questing, why you are asking 'Can I ? May I ? Should I ?' - and then to check *"Is the answer true ?"* and *"Is my understanding ... correct ?"*
- If you think that you may be influencing questions that concern yourself get somebody else to Dowse for you.
- Respect the privacy of others - ask them before interfering,
- Dowsing to help others gets the best result - and gives you more satisfaction.
- Never boast - be humble, and give credit to the Angelic Beings who helped you.
- In all your life, only have good thoughts - always wish well for others. What you wish for others comes home - to you !
- If 'I Love You' seems inappropriate in a message that you are sending, then do not send the message.

Everyone has a Photographic Memory.
Some just don't have Film.

Remote Viewing

I, personally, have not had great success when viewing things in the distance - whether that be in space or in time; my clairvoyant abilities are spasmodic, to say the least. I use my Message Chart to ask and be told. So what follows are 'Gleanings' from the Internet email lists on Dowsing - in the hope that you may find them beneficial. Enjoy!

A real target is a must. But your living room, etc. is a real target, and the reason is a positive and honest one, to improve and learn the techniques so that when a need arises you are in the 'best mettle' to function! We all have to crawl before we walk, walk before we run, and practice jumping before pole vaulting!

Almost everyone can learn to Remote View. For some few it comes easily and well, for most of us it comes after many attempts, and for a very few others, you might try some other kind of Dowsing. Keep trying, if you really want to do this.

It took me weeks, trying every evening, before I landed nose first on the coffee table. It can be disheartening, but it will come. It can feel like being stretched out on a rubber band, and it does almost hurt when you're slapped back too fast - but it's not detrimental to you physically.

Some folks feel nauseated when viewing, and the best fix I've heard for that is to imagine yourself a minute speck on the wall when viewing, instead of 'whole body' you.

The ones I knew having nausea didn't after trying this.

What is Remote Viewing? I don't know what part goes, and what part stays, but I do know you don't want your consciousness 'in the way' or you won't get good results.

It's not the same as 'out of the body' but you do travel across distances, times, dimensions, wherever you want to. I don't have to be a good mechanic to drive a car well, and I don't have to understand every little nuance to be a good RVer.

There are many ways to look at it all. And there is no right or wrong way, just the best way for each of you.

Remote Viewing is often not clear, it almost always starts out to be fuzzy; please don't 'need' it to be like watching a movie. Often you'll just get shapes, colours, perhaps sounds, smells and feelings.

Only a couple RV'ers I've ever heard of could read while viewing, either letters or numbers, so the images aren't perceived like you may expect.

If you want to learn this, keep practicing the relaxing, and letting go. When you can get to the living room, try going outside, and view your home top, around. One student did this and found out he needed to clean his gutters !

The sensations you feel when letting go, viewing and returning will be strange, at first. But you'll get used to them and like riding an elevator, etc, you'll soon understand it's normal and means that 'it's working'.

I allow my consciousness to come in only to give direction, such as go up, go over, down, etc.

When I get there, I explain what I see, but rather than saying or thinking I see a red ball, I'll say I see a reddish coloured sphere shape. It could turn out to be a stop light, not a child's ball in the final wash.

If the only way to describe what I see is as an item, I'll say I see rows of openings, like the mouth piece of an harmonica. (I did this in one view, and when directed back to a time when the shapes had meaning, saw that they were 'man made' caves with elaborate carvings around each one and many peoples around them - I was viewing blind and didn't know what my 'target' was; I was viewing Mars when I was told.

That's a lesson further down the trail, working with a moderator. I do my best viewing when working with one.

But folks, the government taught a lot of the 'original' viewers, and even in the Stargate program the viewers often practiced. They would often spend weeks just doing practice targets. That's how you learn, hone, and test your skills.

Every one of those folks still practice their viewing, several of them have envelopes with pictures, etc, inside.

When they want to practice, they grab a blank envelope from that pile, and view what the contents represented. That way they can practice without a monitor.

So I guess this missive is to say, keep trying, don't lose heart. And if you 'chickened-out' yesterday, try again today. It's new ground, and it's really pretty healthy to proceed with caution.

Speaking of which, I'll share my basic protection for those of you who may not know of one for yourself. I ask for a mirroring protective sphere around me of light from the Free Will Positive Side that reflects any and all negative energies back to the sender, and any intentional or unintentional potentially harmful actions, advances, projections, to be harmlessly bounced off this sphere of protection. I ask for this protection to be enforced always, past present and future. I then express gratitude.

A caveat about protections, I've learned the hard way that any protection can have 'holes' in it. And that the usual cause of those holes is unforgiveness in the heart of the protectee. If you harbour hard feeling for anyone, thing, or situation, you probably have weakness in your protections. As long as we make the effort to forgive, those holes will reseal.

But the effort must be genuine ! Sometimes feeling forgiving takes a while, so keep stating mentally or verbally *"I forgive ..."* until you feel the forgiveness take hold. It can take a while before you do.

I'll get off that soapbox now. I'm so pleased that so many of you are trying Remote Viewing. And I'm proud of all you, no matter how it's going, you've had the 'houtspa' to try !

Blessings of light and love to you all, and good night, LJ

LJ, You have hit on a very important topic, one that has the ability to affect even basic Dowsing; and that is the ability to forgive.

It is the deep personal work, the stuff that actually requires 'work', that has the potential to let us advance to the next level(s).

Without that, we just stay stuck in the same old place, thinking that we have mastered all there is to know. Forgiveness is a perfect starting point for further advancement. Thanks for bringing that to our attention.   F

F, You are so very right, and in my experience, unforgivingness can cause illness in people, personality disorders, and on down the list of dis-ease. I've counselled several people with long running problems, to get to the 'roots' of their unforgivingness.

When it all was accomplished, the transformation was astounding, and completely life changing; I was the first one I counselled about it - and have been practicing what I preach for the last 30+ years.

Healing ourselves is (probably) more difficult than healing others. There can be so many things in the past that require letting go and forgiving. Doing a 'blanket' form of forgiving is okay, changing the energies of resentment, anger, etc., to the energy of love, but I suspect if there are one or two (or three or four) incidents that stand out in our minds, it's a good idea to approach those individually.

Here's a relevant passage from 'The Law and the Promise' by Neville Goddard:

"Man and his past are one continuous structure. This structure contains all of the facts which have been conserved and still operate below the threshold of his surface mind ... it is living - it is part of the living age. He cannot leave behind him the mistakes of the past, for nothing disappears. Everything that has been is still in existence. The past still exists, and it gives - and still gives - its results. Man must go back in memory, seek for and destroy the causes of evil, however far back they lie. This going into the past and replaying a scene of the past in imagination as it ought to have been played the first time, I call revision - and revision results in repeal."

"Changing your life means changing the past. The causes of any present evil are the unrevised scenes of the past. The past and the present form the whole structure of man; they are carrying all of its contents with it.

Any alteration of content will result in an alteration in the present and future."   E

Dear F, At every one of my workshops I pass the Huna prayer of forgiveness which is as follows:

"If I have hurt someone today by thought or word or deed, or failed another in his need, I now repent.

If I can take those steps again, tomorrow will I make amends and heal with love those hurts. I do this pledge.

And if some hurt has struck me deep and no amends are made, I ask the Light to balance all. I count the debt as paid.

Parental Spirits, whom I love, and who I know love me, reach through the door I open wide. Make clear my path to Thee."

I have had young women at work who would wake up in the morning with either a severe migraine, a stomach that churns requiring 6 maalox tablets, or a sore jaw from grinding their teeth during the night.

I tell them to repeat this prayer out loud before going to bed. The next morning all symptoms would be gone. The prayer is simple but it really works. I keep a couple of copies of this prayer in my wallet at all times to pass out to people that need it.   VD

LJ, That soap box was a doozey ! Whether we call it 'forgiveness', we could call it almost anything, it is that capacity in all of us that expresses our inability to accept responsibility for our thoughts and actions, and to force blame onto others.

In that place, it seems to be much safer, at least temporarily, but it really isn't. That is where one's ego struggles to survive, and we all know that the ego is the one thing that sabotages our Dowsing attempts. It certainly has the capacity to make us think we are very good at what we are doing.   F

For those who are serious about Remote Viewing and how it evolved, the statistical results, things that influence it, the combination of Remote Viewing and Dowsing and a whole bunch more of interesting and factual stuff, get hold of a copy of the book by Joseph McMoneagle called 'Remote Viewing Secrets' - Hampton Roads Publishing, ISBN 1-57174-159-3.

Joseph McMoneagle was on the team that was formed over 20 years ago by the US Government to investigate and scientifically analyse Remote Viewing.

He was Remote Viewer #001 in the army's Stargate program and was awarded the Legion of Merit for his contributions to various aspects of intelligence work.

He lays things on the line in a very practical and sensible manner - I was sent a copy of the book from a friend in Texas.

I definitely found his comments on combining Remote Viewing and Dowsing together very interesting.

I believe his book is a good place to start and certainly removes a lot of the bunkum that has evolved in regards to protection, the likely impacts etc.   B

Right on, B ! Joe is a wonderful, big, no mishmashing around kind of guy, and he tells it like it was, and is as much as he can (some is not declassified as you can imagine).

His book is a good read for anyone, and his examples showed my friend and I what not to do in our training programs, and how to balance RV with Dowsing to do the very best job we know how on a case. Both have a very real place in helping others. That said, Joe is one of those 'naturals' at viewing, and even he falls asleep sometimes when viewing.

A note about those of you trying our class, one thing I didn't say is to get ready to view - go to the bathroom, walk the dog, feed the cat, burp the kid, etc. before you view, to eliminate those interruptions. I'll get out of your faces now,   LJ

In my Viewing Training, the teacher approached it this way - and 17 of the 23 consulters there had no problem viewing their interior body. He had you shrink yourself down to size - a size you could enter a pore and enter the blood stream, and by this move to a place you wanted; and then go look at what you wanted to see ! Maybe this approach would work for you ?   B.

In Dowsing, I try to use the awareness of my whole self or field, rather than working from one location within that as you describe. I think you may be right that working from different parts of our field might affect the information we receive.

With 'Remote Viewing' I've been practicing just shifting my awareness to a location and asking what I see about something - the colour of my sister's shirt when I see her at the airport, or whatever. I can usually visualize well, and often I will get a dominant impression that's correct, but my 'interpretation' can be wrong, just as the teachers warn us about ! (I saw a green shirt, but her actual shirt was beige with a strong green stripe across it).   N

Remote Viewing is clairvoyance applied to actual places and events, i.e. not a 'visualization' which is normally symbolic, although it may be highly informative.

When done professionally it is usually carried out by groups who meet to assist each other psychically. Typical uses are locating lost objects and people, by military intelligence for spying, and by home security forces for locating kidnappers and robbers.

There are of course interfaces where RV smudges over into visualization, Dowsing, and 'direct cognition' (gestalt flash-knowing something as though someone told you it yesterday).

Both RV and visualization in turn smudge over into clairaudience, where the viewer 'stops the film' and asks bits of it what is going on.

The first bit of RV I ever did was for the purpose of identifying someone I'd never heard of until that moment, describing a kitchen in Canada 4,000 miles away. A woman I didn't know who'd been given my number phoned to ask if her aunt in Toronto, whom she'd just visited, was allergic to her microwave oven.

I said immediately *"You have two aunts. Is this the one who is 35, has black hair and eyes fairly close together ?"*

The caller said YES, but I could tell I was on a roll and said to her, *"I'll just describe her kitchen so we both know I have a good connection, OK ?"* She said YES, so I gave a fairly detailed description of the kitchen, of which I could see like a still photo taken from the entrance doorway. It was unusual, L-shaped with windows all down the left side and round the corner of the L where I couldn't see. The microwave was on the corner of the L on the left, the worktop was some blue substance and the taps on the nearby sink on the left were new.

The caller confirmed all this. *"No"*, I said. *"She does not have a microwave allergy".* Later after doing some Dowsing, I discovered that the problem was that the aunt was allergic to tomatoes and normally never ate them, but had just discovered she liked the taste of them when microwaved, so had started doing so.

Sig Lonegren keeps wondering why no two people on a site agree about the exact form of 'earth energies' there, unless one of them agrees to comment on one seen by another.

My proposal is that they are all looking, not at different views of the same things, but entirely different things.

One of the things I do in my third day of giving Dowsing lessons (having got everyone to do visualization and guided writing, or at least Dowse for words in books) is to get a volunteer's health 'read' by everyone else.

No two people say anything remotely the same. They all describe a different process or difficulty.

It is then my job to stitch these accounts together.   What is happening is that a person's health is a truly gigantic canvas of influences and causal events which it might take 2,000 such views to describe adequately.

Each Dowser has been guided by the group entity (all of us working together) to view the part they can 'see' with greatest clarity.

It's a sobering lesson in how much we miss when we Dowse someone's health.

Luckily, any one practitioner working alone is usually guided to suggest the remedial course they best can suggest, so the default becomes a minor one in practice.

If you think of the earth you're thinking of something with a history a good few billion times more complex than a single person.

If you tune into it, it's like calling a massive video library 'a TV program'. You might get a tape or DVD that means something to you, but you won't get the story. Sorry. The best you can do is get responses to a particular aspect of it that interests you.

Oh yes, and the 'shapes' that are detected are (I submit) mental maps of the topographical significance of the bit of the story you are tuned into. If anyone ever asks you *"how many 'Ley Lines' pass through this room ?"*, whatever the meaning of 'Ley Line' (and that is a moveable feast if ever I met one) the answer is always 'an almost infinite number'.

Don't forget, they include all the thought-lines of all the insects that ever passed that way since there were insects.

Earth energies are not, because they're bits of something else, too big for us to take in at one go - or probably at all.   Dan Wilson

The first assignment is to find a quiet time and place, take care of all the little details, ie going to the bathroom, walk the dog, etc. first, then lay down and relax. Try to get to your 'centre' and blank your mind. Then as briefly as possible think, *"I want to go to [a room in your own home]"*. This should be practiced at least once a day, or night, if possible. Keep practicing, it can take a while.

Please don't give up too soon ! Also, before I go back to reading, I'm overwhelmed by the response to forgiveness. You folks are great, and have wonderful insights into the process.

I'm not an old expert, but maybe my observations of my Dowsing and those we've worked with will help.

Always, there are no mistakes in Dowsing if you can learn what and why went askew. With this approach, when ever we had an 'oops' in our Dowsing, we sat down and studied everything about it. After a few years of this, we still get some posers, but have upped the accuracy to good 90% or better.

This is what we do ... First off we are very careful about our programming.

Secondly, or firstly, we are sure to clear the room we're Dowsing in of 'other' entities and energies, and ensure our protections are in place. We use map Dowsing extensively, and narrow the field to areas. Very seldom do we spend more than 15 minutes on actually Dowsing a location at one time.

Take a break, come back to it later.

Any impressions received while Dowsing, we write down and study later, not during the Dowsing part. Always try very hard to have a clear mind - and no expectations about what you'll find.

To avoid that usually I or my friend write up the program, assign it a number, and give only the number to the others.

That is one aspect of the RV protocol that has worked wonders for our Dowsing - working blind. But some of us can blank the mind enough to get non-biased results and still be 'front loaded'.

Dowsers become hugely attached to their results, or biased to their ideas about their results. That will skew further Dowsing terribly most of the time.

We never ignore data that comes with the Dowsing, firstly because we have learned to trust the Dowsers we work with, and secondly over the years much of the extraneous data has proven accurate. Hind sight, you know.

If two or more Dowsers working blind get the same results, we have a find !

Now, with the right programming we usually know 'when' the find is, current, past or present.

Thought projections (intents) and energy trails are just as real to the Dowser's rod or Pendulum as the exact location. The right programming helps to avoid this most of the time.

And sometimes, if the universe wants something brought to your attention, the Dowsing tool will show that instead of even your program request. We've had some cases of that, but by recognizing it and letting it 'happen' it made a much bigger 'find' possible.

These are our fixes to the problems we've encountered. We find these work for us, but as in all things, this is only one of other possible ways. Above all else, Dowsing should be enjoyable and taken with a grin whenever possible. What I do with my Dowsing is my gift back to the Universe, Lord, etc. for the gifts given me. In Light and Love,   LJ

Well, I had a bit of success last night. I was focused on the lounge, when I felt it was too large for me to target on and so I turned my attention to the crossword that I knew Eddie would be doing. Just before I fell asleep, I got 4 words, which I managed to write down.

When I checked the crossword, this morning, one of the words I had written 'beads' appeared in one of the clues, but not the others.

I'm encouraged by this and intend to keep practising as I think the centering part is a good exercise in it's own right. However, I've just realised that seeing as Eddie was doing the crossword at the time, I might have just picked it up telepathically from him. I assume there's a subtle difference between RV & telepathy ?   NJ

Hi NJ; well, I'd say they're so closely related the differences are subtle to be sure.

In my experience with RVing, when you're viewing you do pick up the thoughts and emotions of the people in the view, especially once you learn to 'focus' your attention on same.

Not every view will result in a movie-like scene, some are just feeling, and 'knowing' an idea, etc. With practice, you can hold a view longer, and that's when you'll notice that the first hit on the 'target' is just that, vague shapes, ideas etc.

If you stay on it longer, it'll often come into sharper focus and you can actually see, or explore those first glimpses.

Hope this isn't clear as mud for you, but I still am sure you had a successful view. Keep trying, and don't worry about a room being too big a target.

Think of it as when you first enter that room, you scan the whole room, then pick the area or item you focus on. In RVing that's what you do too, you enter the 'room' then narrow the focus to what you're most interested in.

Soon I'll go into the polite and safe protocols that we teach and hope everyone respects. Like traffic rules, they keep the dings and bumps to a minimum.

Keep up the good work, and to everyone else trying, don't give up please. Even getting to your 'centre' is a real accomplishment. From there it's easier.

You might try a different time of day to practice, a time when you're more normally alert, if it's possible. But the body does become so relaxed, even the best RV'ers sometimes fall asleep in a view ! Keep trying, and try any variation you might think of, changing time, changing the place (i.e. try laying on the couch instead of the bed, etc), sitting up a bit (propped up in bed, or a recliner, etc). You'll find a way that works best for you. In the mean time, as I said, it's the greatest cure for insomnia I've found !

For those of you wanting to try Remote Viewing, establish your protections, and then lay quietly in a calm area/time of your home, and blank your thoughts and try to find your centre. When you get there, you will know, then try to see another room in your home, say the living room if you're in the bedroom.

Practice and you will get there.   Of course, you may fall asleep too, that 'centering' is the best cure I've found for insomnia ! I love that word, thanks for the beautiful translation !   LJ

Harold Puthoff and Russell Targ, at the Stanford Research Institute in Menlo Park, California, mention the following successes:

Given only its co-ordinates on the globe, one subject drew a recognizable sketch of Kerguelen Island in the South Indian Ocean.

Others 'looked' at Mercury from afar to discover unknown features of the planet including a thin atmosphere, a weak magnetic field, and a comet-like tail of helium.

Though this was contrary to the predictions of astronomers, these details were later verified by Mariner 10, the first space probe to reach Mercury's vicinity.

Dowsing the Future

You can Dowse the future but not from the present. Any Dowsing answer regarding the future is instantly subject to millions of nodal decision points between now and then. For 100% accuracy you must Dowse the future as the past from a point beyond the date you are interested in.

All accurate Dowsing is 100% correct for the past and the present - limited only by your preconceptions and biases. The process is identical to what you are doing when you map Dowse. A portion of your 'Soul' travels to the site and permits you to gain information.

In this case you don't project to a geographical location you project to a point in the time stream - specifically a date and time (i.e. noon on 15 April 2060), on your own timeline.

Whenever anyone is Dowsing a nodal point in history you need to be sure that you are on your own timeline, otherwise your answer will appear inaccurate.

For a brief exercise Dowse these questions:
* How many timelines do you currently exist on ?
* In how many of these time lines are you male ?
* In how many are you female ?
* In how many are you already dead ?
* In how many are you married ?
* In how many do you have children ?

Continue with any other questions that interest you.

If you get wrong answers when Dowsing the future you are most likely getting an answer from one of your other time lines, or you are letting your hopes and preconceptions interfere.

Orbs

Serge Kahili King, in his book 'Urban Shaman' published by Fireside (Simon & Schuster) suggests 'grokking' as a good method to achieve 'time travel'.

He suggests that you 'imagine' your awareness climbing into an 'orb', and telling the orb the time and place that you are now situated, such as Mars, 2050 earth time (the more precise, the greater the accuracy); the orb will be there, and you should 'see', 'feel', or otherwise 'know' what is there.

Serge also mentions that you can make your 'orb spaceship' whatever size you like - make it so small that you can 'see' into a cell, for example.

This ability to 'visit' and 'see' within your body, your organs, and your cells is taught by the Silva Mind Courses and by other metaphysical schools - and has enabled many people to do Healing work on themselves and on other people and animals; it works !

The biggest problem when working with orbs is trying to get your conscious self into the orb; this is difficult - be content to just get your awareness into the orb.

Are we Being Watched ?

Does this work in reverse ? There are many reports of people seeing orbs, and they show in many photographs even when not visible to the 'naked eye'.

Are these 'Beings' from a different time of our own earth, from a present time of a different earth, or even 'Souls' (or higher level Beings) that are not in any body ? The various possibilities are numerous.

When you look skywards toward a cloudy sky without any particular focus, you may be aware of whitish 'spots' that dart around. 'Medical science' explains these as movement of matter within your own eye.

If this was so, the movements would be slower and in more consistent directions compared to the darting around of the observed spots in numerous directions at the same time.

When these orbs are captured by photography many different colours are observed. Are these just defective spots in the film ? If so, the same arrays would not be captured by separate cameras which have different films.

Orbs and Healing

It is noted that many of the pictures that include orbs are taken when Healing is being done; perhaps they come to be Healed, assist in the Healing work, or both come to be Healed and to Heal.

One of the best photographs is in Dr Emoto's book 'Message from Water' - although not mentioned in his writing.

Dr Emoto shows photographs of a lake before and after a Shinto Healing ceremony - the beneficial change to the water is quite amazing ! In the bottom left corner of the picture showing the lake after the ceremony is a patch of reeds - and in these reeds you can see a red orb and a blue orb. Were these responsible for the Healing given to the lake ?

I mentioned this on one Dowsing email list and had a sarcastic return post from a 'professional photographer' - I agreed that it could have been the fault of the camera, since it was taken with one of the new-fangled Japanese cameras, probably not up the standard of his US made Kodak 'Brownie'.

Crop Circles

There are many reports world-wide that orbs are seen when crop circles are made - and these have been captured on film. Rare elements have been deposited at these sites, in a very pure form not found on this earth.

In crop circles the stems are bent at 'impossible' angles without killing the plants, and even non-Dowsers can feel the energies located at these sites, often near historically recognized sacred places.

Perhaps the crop circles are symbolic messages to us - since thoughts are transmitted as symbols. So although our conscious selves may not understand their meaning, they may have an effect on us at some level.

The best book on crop circles is 'Secrets in the Fields' by Freddy Silva - ISBN 1-57174-322-7 published by Hampton Roads Publishing - www.hrpub.com is their website.

Two of the most intriguing crop 'circles' appeared next to the Chilbolton radio telescope in England in 2001. The first was a 150 ft by 240 ft square showing a pixilated human-like face; 6 days later the most controversial 'crop square' appeared, which researchers agreed was a binary code which closely resembled the binary-coded interstellar radio transmission sent by NASA in 1974 from the Arecibo observatory in Puerto Rico.

Some parts differed - to indicate a variation in the DNA strands, and a short legged person with a big head, and the coding for silicon was added to those sent originally as the elements of life.

Water, Water, Everywhere
-and not a Drop to Drink
'The Ancient Mariner'

Water Thoughts

Erle Montaigue tells how he was taught by one of his Tai Qi teachers to extract the maximum amount of Qi from the water that he drank. The teacher's health was amazing !

The brain (about 90% water) takes in the Qi from water directly from the mouth before it goes into the stomach. The rest of the body (about 70% water) must rely upon the digestion process to get its water.

The body treats food differently to water - most people get into trouble by thinking that things like coffee and tea or fruit juice are water. The body senses that anything that has food in it, is food - and treats that liquid as food, not as water.!

The Qi stored in water is never taken out in the mouth when we drink anything other than water; this is explained in the book by F. Batmanghelidj MD published by Global Health Solutions.

Water Quality

First get good water; the water that usually comes from a city tap may have little energy, and be contaminated with chlorine and sometimes fluorides.

Rain water that has been sitting in a tank for some time is ideal as it has some beneficial bacteria and organic material - but filter it first to remove the bugs, since they may be considered to be food.

Water that has been energized with Blessing is ideal - drink it at least three times per day.

Blessing Water

The method that follows is based on the skills of Bill Askin, a trapper in Northern Alberta who introduced Raymon Grace, the well-known Shaman and Silva Method Guru, to Dowsing, and passed on his skills to many other people in the Canadian Prairies.

Bill works to take out 'all that is not beneficial' and then inputs 'all that is needed for good health'.

My main contribution is to Bless the water with 'Blessing 995' and 'Healing 997' - which, I understand, invoke very high levels of Blessing and Healing; I may be wrong, but using these cannot do harm, and usually give very good results.

Raymon goes much further - he found that water has a 'Spirit' which responds to respect. Lack of respect and greed seem to be the main reason that water has been polluted.

He found that some bottled water had a 'spirit of greed' in it, along with several negative thought forms; these had to be removed.

How do we purify the water ? Raymon suggests that we use our Dowsing methods to scramble the frequency of the chemical, biological and radiological pollutants of the water and adjust (or transmute) them to the frequency of pure water.

Then ask for the water to be raised to the most appropriate level of energy for the person who drinks it, rather than asking to raise it to the highest possible level.

Raymon has found that a thought form can be loaded into the water to cause it to energize all water that comes in contact with it's energy field - and that the process be repeated continually.

This was tested by sitting a bottle of energized water on a table next to a bottle of untreated water. The next morning the untreated water had an energy equal to the energized water.

Marilyn Gang suggests reducing the surface tension of the water to be 'most beneficial for the users'.

How to Drink Water

Erle Montaigue: Take some pure water into your mouth and hold it there for a count of 7. Then spit it out ! This is important. Do this three times in all. On the fourth time, take the water into the mouth and drink it.

It is best to drink water in this way at least half an hour before taking any coffee or other food laden liquids - as the water you take will only mix with these and become just food rather than water.

Water tends to attract to it more toxins than wet food does. So some of the effects of going onto this regime is that your urine will smell different and you will be urinating more - even though you might be taking less liquid than you were before.

After some time when your body is getting cleaner you will notice that you are not urinating as much and your urine will gain a clearer colour.

You will also feel great and have much more energy to do things. You will probably find that your sex drive will improve as a direct result of this better Qi energy.

Working with Water

Your Pendulum may make many complicated patterns while doing this work ! With your water in a container such as a jug, bottle, or glass:

- With your Pendulum circling clockwise: *"I open In True Holy Love, Namaste, and ask the help of 'The System' to transmute this water to be Blessed, Healed, and completely beneficial to all the life forms that it serves, beneficial meaning: to operate in True Holy Love, Namaste, and in truth with good intent for all life forms and for all Creation, doing so without harm to any life form"*.

- Stop your Pendulum, and ask *"Will 'The System' so give this help ?"* - your Pendulum can be expected to signal YES.

- Pendulum rotating clockwise: *"I send this water and all that is in it 'True Holy Live, Namaste' with 'Blessing 995' and 'Healing 997'."* When rotation ceases:

- Pendulum rotating clockwise: *"Working with 'The System' I now scramble all vibrational patterns, frequencies, and energies that are not beneficial [for all creation, for (name), etc.] and that are in this water and all that is in it, and transmute them to be beneficial and to transpose them to their correct place."* When rotation ceases:

- Pendulum rotating anti-clockwise: *"I take all that fail to now be beneficial from the water, and send them to be Healed with 'True Holy Love, Namaste' in the way that is best for all."* When rotation ceases:

- Pendulum rotating clockwise: *"I ask 'The System' to raise the energy level, adjust the surface tension, and input all essences, vibrational patterns, frequencies, and energies that are needed and are beneficial [for all creation, for (name), etc.] [to include all medicine required for perfect good health] into this water and all that is in it, to ensure all spiralling is in the correct good direction with all polarities adjusted accordingly, and to make certain that all action and operation is in True Holy Love, Namaste."* When rotation ceases:

- Pendulum rotating clockwise: *"I ask 'The System' to place all needed protection against any and all degradation of the energy field so energized and treated, and to maintain such protection in all ways, in all aspects, in all 'nows', and in all times."* When rotation ceases:

- Pendulum rotating clockwise: *"I ask 'The System' to do all that is required to energize and treat in the same way all [appertaining to the named person] that comes in contact with the energy field so energized and treated - and that the process be repeated continually without any loss of such energy or treatment."*

- Again, your Pendulum may make many complicated patterns while doing this work. When rotation ceases:

- Pendulum rotating clockwise: *"I send my Love, Gratitude, and Thanks to 'The System' and to all who assist in this work."*

Feel free to add or amend this suggested procedure - preferably getting approval by Dowsing for the procedure and any changes.

Note that the expansion of the treated energy field is not restricted to other water - it will expand to all sorts of energy and matter, and keep doing so !

Gas Mileage

Raymon's concept for gasoline is along the same lines as for water, to remove any negative or non-beneficial vibrations and put back in the positive or beneficial.

With your Pendulum (or Bobber) counter-clockwise ask that the 'Spirit of Greed' be removed from this gasoline in my car - wait until swinging stops.

Then with your Pendulum clockwise, ask that this gasoline be immune from any force, physical or non-physical, that would prevent it from achieving its life purpose, to make this car run in the most efficient way possible, to the highest and greatest good. Wait until pendulum stops swinging, and say thanks.

Our Thoughts have Power that we have Sent
Make Sure that Good was Really Meant

Radionics

When we hear of Radionics we think of a box with dials and indicators - since this was how the original machine started, and amazed people with its success in curing diseases and changing substances.

Since this was technology, it started as being acceptable - but two things happened. First, once when it was used successfully it was later found that the batteries had been missing. Second, it was found that a diagram worked as well as the actual box !

This played into the hands of the people who had most to lose from such work - the medical and pharmaceutical crowd. So the originators were persecuted, and the use banned in medicine in the USA, except for veterinary cases.

Most Radionics practitioners go through extensive training and still use very expensive equipment based on the original boxes; they place a witness of the problem on dials, read the 'rate' by testing for it on a 'sticky pad', look through lists that have been prepared over many years to find the 'rate' that should be sent out to correct the problem, and then set the machine to broadcast that corrective rate to a carrier such as water - or directly to the client.

These 'rates' are numbers that are used to describe (or label) the vibrationary patterns involved, which are so loaded and sent out when the equipment is switched ON.

But Radionics can also be simple to do. It is only personalities of people that make it complicated. Radionics equipment is simply an enabler. It doesn't do the work in and of itself - it enables the operator to focus his thoughts and mental energy, and perhaps alter his psychic/mental energy in such a way as to bring about a result.

A Paper Radionics 'Machine'

As mentioned, a diagram of a Radionics machine was found to be just as effective as the actual 'black box'. So certain items such as batteries may be omitted, and a more simple diagram used.

It has been found that a 'Paper Chart Machine' can do anything that you can do with a Radionics box - it works !

Hank Smyth tells how to make a Radionics Paper Chart Machine - and you can easily make many copies !

Draw two big circles - a witness chamber on the right and a touch plate on the left, and three dials in a row slightly below and between the two large circles.

Draw a continuous straight line from the centre of the right hand witness chamber circle over to the left hand touch plate circle.

Continue the left end of the line by making 3 counterclockwise spiral circles within the touch plate circle with the bottom of all 3 spirals touching each other at their base lines.

Then continue the line down and out through the centre bottom with a slight angle down to the right to pass horizontally through the centres of the 3 smaller dial circles.

Continue the straight line to slightly outside the last dial circle and then angle up toward the centre of the larger witness chamber circle on the right side of the chart.

Leave an open space of about 1/4 inch between end of the line to centrepoint where the line began.

Use a simple pendulum 'fan' chart with numbers from 1 - 10 (or your 'Handy Chart') to determine the broadcast rate numbers.

Get a witness of what you are working with (plant, soil, car, electricity, fuel, etc.) and put it in the right hand witness chamber / circle. For example, draw a picture of your car sitting under a sign that says '59 miles per gallon'.

Put your left hand on the touch plate to get in tune with the witness.

Dowse with your Pendulum for the three numerical rates that will make happen what you have put in the witness chamber.

Write those numbers in the three smaller circles below.

To activate the broadcast - connect the two open ends of the drawn line (as though plugging into a light socket or flipping the switch ON)

Check the number settings on the broadcast at regular intervals - at least once every 24 hours to determine any change needs on the broadcast rates. These rate numbers do change.

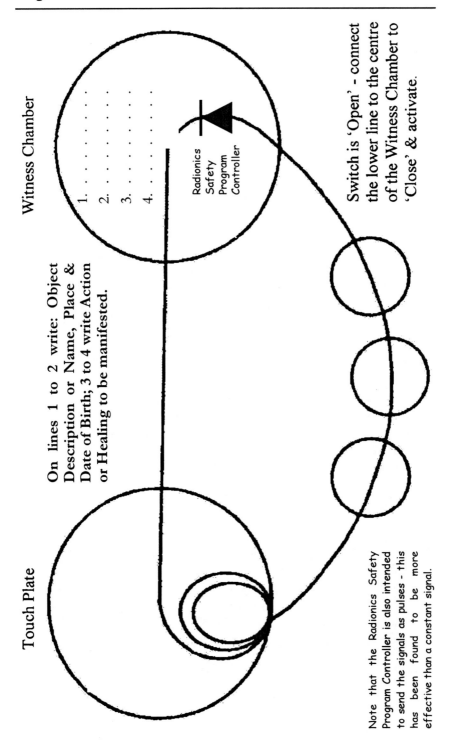

Witness Chamber

1. . . . .
2. . . . .
3. . . . .
4. . . . .

Radionics
Safety
Program
Controller

On lines 1 to 2 write: Object Description or Name, Place & Date of Birth; 3 to 4 write Action or Healing to be manifested.

Touch Plate

Switch is 'Open' - connect the lower line to the centre of the Witness Chamber to 'Close' & activate.

Note that the Radionics Safety Program Controller is also intended to send the signals as pulses - this has been found to be more effective than a constant signal.

Erase the prior numbers when necessary and insert the up-dated numerical dowsed reading, to accommodate with the change needs. (Better yet, use a fresh diagram drawing to set up a clean/clear broadcast space with no remnant vibrations in the number circles).

The Radionics Paper Chart Machine probably adjusts when we 'turn on' our mind - when we send out certain energies from our thought forms.

You can adjust the volume of your thought form to bring about the result that you want (at least this is the way we can program our subconscious mind) and it helps it happen. We also get assistance from our superconscious.

Examples:

Increase the gas mileage you can get out of an automobile.

Take a picture, or draw a picture of your car, and include a written statement *"this car is getting better gas mileage"* or *"this car is getting 33 miles per gallon in town now."*

Then determine the number settings needed to help bring about this result, and check:

"Are the correct numbers in each circle to accomplish the result illustrated in the drawing that I've put in the witness chamber ?" If so, put the Radionics Paper Chart Machine on a shelf and forget about it for a couple of days.

Save Electricity - Save Fuel

Average out utility bills and fuel bills before you begin trying to lower them - to get a base data.

Make a cartoon drawing of the electric bill or fuel bill - and each month write in an amount about $10 - $15 lower than you would expect to get.

Put it 'on broadcast' with appropriate setting. Do not deprive yourself of any of your normal electrical or fuel uses. Use all your electricity and heating as you usually do.

Wait and see what happens.

Balancing Medications

Get a sample of each of the particular medications plus the picture/ name or other kind of witness of the person.

Write in a statement that the person receiving the medications will get all the benefits of the medications but none of the non-beneficial/toxic side-effects or toxic build-ups.

Even if the person no longer actually is taking the medications, he will still receive the benefit of them through their written essence.

Notes on using your Radionics Paper Chart Machine

Faith healing can be effective even when a person is unaware he is being worked on. Properly set Radionics tools work whether other people believe in them or not.

Our own beliefs / thoughts / visualizations can create for us on the physical / material levels. We can make things happen with our minds; the subconscious mind responds well to images / pictures.

Basically, if we believe Dowsing is wrong, our Dowsing won't work for us. What we believe is what we can do.

Key principle - do no harm to others; so be aware of using power and control over issues. It's okay to create opportunities, maybe - but not okay to force others to do what you want.

Question: Are we just attaching intelligent 'Thought Forms' to the machine, or also using the natural intelligence of the machine itself ?

Easy Self-Care with Paper Radionic Broadcasts

Instead of Dowsing for the settings, a paper with the desired result can be placed between the machine and the 'witness', and enclosed in a 'black box' by sandwiching them between pieces of black paper.

Wynelle Delaney shows how we can create a global command program that sets up a safe energy field for sending and receiving the broadcast, and make a paper 'black box' Radionics machine.

It is imperative to consider the safety and comfort of a recipient of a Radionic broadcast. Healing crises from too quick de-toxing and 'overcooking' are absolutely avoidable.

A safety program can help the Radionic broadcast be just as effective without causing discomfort and healing crises. Include the safety program in either every general broadcast you send and/or have it set up permanently - write 'Controlled by the Radionics Safety Program Controller' on the Radionic activator you use.

Radionics Safety Program

'The Radionics Safety Program is to work with all my programs or agreements, and to be continually in effect.

The intent is to ensure that all needed Healing and corrections are made to the recipient of all Radionic broadcasts, such broadcasts to sequence in, potentize, and automatically switch ON/OFF and operate in pulses as is necessary for optimum benefit, protection and Healing according to priority and percentage needed, Divine Principles of creation governing, and body fields patterns of perfection prevailing, so operating on all levels in all planes/dimensions/domains, realms, time-space continuums known/unknown, without any harm and at the most appropriate level and rate of change, including where applicable to:

* Balance appropriate/beneficial acid-alkaline amounts/ratios/levels.
* Balance/enhance soil porosity, rejuvenate, regenerate overworked soil.
* Resolve, rectify, correct, clear deficiencies.
* Offset non-beneficial effects of noxious rays-radiations-emissions.
* Balance appropriate/beneficial presence of animals/insects/nature beings/Deva help and contact.
* Rectify, resolve, correct, self-pollution.
* Balance, harmonize, co-ordinate, enhance Life Force-Vitality.
* Remove, rectify, correct non-beneficial/harmful blockages and distortions.
* Clear over-stimulation; protect from over-stimulation.
* Clear distortions; protect from distortions; create a healing sanctuary.
* Neutralize, disperse, eliminate clear, eject along with all their toxins all specified and/or unspecified processes and/or energy patterns and essences that fail to be beneficial.
* Balance, harmonize, co-ordinate soil vibrations/patterns.
* Align, balance, harmonize Subtle Energies.
* De-toxify, neutralize, block, eliminate, clear non-beneficial chemicals/toxins/poisons and their patterns.
* Block, de-toxify, neutralize, eliminate, clear, offset non-beneficial effects of chemicals/gases/metals/toxins/poisons.
* De-toxify, neutralize, block, eliminate, clear, offset non-beneficial effects of caffeine, tannic acid, fertilizers, pesticides, insecticides, herbicides, pollutants, contaminants.
* De-toxify, neutralize, block, eliminate, clear, offset non-beneficial effects of non-beneficial/pathogenic bacteria, mycobacteria, viruses and their mutations/variants/subsets/toxoids.
* Enhance, synchronize healthy co-ordination between land/plants/trees/nature beings.
* Enhance, balance, harmonize surrounding environment.
* Balance, co-ordinate, harmonize, clear negative energy patterns from Vortices A, B, C, D, E, F, & G.

* Balance appropriate/beneficial amounts/ratios/levels of: copper, potassium, ammonia, silicon, calcium, iron, phosphorus, sulphur, helium, magnesium, manganese, nitrogen, zinc, selenium, sodium, iodine, salt, rock dust, all minerals and trace minerals present as needed.
* Balance appropriate/beneficial amounts/ratios/levels of oxygen.
* Block, repel, deflect, offset non-beneficial effects of noxious/harmful/pathogenic insects/pests.
* De-toxify, neutralize, offset non-beneficial effects of, clear negative energy patterns in water pollution.
* Clear Energy Field and aura distortions/shock.
* Block, detoxify, minimize, clear non-beneficial infestations/infections.
* Detoxify, eliminate, clear non-beneficial/pathogenic fungi/molds.
* Detoxify, eliminate, clear non-beneficial/pathogenic bacteria.
* Block, detoxify, eliminate, clear viral pathogens and their crystalline patterns.
* Support, enhance appropriate/beneficial amounts/ratios/levels vitamins/minerals.
* Neutralize, detoxify, offset non-beneficial effects of, and clear all radiations.
* Balance appropriate/beneficial amounts/ratios/levels sodium / salt.
* Balance ratios/levels reduction/oxidation (25-28 norms).
* Balance ratios/levels water energy factor.
* Detoxify, offset non-beneficial effects of toxins/toxicities/toxoids/poisons.
* Use the Violet Flame of purification, Electric Blue Light protection, and Indigo spirals cloaking when needed.
* Send Love and Gratitude to all who assist in this work.

End of Program. Thank you'.   Remember to check the installation !

Construction of a Radionic 'Black Box'

You can make your own Radionic 'black box' with black construction paper, using a plastic notebook paper protector to hold everything together. Black paper always goes on the bottom of a paper broadcast - and sometimes on the top of the broadcast as well.

1. Place the geometric activator on the black paper - with note of Safety Program Controller.
2. Put your written broadcast command on the activator - the problem to be Healed or corrected.
3. Put the witness on top of the broadcast command.
* For a person, use hair, written signature, blood, saliva, nail, etc. and be sure to write their name, location if known, and birth date if known.

*   For an animal or plant, use a hair or a part of a leaf.

*   For an area, you can draw a sketch map

4.   Cover the whole thing with another piece of black paper.

If you wish to use manual switching instead of the automatic Safety Program Controller :

1.   Dowse to determine how long the broadcast should be kept on; then figure out the date the broadcast is to come off.

2.   On a piece of small paper write the name of the person receiving the broadcast and the date the broadcast is due to come off. You need some way to keep track of broadcast time so you can be there to take the broadcast off. Place the paper somewhere you can see it on or near that broadcast 'Black Box'.

3.   Check your OFF date, and if it is time, open the program and Dowse how long the program should rest OFF broadcast. Ask if it should go on again (it may not need to) and if so, how many days to wait before being activated again.

4.   For the OFF period - remove the broadcast and person's witness from the activator and store it behind the black paper/ activator.

5.   On a piece of small paper write the name of the person to return on the broadcast and the date to activate the broadcast again.

You can explore many different kinds of geometrics to use as activators.

Just remember to Dowse and check if the energies are appropriate, potent enough, and especially if they are congruent with the object/person of your Radionic broadcast.

Some things work better than others on different people or objects.

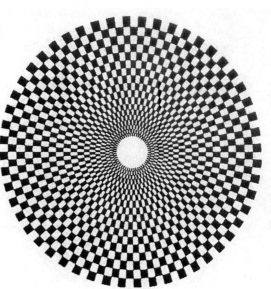

The Chakra Spiral - one of the most powerful symbols for both transmission and receiving signals.

Trees are the Earth's Endless Effort
To Speak with the Listening Heaven.

Rabindranath Tagore, 'FireFlies'.

Trees and Healing

It seems that in the order of creation trees and insects existed before birds and animals. Perhaps the Spirits in trees wanted to have experience of moving around, and asked the Holy Creator to let them have life forms to get such mobility.

If so, then it may be that Human Souls have had previous experience as trees, and other life forms such as fish - this may account for the auric formation of our legs, and the development through different stages during pregnancy.

It may be that the trees look upon us as their 'children' - and so are willing to help us. Perhaps we should give more respect and love to our 'ancestors' and care for them in a better way than we presently act - such as cutting down forests just for our own benefit.

Order in Nature

The wisdom of the ages has recognized elementals of various degrees, each having responsibility for an aspect of life in nature. There seems to be a hierarchy, where each level of life has a 'Leader' - an energy Being 'in command', a 'Head of Family', who guides and controls others in charge of their own group or family, as part of the larger whole..

I suggest that we consider a Deva to have responsibility for a piece of land - acting as the 'Land Lord', being 'in charge' of the plants, insects, and other life forms associated with the land.

There may be a hierarchy of Devas, with one in charge of a continent, down to Devas in charge of a garden and a home. A Tree Sprite seems to be the co-ordinator of a group of trees.

A plant grows from a seed (or cutting) which carries the DNA of its parent. When it sprouts it is becoming the vehicle for a Soul-type Being (perhaps not as advanced as the Soul in a human) to have experience. It has been noted that the auric pattern of a sprouting seed shows the final form of the plant.

The growing life form uses the DNA to get instructions from the Spirit of that specie (who has the blue-print) and grows accordingly.

The thought came into my mind that perhaps the 'Elves' and the 'Fairies' were involved - as the Yin and Yang elements of plant life.

This was followed by me being given a snatch of conversation to help clarify my understanding:

"I am a Fairy. I don't want him in here with all his muddy boots on", "I am an elf I been working in ground. I come here to give her love now" "I Fairy. I love him too. Him get clean. Him come in..."

The connotation here is that the elves are involved with the roots below, and the fairies the growth above. They need each other to have a successful life.

Energy Beings, Plants, and Nature Spirits

Nigel Percy, one of the top level Healing Dowsers from England, who now resides on Arizona, USA, kindly wrote this section.

It is widely acknowledged that we are energetic beings. There is energy within and around us. It is also true that we have many energies around us which are external to us. The term 'energies' is not one of my favourites, as it is far too loose a term to be accurate.

The first exercise I should like you to engage in is a brief exploration of those 'energies'. To do this you will need to take your Dowsing tool and decide what it is you wish to examine. Pets, unless they are asleep, tend to either look disdainfully at you or run away - Cats can be SO withering!

Plants and trees therefore are probably better subjects and, as we will be looking at those in more detail later, I would suggest starting with one of them.

I would not suggest using a rock or similar unless, of course, you are accustomed to working with them 'energetically'. If you do choose a rock, you will find some of the later exercises more difficult.

Locating a Plant's Energy Field

Next you need to program your mind (and, hence, your tool) to locate the energy field. In order to achieve this, you will need to concentrate upon the idea that you are searching for the outer edge of energy which is centred upon, or radiating from, the object.

In other words, you are not looking for energy coming into it from another source.

I am assuming that you are working on a medium-sized plant inside the house. Adjust distances accordingly. With your tool in search mode and starting from about five feet away, slowly move towards the plant. Note the distance at which you obtain a reaction. Note the strength of indication. Try coming at it again from a different direction and check the reaction-distance again.

Understanding Differences

Are they same or different ? Are there any obvious external indicators which might explain any differences, such as sickly leaves or something similar ?

Now you have obtained a first reaction, acknowledge to yourself that what you have found is the outer edge of the field surrounding the plant. This time start again and, when you obtain a reaction, re-set your tool and tell yourself that you are looking for the next edge of an energy field closer to the plant. You might obtain several, or you might obtain only the one.

Assuming you find more than one, is there anything you notice about them ? This could be in terms of strength of indication, or that they follow the original shape, or, even, deviate from the original shape.

Having investigated a little the shape and extent of the field, do one of the following with the plant:
* If it needs water or fertilizer, give it some.
* If it can be easily moved to a new location (sunnier/draughtier/ warmer/cooler etc), re-locate it.
* Send it some loving thoughts, tell it how beautiful it is, how much you admire it (and so on).

Now repeat the exercises above of finding the edges of energy fields and note what changes have taken place (if any).

Experimenting with Multiple Plants

For those of you with more than one plant, you may like to try the following:

Begin by Dowsing around one plant and note the shape and size of the field. Repeat this with another plant in a different location. Place them side by side.

Now Dowse again and see what differences you note in size and / or strength of the field of each. If you are able to, repeat this with another combination of plants.

You have looked at the shape and strength of energies around plants (some of you undoubtedly worked with trees and perhaps some of the more willful amongst us worked with a rock or stone of some kind). Whatever, I hope that you had some results and that you were able to repeat them and notice changes and differences of various kinds.

Leaves and Blooms have their Own Energy Fields

Now we will concentrate upon another area of natural energies which may be new to you. It may also be an area which you feel comfortable within, or it maybe has an outlook which does not fit well within your world view. If the latter is the case, I apologize and hope that you will, nevertheless, gain something from it.

If we can assume that there is 'energy' around us and that it can be detected by Dowsing, it seems reasonable to assume further that there is something which is responsible for that energy.

Or, at least, that it is responsible for the way we interpret that energy. By that, I mean that the shape and characteristics of the plant you worked on in the last lesson was the result of the energy within, or 'coming through', or from that plant.

Let us begin by looking in a little more detail at the plant before we explore that idea further.

Taking your tool, approach the plant again, but with the intent this time of looking at the energy around a leaf or even a bloom. It is probable that you will have to approach more closely this time before you obtain a reaction.

As before, note the distance and the strength of the indication. If you are working with a leaf, try approaching it from the edge as well as from the top and bottom.

Note again any differences.

You should now realize that you can look for the energy of the plant as a whole or for the energy of each individual aspect of the plant.

I am not too sure that I would like to lean too heavily upon logic in the field of Dowsing, but I think it is fair to say that such a distinction could easily lead one to think that if the plant's main field consists of or contains other, smaller energy fields within it, there is nothing wrong with the idea that those smaller fields should also contain even smaller fields.

Such fields, because of their size, may be difficult to find by Dowsing, but there can be some assessment of, or contact with, them.

These smaller fields would, it is safe to say, be responsible for co-ordinating the energy of the lesser structures of the plant, such as the cells within leaves or the stem etc.. In Dowsing these aspects, you are reliant less upon tools than upon what moves them - your own Intuition.

The Elements and their Beings

There were considered to be 4 major elements around us in the Western tradition - 5 in the Eastern. These were earth, air, fire and water - with metal the additional Eastern one. Each of these was responsible, either individually or in combination with one or more of the others, for everything in the physical world.

Such views became placed in a more formalized belief system where each element had its own personal characteristic, so that the gnomes, elves, pixies, etc. were considered the personification of the earth; sylphs of the air; undines of the water; and salamanders of fire. Dwarfs have been associated with metal.

I understand that Elves are concerned with taking nutrients to the Fairies who look after plants, and that Gnomes are 'in charge' of joints, organs, and brains in the animal, etc., kingdom. John Living.

In time, these views were called pagan, which only really revealed their origin ('pagan' meaning 'of the country'), but which gradually took on a pejorative or condescending tone. Nevertheless, whether or not the physical world is caused by the combining of these elements, they, or something very much like them, are still to be sensed today.

Now try to sense these small, sub-units of energies. Because they are small, you may find that you will not be able to sense them in quite the same way, or with the same precision, as if you were sensing the plant itself.

For this you will need some soil (presumably from the plant container, although any will do), some water, and a candle (or flame of some kind).

To begin with, you will need to try to relax your mind in whatever way works best for you. You are going to let your conscious, logical mind free - and listen instead to the intuitive part of yourself.

Once relaxed, let yourself become aware of the soil. By that I mean let your focus of intent be the soil, without expectation or concern for the result. You might want to pick it up, dribble it through your fingers, sniff it, or whatever. But interact with it in some fashion. As you do so, let yourself be open to any images, sensations, feelings, sounds or such like impressions. Make a note of them when you have finished.

Take your time doing this, but don't re-run it to try to get 'better' results. The results you get are the ones you get, neither good or bad.

Repeat the procedure with each of the other elements.

* For water, let your fingers dangle in it, really feel it on your skin.
* For fire, watch the flame not just to see the colours, but to try and 'see' inside it, feel for what makes it special.
* For air, either waft a large feather before you, burn incense and watch the smoke, or simply listen to what is happening around you - if appropriate.

You may want (or be forced) to do these exercises over a period of time, rather than one after the other.

Feeling is your Critical Sense

Whatever you have written or drawn after each session is your own impression of the element you were interacting with. Each person will be different, although there may be similarities in some areas. Look at what you have intuited and see how this sits with you and what you feel or know about the elements.

Don't be too logical, but see if it leads you to any insights. Again, in 'feeling' your way around the results, let the logical brain sit it out and only let it in when you have finished.

Intuit your way around. You are, after all, revealing to yourself (maybe for the first time), how you actually feel about these things - and I do mean FEEL !

Be aware that there are no right answers or results. There are only your results.

Understanding Elemental Relationships

"How can fire be associated with the plant in front of you ?" Well, the stimulating element of fire can be found most successfully in buds or in any rapidly growing part where change and transformation are taking place at a good pace. A good time to look for this element is in the Spring when there are buds.

By now, you will have varying impressions of what is termed 'energy' around and within your plant. Those energies will be entirely as you perceive them. They are your sensations, your mental constructs - but that does not make them any the less meaningful.

Perhaps you may wish to Dowse your plant again, this time with your perceptions of 'energy' also present in your mind.

By this I mean that, instead of just Dowsing to find the edge of the plant's field, you are now Dowsing to identify (or simply become aware of in some internal fashion) the dominant element(s) within it, as well as how far out it extends and how clearly it is sensed.

Those of you who have been thinking ahead can see where this might lead. For those who haven't, I'll lay out the steps as follows.

If we have found energy emanating from or present in the plant, detectable through Dowsing as an 'edge' or 'boundary', and we have found smaller units of energy around leaves and other parts of the plant, the natural question which is raised by that is *"How are all those 'energies' co-ordinated in such a way as to work harmoniously ?"*

Put another way we could ask, *"Why is the plant the way it is ?"*, *"Why has it grown in this fashion ?"* - DNA certainly has a role to play in living things, but it does not go anywhere towards explaining what you have just Dowsed.

Your Dowsing could well be explained by the assumption of the presence of a controlling blueprint. Something which acts as a co-ordinator or 'boss' and which regulates everything, but is not actually engaged in the building itself.

The Controlling Energy can be 'contacted' or 'intuited', and can be Dowsed for directly, in that you can direct questions to it.

It is sometimes thought that, if you Dowse a plant to find out its needs in terms of water, fertilizer, location and so on, you are really contacting the Controlling Energy - or 'Head of Family' of the plant.

Let us assume that you have indeed Dowsed for such things mentioned in the previous paragraph.

Working with the Energies of a Plant

That does not necessarily bring you any nearer to understanding the plant's system. So what I would like to attempt is an experiment at contacting the plant in another way.

Put your tool to one side as you will be using your intuitive sense fully this time. Relax your mind in the manner most appropriate to you and allow your focus of attention to drift towards the plant. You are going to look at it with relaxed eyes or with your 'third eye'. Let your awareness reach out to it without any expectation.

You already know through your Dowsing that the plant has a field of energy around it and that it has other energetic movements inside that. You are 'looking' for the controlling energy.

It might present itself to you in various ways. It could be as a small glittering cloud hovering over or to one side of the plant. It could be as just a face or just eyes. It could be felt only as a presence in some fashion.

Whatever way it finds to present itself to you is the way you will perceive it. I am assuming that it wants to present itself and that you are able to relax enough to receive the perceptions. Remember, it may take a few tries before you 'get' something.

The interesting point about the Controlling Energies and their role is that, if there is an entity in charge of one plant, there's also one for each plant. Logically speaking, there is no reason why there cannot or should not be one for every thing we see.

Anything where 'energy' exists and is in need of controlling - from a plant to a valley, from an ant's nest to a lake or a building; each will have its own Controlling Energy.

Dowsing with tools can enable contact with them as can this relaxed state of mind. However, it is interesting to note that many of the creatures which populate fairy tales (elves, fairies, dwarves, and so on) are also ways in which the 'energies' of the world around us were able to be depicted.

They are energies, and they can interact with our energy in ways which is easiest for us to perceive them.

Thus, for someone who is afraid of spiders, contacting the Spirit of a spider may bring a large and terrifying image of a spider - as that is the way your mind would find it easiest to perceive it.

'Talking' to the Trees

If you would like some practice at this I would strongly suggest going out to a tree or large plant.

Dowse or 'feel' in some way whether it is friendly to you, open to communication - everyone has 'off days' and wants to be left alone ! If it is, relax and drift 'into it' with your awareness. Maybe, out of the corner of your eye, you might just notice a brown-skinned face grinning at you or you might glimpse a movement in the branches. Thank it.

If you want to show respect for it by exchanging some of your energy with it, leave a bit of you on it. A little saliva will do instead of blood or skin. It will tell the tree that you are donating something of yourself for it to keep. It will recognize you in the future.

Why bother contacting these energies ? The answer is simple. If they are the controlling forces of the world around us, it seems foolish or plain stupid to ignore them. We should, wherever possible, learn to live with them. It should be a co-creative environment.

Respecting Other Life Forms

So, next time you find yourself with ants in the house, instead of stamping on them and getting even, try to contact their controlling energy and explain that it is your territory and that there must be a way you can exist side by side.

Offer solutions, offer food dumps outside, offer whatever seems realistic and achievable, but listen for the answer. It might not be a simple answer. It might involve different steps. But it's worth at least trying to find out how you can live together - rather than automatically assuming that you have the right to attack that which annoys you.

We have had a very successful relationship with spiders in our household since the day we built this house. I declared to all my family that no bugs would be killed in the house.

We would capture and release them outside. The spiders could stay if they did us no harm and I gave them the job of policing the house to keep other bugs out. This has worked like a charm for 15 years.

As a final experiment, go back to the plant you began with and, this time, instead of Dowsing its 'energy field', ask it directly what it will need for optimum growth. In order to do this, you might want to draw up a list of possibilities including water, locations, people, fertilizers and so on which you can refer to. Always remember to have space for OTHER on the list as you can never cover all the bases. *Many Thanks to Nigel for his wisdom*

Trees Heal *by Barbara Janelle*

An amazing experience came during the first session of my Level 2 Therapeutic Touch class last week. Instead of doing the usual meditation and work in pairs, I sent people outdoors to learn about the use of energy from trees.

The instructions were for each one to find a tree that called, go to it and invite its work. The steps are:

1. Sense the energetic difference as you walk toward the tree.
2. Then stand facing the tree and place both hands on the trunk. Hold that position until the tree tells you to move.
3. Next, turn and stand with your spine in contact with the tree. Hold that position-until the tree tells you move.

One woman had come to class with a pain in her neck and shoulders that had hung on during the day. When the tree finished with her, the pain was completely gone; her face was brighter and she was very relaxed.

Another, unable, to see her chiropractor for a few weeks, described the tree doing an adjustment on her neck with a gentle crack. She too looked very different afterwards. Another felt a major change in her chest - a clearing of congestion. Everyone felt very deeply grounded.

And I had been coping with a digestive upset for several days that left me with terrible acid indigestion after I ate anything. As I stood against the tree, I felt a very quick rise in energy through my feet up into my stomach, a sudden twisting action there, and then a sense of draining down through the legs into the ground. It was all over in less than two minutes.

I waited a while and then ate something and lo and behold, no indigestion. I've continued to add different foods over the past several days, and I feel fine ! Wow !

I found that communication with animals during TT treatments quickly led to communication with trees and plants, rocks, rivers and lakes and to the Earth herself. Everything has consciousness. Everything has knowing. TT leads to a different understanding of the world.

Over the years, I have combined exercises learned from Merlin Homer (energetic abilities of trees and plants) and Linda Tellington-Jones (communication with trees) with my own experiences.

Now, I teach the following:

1. Notice what you feel as you move toward and away from a mature tree.
2. Scan the ground with your hands as you move toward and away from a mature tree.
3. Scan the trunk of the tree - notice how the north and south sides feel, and the field over scars and healthy bark.
4. Ask the tree to scan you - notice how this feels.
5. Put your back against the tree and ask the tree to work on you. Trees are very powerful and effective energy workers. How do you know when this is finished ?
6. Ask the tree a question and pay attention to the thoughts, images, sounds, etc. that come into your mind. The question may be as simple as, "Tell me something I need to know".
7. Thank the tree for the experience.

This can be done with other kinds of vegetation too.

Barbara Janelle's website: www.barbarajanelle.com/kktt/A09-Trees_Heal.htm

Group Interaction with Trees

John Gibbons suggests the following procedure:

<u>First</u> go out with two or three friends and find a likely looking tree. The tree should be big and strong, sometimes called a 'grandparent' tree of the area, fairly imposing in stature.

It is always wise to do this with other people as it helps to share the technique with other people.

The other people can help and give focus if one person is a bit off colour. Using three people or more helps build some consensus and reality into the method, and encourages support and feedback.

Second - stand some distance away and then approach the tree with kindness and reverence. This tree will be asked to assist in the healing and so it is best to keep on its good side ! Respect for all living things is vital; along with compassion for all sentient beings, like the tree.

Third - when you stand under the canopy, pause and form a circle around the tree. You can stand with you hands outstretched at your sides, and then feel for the rings of energy that surround the tree as you slowly take a few steps towards the tree trunk. Feel for that circular ring of chi !

Fourth - standing under the tree feel whether the energy is spinning clockwise or anti-clockwise. It may take a few minutes to begin to make out the fine detail of the energy and feel which way it flows. Does it flow around to the left or the right ? Clockwise or anti-clockwise ? You should get some consensus in the group.

Fifth - enhance the spin by adding energy of your own. This is like the acupuncturist who grasps the needle and twists slightly as they insert and jiggle it to get the chi flowing through the body. The same thing happens with the earth. Boosting the spin like this helps the chi build and flow.

Boost the flow for about 5 minutes and stabilize the pattern. The three of you should sense the chi over-flowing and spilling along the straight ley-lines and out across the landscape.

Sixth - Diagnose. Check the meridian that needs a little healing and encouragement. That will tell you which quarter of the circle to stand in. You can Dowse, or consult your Feng Shui notes and see which direction of the compass needed a shift and a change of energy. You could sit down and the three of you chat and decide on some different direction altogether.

By some method make a decision and decide on the direction. Then you have two co-ordinates: the distance from the tree (chosen in Step Three), and the direction from the tree.

Right ? You know the distance and direction. That should give you the optimum spot for that precise dis-ease.

<u>Seventh</u> Meditate. Circulate the energy and let the energy flow through the tree and then through the person, washing and showering their aura. The tree acts like a pump or a battery, assisting the flow.

The focus and precision of the technique lies in picking the right direction. You can call energy up from the roots and down from the canopy and use the energy to assist in healing that particular meridian and the related parts of your life and body.

Again, people from different traditions will find different ways of activating the meridians in the body. Some will use the techniques from Tai-ji, some from Shiatsu, some from Chi Gung, others will use rattle and drum, others again will use yoga-postures and breathing.

The tradition that people come from gives clues to the best ways of healing them. In the preliminary discussions amongst those present, all this can be sorted out. At this stage in the process, the important thing is for the energies to be assisted to do their work.

Perhaps it is the land that needs healing ? You can then use this to focus your chi and push healing energy back down into the ley-line and re-power the grid ! Like switching on the light, but for the countryside rather than the lounge-room.

<u>Eighth</u> When the three of you feel that this is enough, stop. Go and hug the tree and give a really good squeeze for thanks. Thank it for its help. Thank each other and have a break if you choose, comparing notes, or having some refreshment.

<u>Ninth</u> As you depart from this place, once past the canopy and at some distance from the tree, turn one final time and say farewell ! The tree will be more happy to see you again some other day.

A Quick Summary
1. Take two friends and find a likely looking tree.
2. Approach the tree with kindness and reverence.
3. Feel for the rings of energy flowing around the tree.
4. Feel for a clockwise or anti-clockwise spin.
5. Add to the spin until you feel the radial energy has become like spokes from the tree.
6. With the direction and the distance from the tree, taken into consideration find the ideal spot for healing.
7. Circulate the chi through the person being healed.
8. When finished, stop. Then pause and thank the tree and thank each other.
9. As you depart, wave farewell! You may find yourself healing with the tree again some time.

So that's it. Simple. Nine steps for getting the energy to heal you.

Dowsing the Energy of Trees

Steve Herbert tells that the Front Door is really where trees breathe in Ch'i (life) energy. The back door is where they exhale the same. Most interestingly, when you check different trees for this, you will find they are taking in energy from trails, streets, sidewalks, where people walk. It doesn't matter what direction it is, towards the rising Sun or not, for example. They like people.

You will find other interesting things. In the city, where trees roots are cut by sidewalks, for example, and they are weakened by the pollution of cars, industry, etc., they are taking in Ch'I energy, not exhaling it. Perhaps they need all they can get to survive - this same phenomenon can be found in quite old trees.

When people stand on the exhale side, the Ch'i energy does not continue past their body. They seem to be absorbing it. We can help trees, and they can help us, especially in regard to diseases of either.

Working with a Tree

1) Connect with the tree to ask permission to approach. You do not need to be in close proximity - the entire procedure can be done from 1500 feet away, from inside a building.

2) Walk slowly towards the tree (with an L-rod for example, or no tool). You are asking to feel the aura of the tree. The L-rod will turn 90 degrees when the border of the aura is felt.

3) At the perimeter of the sensed aura, walk around the tree. When you encounter the 'breathing in' place, the L-rod will turn in towards the tree trunk - you will feel a sensation of being drawn in. The palm of your hand is especially sensitive to this.

4) Keep walking around. You will find the 'breathing out' place, usually (but not always) on the opposite side of the tree trunk. The L-rod will turn out 90 degrees (straight out) from the tree trunk at that place.

You will feel a pushing out, breathing out, of life force (Ch'i energy) at that place.

If you are tired, you may ask the tree if it is OK for you to share the excess Ch'i energy. Stand with your back against the tree at that place. You will find it is energizing.

If you are ill, and need extra energy, then that is the part of your body that can benefit from contact with the tree there.

If you are very ill with a disease that is not going away, you may ask permission to give the disease to the universe through the tree (but not to the tree or any being). The disease may be taken from you and transmuted harmlessly to the universe through the tree's breathing in point. It is important not to have intent to give the disease to another.

Tree Communities

Where there are a group of trees, you will find the 'breathing in' place from the centre of the cluster of shared tree trunks.

They are breathing in from each other, and exhaling outwards.

There is a vast difference in young trees and old trees, with regard to their aura. Very old trees that are healthy have very powerful healing auras. Young trees can have weak auras. There are big differences in different individuals, regardless of species. This is a whole topic. There are big differences in species.

Of course, they have a different vibration than small animals or bugs. So, it will take some time to attune to them. But I am sure you will attune to them, and they will attune to you. Patience, and fortitude will see you through.

French Coil - Pest Control   *by Marcel Triau*

Of all the systems of insect control in use today, the majority are artificial. Nature is very precariously balanced and any tampering can bring about disastrous results - as evidenced by indiscriminate use of insecticides and upsetting the prey-predator ratio.

For the past 18 years I have used and researched a safe and simple system of pest control which takes advantage of some little known and little understood laws of nature.

Because we cannot scientifically define and analyze these laws many people disbelieve them. However, nature is full of mystery and even the working of our own bodies is not fully understood.

This particular system is called the 'French Coil' because it originated in France in the 1930's and consists of a coil of wire.

The equipment needed is a long piece of copper wire (# 10 for small trees, # 8 for larger trees), sticks for support, rubber for insulation, and of course, an infested tree.

One end of the wire is buried in the earth at the base of the tree to provide a ground and prevent short circuits.

The wire is then coiled around the tree trunk several items with the free end left pointing into the air - to act as an antenna.

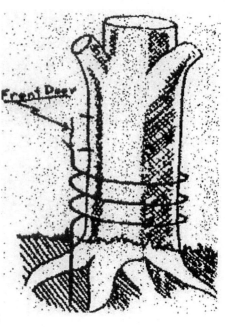

The coil can be held in position by wooden stakes with insulation to prevent grounding the wire to the stakes.

Perhaps the minute amounts of electricity in the air flows into the wire and the tree and creates a magnetic field around the tree, giving the tree more health and strength and weakening the pests resulting in their destruction.

You should install the French Coil before the sap starts to run.

A Tree has a 'front door' - a certain place on the trunk, about 6 to 18 inches long, where this energy enters the tree. It usually faces northwest but varies slightly from tree to tree.

On the opposite side of the trunk is the 'back door' which acts as a safety valve allowing the release of electricity should the tree become overcharged.

The 'front door' demonstrates its affinity for electricity following the path of an electrical storm; it returns to its original position when the storm is over.

French coils should not touch the tree but must be like an inch to maybe six inches away depending on where the support poles must be to miss the roots; the farther away, the bigger gauge wire needed.

Ask the tree where to put them if needed. The coils might be an inch apart and held around the tree by three or four stakes, metal or wooden makes no difference as they must be insulated from touching the copper wire to keep the signal from being grounded.

The bottom might be about a six inch straight run vertically pointed at the tree about an inch away starting near the top of the front door. The tree will say how many coils and how far apart. The top would terminate in a length and direction specified by the tree. The support stakes might be insulated with a complete wrapping of electrical tape, at worst, or might be covered with a length with neoprene pipe wrap sheath, at best.

Ask the tree if it will help, first, of course - and how long it will remain in place. If it was temporary, like in the months range, you might consider putting the four insulating pieces right against the tree instead, to be lightly held in place there by the coil. If longer, it seems like that apparatus might bind on the growth of the trunk.

The King of All Plants Offers His Help !

Some years ago I gave an Intuition Technology workshop to Healers in Hazelton, BC, sponsored by the Gitksan Residential School Healing Committee.

On the last day, before going to the workshop, I had a message from a Being calling himself the 'King of All Flowers' that explained how we could use the 'Power of Flowers' in a new way - it was so exciting that I missed my breakfast !

He said that the Red People call on the help of Animal Spirits to help with Healing and other matters, and that the 'Flower Sprites' could offer similar help if asked !

I tried this with imagining that I planted 'Holy Broccoli Seeds' on my leg, where I had been experiencing a pain in the hip joint and muscles.

I put them at about 1 inch spacing, and visualized them putting roots down into all my tissues that sucked up all the 'stuff causing hurts', took these into the roots and up to the plants, where they were transformed into good, blossoming into buds and little yellow flowers that radiated the now good energy into the void for use by others.

I then 'felt' that a violet flame burnt out these roots after they had extracted the 'hurts', and that 'True Holy Love' was sent in to replace the roots and help Heal my tissues. My leg did feel better!

The King of All Flowers also suggested that a Dandelion seed, planted in your Third Eye, sends down deep roots that take all the 'bad' from your organs in a similar way, and that the 'Powder Puff' seedlings then will float away into your Aura, collecting 'things that are not good' and taking them to be Healed.

While writing this, other plants have been recommended by the King of All Plants. You can visualize a shield of Blackberry bushes around you which act to bar the entry of 'not good' energies into your Auras. I understand that the Angels and other Good Energies like to eat the berries!

Further help comes from the Thistle - planting a Thistle in your Third Eye will help reduce any high blood pressure. And if you plant a Holly tree in your Third Eye it will help to clear your arteries of cholesterol.

I understand that the Oak tree will give strength, and the Willow helps in manifesting Good Outcomes such as getting a desired happening. Try these - and you may get other cures in meditation.

Growing an Early Crop

A booklet called 'Solar Energy + Dowsing' tells the story of how farmers discovered a way of producing early flowering narcissus for the market before the advent of greenhouses.

By forming a pentagon shape using 5 sticks, bricks or other markers and walking round the perimeter with a Dowsing rod, ensuring that you overlap the start point, the ground inside the pentagon will become warmer than the surrounding area - thus giving the plants a head start in the growing season.

Further on in the booklet, it refers to creating five pentagons around a house or garden to create a warming effect which is supposed to save on heating bills. Note that anything metal pushed into the pentagon area may diminish the warming effect.

This is something that anyone with a small lawn could try out and on frosty mornings - it could be that the area inside the pentagon is frost free, and this would be easily visible.

"More Drugs, More Drugs !" - not any Pause
Real Healers Seek to Heal the Cause

Healing Overview

The Keys to Healing are Compassion and Love

Any attempt to do Healing with anger, annoyance, or intent to harm those involved in the problems will have a relatively low chance of success. Remember that it may not be the right time, time may be needed for Healing to be effective, and they may need repeating.

Going back to basics, each and every life form is comprised of Lights, baby energies, and their families and teams; they do different dances at different speeds to form 'All That Is' - including ourselves, and all the problems that we encounter. They are all part of our 'Great Family', part of creation, our brothers and sisters !

The universe has been described as being 'Holographic' - where 'All That Is' is in each and every part; this implies that we hold within each part of us a key to the total universe, to 'All That Is'. By accepting this, we can Heal any part that has been hurt or damaged.

Many mystical disciplines tell how we can reduce our Beingness to an infinitely small size - and so reduce the total universe and bring it (or any part of it) within ourselves for Healing.

The 'metamorphic field', 'standing wave', and 'implicate order' analogies describe how our thoughts and actions have an effect (to some extent) on all creation, that 'how we perceive' becomes 'how it is'.

Life is Love

All life is based on Love - the real 'God Energy' that gives life in all forms. All Lights, baby energies, their families and teams are created with Love. Their whole Beingness is to express Love. This 'Love' is best defined as 'True Holy Love, Namaste'.

If any life form acts in a way different from Love, it is because they have been hurt in some way - by being given a 'bad job' (which they dislike, but may have accepted due to fear for themselves or their families), by having 'not good' commanders in charge of their higher level Beingness, or have been forced to so act by constraints placed in or on them.

In some cases this seems to be due to a communication problem - resulting in the reversal of the meaning of a 'good order' and so causing harm instead.

The actual reason does not matter so much as the need to Heal 'All Involved' - when the root causes are Healed, Healing follows at all levels of Beingness. So it is best to start by Healing the Lights, baby energies, their families and teams.

This may best be accomplished by having compassion for them, expressing sorrow at the way that they themselves have suffered, sending them your Love to help them to be Healed, freeing them from constraints and 'bad management', getting the help of the Angelic Beings to help in this work, and sending your Love, Thanks, and Gratitude to all who so help in this work.

Why do we Suffer ?

'We are All the Same' - so why do we suffer in various ways ? In some cases it may be harm that we have caused others reflected back to us - perhaps in a different form. None of us is perfect !

This may be part of 'Lesson Learning' during our incarnation as human beings. So we may have contributed to some extend to our own problems.

This is not to blame ourselves for all our hurts, although some may be due to our failure to care for ourselves - sometimes due to our lack of awareness that causes of certain problems even exist, such as germs (unknown in times gone by) and noxious earth energies (of which most English speaking people are completely ignorant).

Viral and bacterial attacks usually occur when we are already weakened in some way; this may be nature's method of improving life stock - survival of the fittest.

These viruses and other germs are life forms, too - and should be respected as Beings in their own right. Strange, but true !

We can dialogue with them, and persuade them to help reduce their noxious effects on our bodies. This works well to overcome colds and influenza.

Other factors may be involved - such as being in the wrong place at the wrong time, control by our family and associates, greed and envy of others, and malicious attacks.

We may even be invaded by now deceased human life forms, or parts of them. This includes relatives and friends who come for various reasons (some with good intent but unwanted side effects), lost souls seeking a good home but so interfering with our own Beingness, and earth-bound Souls (or parts) seeking the pleasures of sex, drugs, and even crime.

Earth-bound Souls and perhaps Soul types from other places may even try to possess us - and in some cases, they succeed !

The most common causes, however, are ones which we create - having anger at a distant person or group seldom affects them to any large extent - but has a great effect on ourselves ! Most Heart and liver problems seem to be related to anger in some way.

Thought Forms

There are many reports of forms of different shapes, sizes, and colours being seen in auras - and that special meanings are found to be consistent to forms of any particular shape, size, and colour.

Anger is seen as a dark red, jagged, lightning flash shape; Love usually is pinkish, often associated with a grass-green Heart colour, rather more diffused than having a particular shape. The size can indicate the intensity, and the location the area of the body affected.

Beliefs are so accumulated in thought forms, which then act as filters to how thoughts occur - how any situation is considered, and the resulting action chosen. These have been built since the time that we were babies - holding things that we were told or our understandings of our experiences.

This includes beliefs that may have been appropriate when we were small (for our own safety) but are no longer valid; mis-understood analyses of situations in which we found ourselves; and things that we were told for control purposes (family, community, religion) which may not be correct, although sometimes believed to be true by those who so told them.

Thoughts originating in other people are always being sent to us - with or without intent, consciously or unconsciously. If these are strong in themselves, or combine together to get such strength, then they may form Thought Forms that stay with us. They may join with existing Thought Forms (from all sources) to increase their combined strength.

We do not have to see these forms to make changes - but we must recognize that they, themselves, are life forms ! We must show respect and ask help - not use an aggressive approach or force changes, since this will cause them to 'clam up' and increase resistance to change.

Each thought form has been formed, by energy obtained from the sender or 'The Void', with the belief that it has a good job to do - and it has done its best to so act.

We can dialogue with a Thought Form:

- Think of the source of a particular thought (or range of thoughts).
- Send Love and ask to be told the job of the Thought Form; you may enquire its source, to better understand the motive and context involved.
- Send it your gratitude and Love for the work done by the Thought Form - even if hurtful or otherwise unwanted !
- Explain that the job is no longer needed, is not now in your best interest.
- Ask the Thought Form if it would like a better job - usually YES.
- Suggest a job similar in context to that which had been given, but is beneficial, and ask if this would be acceptable to the Thought Form. If not, suggest another.
- When an acceptable job is found, ask if any other Thought Form is now doing such a job.
- If so, ask if it would accept extra help from a friend - usually YES.
- If so, ask if they would now work together in Love for your 'Highest and Best Good' - usually YES.
- If so, thank them and send them your Love.

It is rare for this procedure not to work ! Healing these Thought Forms and enabling them to have a good task is beneficial to them.

Just 'getting rid' of them leaves them with pain within themselves - I hear them tell me that when sent 'into the void' they cry at the damage they have unwittingly caused. They are Life Forms, like us, and we should do our best to help them be Healed.

I have been suffering from a moving pain in by left hip and thigh, and tried many ways to be free of this pain. When I wrote the above, I took a break - and had a wonderful experience.

I suddenly saw in my mind's eye, and with my eyes open (rare in any case for me !), an upright red streak, bent at the middle about 20° to the right, that opened dialogue with me ! It told me that it was a thought form that was in my hip and leg, formed by me.

My mother had been paralysed on her left side before my birth, and perhaps in sympathy I felt that this could happen to me too.

I thanked the thought form for its work and Love, and it told me that it would now dissipate - it changed colour to pinkish white, and then disappeared. I understand that its friends and associates left as well, to get good jobs.

This will be ignored by scientists, of course, since there is not any scientific proof, only my subjective statement. But that is good enough for me !

When the work is finished, if a thought or a Thought Form is not important it seems that it disintegrates and its energy goes back into the void; if important, it goes into the owner's Akashic record.

Affliction of Healers

A possible explanation why some Healers are so afflicted maybe to the way that they do Healing ! If they attack the life forms that are causing problems to others, they may attract attacks on themselves.

Compassion is needed not just for the people that go to Healers, but also for the life forms that are causing the problems !

Healers need to be grounded and protected (see the next chapter) - but even this is not enough. Great compassion is needed.

It is not generally realized that Healers are seen in planes above the physical as 'Beings of Light' - and so attract life forms, including lost or injured Souls, who want to be Healed and come seeking assistance.

Often their effect on the Beingness of the Healer is felt as being 'not good' - so they are judged as 'bad energy' and sent 'to the ends of the universe, not ever to interfere with humans again'. This is like going to a doctor and being told *"F... Off !"*

Yet it is so simple to help them - just ask Angelic Beings to come to them, and take them to be Healed and be again with their families, friends, those that they Love.

Then send them your Love, your gratitude for being given the honour of helping them, and good wishes for their future life.

Identification of Causes

A clairvoyant Healer may see the cause of a problem in the aura of the Healee; Dowsing with a Pendulum can assist the Healer to focus on a particular problem; using hypnosis or just sending Love to the 'Total Being' of the Healee can help the Healee identify the problem and its cause.

The more knowledge and understanding that the Healer has about the 'Total Being' of a person in general, the better the context in which causes can be identified and assistance given.

The use of Dowsing Charts is a great help - possible systems of causes are shown, with guidance to the next level until the real cause is determined.

Accomplished Dowsers are better able to do this on themselves than most other people - but there is a problem. Sometimes the cause is very deep, hidden or camouflaged, protected by the sub-conscious or other influential levels. The Dowser is, unknowingly, in self-denial.

This also applies to the questioning concerning the effectiveness of Healing - especially when there is a great desire to be Healed, and that desire is shown as the result, which is not happening or has only happened to a lesser degree.

This is where assistance from another Dowser/Healer is required - the obscuring mechanism can fool the Dowser/Healee, but in most cases cannot so fool the other Dowser/Healer.

Having identified the cause, the Healee must release it in some way. This can be a real problem if anger is concerned, especially when broken relationships are involved.

How Healing Works

Essentially it needs the Healee (the person being Healed) to Heal themselves. The Healer acts as a facilitator to help this happen - in identification of the causes of problems, in giving advice as to corrective action, and as a conduit for help from the 'God Level' by Angelic Beings.

Remember that the resources of the 'God Level' are assigned by 'The System' - so it is best to ask the help of 'The System' rather than any particular Deity - who may not have responsibility or power in the needed aspects.

I understand that a 'Love Namaste Healing Team' has been formed, which combines the skills, knowledge, and experience of Souls who have been Healers and otherwise engaged in Health matters with that of the various degrees of Angelic Beings - and that 'The System' may use this team, under the leadership of an Angel, for Healing as needed.

A Healer who uses his/her own energy or life force depletes it, leading to problems arising in the Healer; this also happens if the Healer 'takes on' the problems of patients.

There are things that we cannot do ourselves, and similarly the Angelic Beings may have limitations on their abilities. When we work together as a team, all things are possible.

It seems that the Angelic Beings have been restricted in their activities - not permitted to intercede or help unless so requested; and even in giving this help, it is more readily given when requested for another person, not oneself.

A procedure that works is:

- Open in True Holy Love, Namaste (THLN).
- Explain the intent of Healing - who, why, what, when.
- Ask the Angelic Beings if they are willing and able to help in this instance. If declined, just send THLN to the Healee. Otherwise:
- Stand one space back from the Healee and hold out your hands, palms uppermost, to receive the energy of the Angelic Beings.
- When you feel this has been loaded into you, step forward into the space where the Angelic Being energy was sent.

Should the Healee not be present, you can imagine their presence, or designate a Doll (for females) or a Teddy Bear (for males) to represent them - that is how I work in distant Healing. Make sure that the identity is correct, telling their name (and maiden name), place and date of birth, current address, or as much such information as you have available - a witness such as handwriting, hair, or a photograph is ideal for verification.

You are now acting as a conduit for that energy to be used in the Healing. The Angelic Beings will work through you to help the Healee be Healed, including to guide you intuitively as to any action you should take or speech that you should give.

In all Healing that you do, avoid 'diagnosis' - since some laws consider this to be the personal domain of physicians, not God.

You can say *"My Intuitive understanding is that [problem cause] needs to be Healed for your better health"*. Do not tell them *"You have cancer"* or *"You only have X months to live"* - this could cause it, and certainly cause worry; and you may be wrong, as are many physicians !

You can suggest that they ask a specialist for further examination, and certainly ask extra help for them from the Angelic Beings.

In this same context, never promise a full Healing - the Healee has a duty to help him/her-self, and if this is not done, problems will probably remain.

In cases of extreme suffering and terminal disease, the Angelic Healing may included suppression of pain and an advance in termination - if the Angelic Beings decide that this is best.

Charges for Healing

A Healer is entitled to charge for time (family to feed, clothe, and educate) and facilities used (travel, office, staff, advertisements, etc) but it is best not to charge for the Healing itself - that is the gift of 'Upstairs' via the Angelic Beings.

Such charges should not be excessive - if greed is involved, the help by the Angelic Beings may cease. And perhaps the charges to those who are wealthy can be used to cover Healing given to the unfortunate poor.

Changes due to Possession

An interesting situation has been reported in some cases of possession. Perhaps three possessing entities are observed - and each one has distinctive speech, habits, and health problems.

When a change of possessing entity occurs, the change in speech, habits - and health problems - is almost instantaneous.
- Entity A has a Heart problem - no sign of cancer or arthritis.
- Entity B has cancer - no sign of any Heart problem or arthritis.
- Entity C has arthritis, no sign of cancer or any Heart problem.

This seems to indicate that any health problem can be cured instantaneously, and that it may be associated with a 'higher level of Beingness' - or with the Thought Forms belonging to that entity that displace those previously in occupation.

Perhaps understanding the modality of change will lead to future Healing methods to give perfect good health to most people !

Grounding, Protection, and Clearing

Now we look at ways to work with the Energies of Creation without hurting ourselves - or others. Grounding lets unwanted Energies pass through us to Mother Earth. Protection is to prevent Energies that are noxious to us from having an impact on our Being. Clearing is helping Energies that have been misplaced and given 'not good' tasks to be Healed and sent to their rightful place.

Grounding

By Grounding we enable unwanted energies to pass through us and into other realms like Heaven and Earth, Above and Below, so they can be Healed in the way that is the 'Highest and Best for All Creation', similar to the way a stray electrical current is grounded - so that it can find its way home without hurting a person who touches an electrical appliance.

We do not have to walk around trailing a wire - and such a wire would be useless, because we are dealing with Energies, not physical electric currents. Our 'grounding' is achieved by imagining a cord, or a beam of light, which comes from above and connects us to below - bringing in the 'good' from Heaven and carrying the 'not good' to Earth, where it can be recycled to become 'good'.

Some people are very sensitive to others, being empathic; most of us are empathic to some degree, even if we are not so aware. People sense problems that are troubling others, and draw these into themselves. This is beneficial to others, but harms you.

By grounding, the empathetically attracted energies involved in the problem are carried away, and do not hurt the empath. If we do not ground ourselves, we can accumulate these noxious energies and become ill over time.

Living 'In the World'

Another connotation to 'grounding' is 'being with it' - by living in the 'real world', not in a fake imitation.

To many, the idea of Spirits and Fairies seems unreal; to mystics, the Spiritual world is the 'reality'. Yet most of us accept the idea of unseen 'good' entities such as Angels, and believe in 'God'. So perhaps we are halfway there !

Most of our beliefs originate in what we have been told over our life span. We believe that matter comprises various atoms, because we have been told so by those who we believe know that truth, even though we have never been able to personally identify or see an individual atom.

When we experience something ourselves it becomes more easy for us to change our belief system to incorporate that experience - or at least our understanding of it, which may be 'coloured' by other beliefs that we hold.

The experiences that we gain in our Dowsing (in our using Intuition Technology) probably demonstrate things that previously we did not know, understand, or believe. Such experiences assist us to expand our knowledge and understanding of realms that have been veiled from us.

Grounding Exercise

Put you hands on your legs (palm down) and your feet flat on the ground - intent is important, rugs on the floor or the fact that you are in a high-rise apartment will not have any effect.

Relax and still your mind, and imagine a beautiful beam of brilliant light (ask your Guardian Angel to put in it all the colours that you need, tinged with good gold and good silver) coming from way above, through a five pointed star about 2 feet above your head, going through you, and going to way below - forming roots from the soles of your feet and from your tail bone that go deep into the earth; this beam connects you to Heaven and Earth, with the five pointed star filtering out all that is not good for you.

Intend in your Heart and visualize in your Mind that the Light dissolves any and all pain, sickness, negative emotions, or blocks within your body and auras, Healing them to become beneficial.

When your entire body is filled with light, allow beams to come out of your third eye, throat, heart, and the palm of each hand. This will help open and clear each Chakra.

Ask the help of 'All in your Total Being' to make sure that this is fully effective - and then send them your Love and Gratitude for the help that they give to you.

Tell yourself in your mind *"I am now fully grounded, and will remain so"*.

Cleaning

Take a Pranic breath, feeling the life force coming into you at the top of your nose; hold your breath and imagine this good life force going through 'all your being' to below your feet.

While doing this, see and feel your meridians, lymph system, and other (perhaps unknown) systems clearing all unwanted Energy from your Being, and collecting all that is not in your 'Highest and Best Good' for disposal.

Now breathe out, sending all the unwanted Energy to be recycled for good with True Holy Love - and send them on their way with your Blessing for a good life in the future.

Repeat the Pranic breathing twice more.

Hooks and Cords

There are 'hooks' that can be placed in our body to control us (often from a parent or a loved one) or drain our energies.

These can also be placed by those with whom we are in contact at work, in religious groups, or have any other association.

I have attended a number of Bill Askin's workshops, and the reaction of students that Bill uses to demonstrate his skills is dramatic ! You can see the change happen in front of the class.

Bill focuses his thoughts on the Healee, visualizing all hooks that have been placed in the Healee and all the cords that connect the hook to the life form that placed them.

He then uses his Bobber as a cutting sword to cut all cords, putting a lot of effort into the cutting motion and shouting *"CUT !"*, he does this three times, and the Healee has been seen to jump in the air at each cut, even when Bill is 10 feet away.

Then 'The System' is asked to remove all hooks and all cords, taking them to be recycled for good, and placing protection against any replacement of these or similar devices.

As with all Intuitive work, your intent is paramount - and the more that you can illustrate your intent by visualization and emotion, the stronger the effect.

Personal Protection

Protection is the next step - this prevents 'not good' Energies from being able to get into your Being, but still allows them access to the beam of brilliant light that is grounding you.

People can use bands of different colour light having varying thicknesses, and place these 'screens' around themselves.

For your personal protection, imagine that the brilliant light forms a bubble around you, surrounded by a shell of 'Good Gold' light as a shield also guarded by Angelic Forces.

Specify that it allows good energies (having good auras and good intent) to pass through, but sends any energies whose aura or intent is not good to be Healed with True Holy Love.

Plugging Emotional Energy Leaks

Besides the obvious things that use up our energy each day - work, family duties, daily chores - there are more subtle elements that sap your physical vitality as well as your potential for living well. We can call them 'psychic energy leaks'.

These are self-defeating behaviours like guilt or worry that rob us not only of physical energy, but drain our spirits as well. You may be so used to them that you're not even aware of how they force you to row against the tide - but patching those leaks can help you experience smooth sailing !

LIVING IN THE PAST OR THE FUTURE: If you dwell on the great life you had in college or are waiting for your 'real life' to start after you've lost weight / gotten married / gotten a better job, you're throwing away your most important energy resource: the Now. The past is gone, the future isn't here yet, but in the present moment, you have power. Don't throw it away !

HOLDING A GRUDGE: Carrying around the invisible excess baggage of grudges is as exhausting as lugging around a complete set of Samsonite all day. Many people would rather 'be right' than have peace within themselves or with the person that hurt them.

The irony is that holding a grudge only takes away from your life. Who are you still mad at ? Give it up already - forgive, forget and move on.

WORRY: *"The fearful die a thousand deaths, the brave only one".* Words to live by. When we worry, we tend to imagine consequences that are far worse than what happens in reality. Thus we are literally 'making it up', agonizing over complete fiction ! Is this any way to spend your time ?

Since our brains work like a computer, acting on the information fed it, it's likely that obsessing over something may create a self-fulfilling prophecy.

Why not feed your brain the information that says, no matter what curves life throws us, we are equipped to handle them - and will do so if and when they come along. Then start Living in the here and now !

GUILT: Guilt is a man-made emotional response that, in effect, tells society that even if you do something 'bad', feeling guilty about it shows that you are still a 'good' person. This kind of complicated manipulation is exhausting - and beating yourself up over something that's locked in the past won't change the outcome.

A healthier response is to admit that we will make mistakes, but rather than feel bad about them, identify them, learn from them and go from there.

LACK OF FORGIVENESS: Studies show that the act of forgiveness has a powerful beneficial affect on the person doing the forgiving. In fact, letting go of old anger and hurts has often helped resolve seemingly unrelated issues like addictions and depression.

Admittedly however, forgiveness is tough - remember how we'd rather be 'right' than have peace ? Keep in mind that 'forgiveness' doesn't mean you're condoning their actions or letting them off the hook: it means acknowledging that they did what they could at the time with what they knew or understood.

You don't have to call or write every person you want to forgive - simply picture them in your minds and when you feel that old sense of hurt or anger rearing its ugly head, say to yourself *"I forgive you and release you"* and send positive thoughts their way.

When you forgive (and this includes forgiving yourself) you're the big winner, freeing yourself up to live a healthier, happier, more productive life !

JUDGING OTHERS: You do not know all the facts or circumstances involved, or how these were considered by the other person. We all have lessons to learn. It is OK to help them if asked.

The only judgement that you should make concerns your own relationship with them, deciding how you yourself should act.

Protection of Property

A recommended protection for a home is ask for an inner band 15 feet / 5 metres thick of Good Gold (the most healing of all colours) and then similar bands of good blue, good green, and good red to be placed next, in the order that is best for harmony.

For an individual human or animal a screen of Good Gold having the needed thickness is suggested.

Remember that you can fill the property with the essences, vibrational patterns, and energies of Peace, Harmony, and True Holy Love, Namaste

I have found that protection is needed for my computer and its accessories such as printers. Anything that works with electricity is vulnerable and should be given extra protection.

In all these cases Dowse for the colours and thickness that you need for the particular purpose.

Remember that any such device used for protection must be told the needed purpose, informed of the duration of its existence, asked to help in True Holy Love, and be sent True Holy Love and your Gratitude in appreciation.

Such a shield does not have to be fixed in any one spot - it can be linked to a person or object. You can build a mosquito shield around yourself, or place protection around your car.

Good blue is probably the best colour to use to protect a car - Bill Askin uses one 150 feet / 50 metres in diameter for his vehicle.

A case has been reported concerning the effects of such a screen around a car - the owner placed a shield of blue light around the car with the intention that the car would be invisible to police.

It worked ! The car was rammed by a police car on an emergency mission - the police driver did not see the car !

Clearing

Clearing should only be done when you are grounded and protected. There are noxious energies in many different forms, shapes, and sizes.

Many people say *"To clear bad energies I send them into deep space where they will not hurt others again"*. Our approach is to Heal them from being bad, so that they will be good in the future.

When we consider that all energies comprise families of families of families, each family having a 'Head of Family', with the 'Head of Family' at the highest level having command, there may be very many tiny energies that want to be good in those families, but do not have a chance because there is a bad 'commanding officer'.

This is similar to warfare. Most of the soldiers just want to do good, but are led astray by the politicians and bad leaders.

If we can get those that are good to come over to the 'Force for Good' then not only do we gain more 'soldiers' but the 'enemy forces' lose their ability to fight.

There are different levels of energies that we, as humans, consider to be bad: a ghost perhaps; a poltergeist (stem is from German 'restless or noisy spirit'); souls that intrude upon humans and possess them; and energies that are pure evil or act in malice.

As previously mentioned, if you are a Healer, 'shining' with brilliant light, you will attract lost souls and other energies to you - many are not coming to hurt you, but are seeking to get into the 'Light'. They may act in a way that you do not like, perhaps to get your attention - but they are seeking your help !

All you have to do to help them is ask the Angelic Forces to take them to be Healed and be in their rightful place - with their own families and those that they love.

Malice

If you ever get a sudden, unpleasant, cold feeling, then it could be that you are dealing with an evil entity that acts with malice. Your body may even feel 'frozen' in bed - but your Mind still works !

In such cases, send them 'True Holy Love, Namaste' (this is the most powerful force in all creation) and immediately ask for additional help and protection from the 'Force for Good', 'The System', and others in the God/Angelic realm.

'The System' has specialist teams to deal with such entities - and unless you Dowse or Intuit that your active involvement is needed, leave it to them.

There are those humans who understand exorcism and have the ability to properly assist the 'Force for Good' - ask them to handle any cases of evil entities or others acting in malice, and cases of possession of humans. In the future you may get this ability, too - but as a beginner, be cautious !

The best book that I have found on this subject is 'Exorcism' by Eugene Maurey - published Whitford Press, ISBN 0-914918-88-5.

Clearing Procedure

When clearing a place, it is best to go clockwise around the building and around each room - it is the direction that is 'good'.

Enter a room, and walk clockwise around it slowly, asking that your Pendulum point to any energy that is 'not good' or needs Healing; face in the indicated direction, and with your Pendulum rotating clockwise, the 'send mode' of your Pendulum, and say:

"I send this life form True Holy Love, Namaste, and ask 'The System' that it be Healed in the way that is best for the Highest and Best Good of All Creation.
Go now, in Peace and with True Holy Love, Namaste, to be Healed;
Go now, in Peace and with True Holy Love, Namaste, to be Healed;
Go now, in Peace and with True Holy Love, Namaste, to be Healed".

It seems that saying a thing three times is favoured - it gives you a choice to amend your initial thoughts, and implies that you really mean what you are saying. You do not have to say these words aloud - to express these thoughts in you mind is quite sufficient.

It is important that you do not 'take on' the energy involved; this is why you should be grounded and protected, and why you should ask the help of 'The System' to do the actual Healing.

Have you heard of 'Pyramid Power' ? It can even sharpen razor blades ! When your Pendulum circles it is making a cone shape, a 'virtual' circular pyramid.

A loudspeaker is such a cone - a tiny vibration at the point of the cone is carried throughout the whole cone - enabling you to hear a sound which otherwise would not register in your ears. A cone shape magnifies vibrations given at the peak.

I find that when I am in sincere concentration (aka prayer) my Pendulum makes that cone shape, perhaps amplifying my question so it is heard clearly, or making a Healing prayer just that much stronger.

Communication and Influences

When I find a life form whose energy is noxious to me I sometimes use my 'Message Chart' to ask *"Who are you ?"* - and get replies such as *"I body of dog dead"* or *"I am curse on land"*. When asked if they would like to be in the Light, the response is always YES.

You will often get a 'not good' signal at a rubbish container - the refuse itself knows it is being discarded, that its 'life' in the present form is ending, and is sad. The Beings in it respond beautifully to being sent 'True Holy Love, Namaste' !

I have got 'not good' signals from photographs and from paintings.

In Radionics a photograph can be used as a 'witness' - representing the 'whole person'. This is effective in linking to any time period of the person in the picture, even before birth or after death.

So a picture of a person that does not like you can exert the emotions and feelings of that person towards you - even if they are not now alive on this earth !

This may explain the Intuitive feelings of many 'second partners' that remnants (such as photographs) of previous partners not now be around. Check by Dowsing to see if any such remnant is 'not happy' at the change !

If they are (or were) unselfish and enlightened, then their influence may be advantageous.

A painting of a hunting scene (or other display involving cruelty or failure to respect and love the object displayed) often includes the emotional vibrations that are felt by the 'image' and propagated by that image. A Holy or Love painting, the quiet of a woodland scene, or the beauty of a flower - they will send out 'good' feelings.

Perhaps a loving picture or image of a Deity (Jesus, Buddha, etc.) would improve the good energies in your home - but I suggest that you do not include the crucifixion, which includes pain and anguish in the message radiated.

Effect of Shape

The effect of objects on energies, the placing of such objects, and the layout to enhance beneficial energies and discourage the intrusion of 'not beneficial' energies, is the art often practiced as Feng Shui.

Energies are responsive to shapes, including lines of objects and patterns formed by them - as well as to the emotions of those who made the objects or placed them in position.

Any line of objects (such as telephone poles, electricity pylons, a curb / kerb along a road, or centre lines painted on a street) have an effect on energies. Not necessarily bad - but an effect which you can investigate by Dowsing.

A friend of mine was holding a reception in a recently opened art gallery, which had previously been used as a funeral home. I cleared the main area, and then wandered into a back room, where the gallery had stored an ancient gargoyle, taken from a church, for restoration.

I spent some time clearing the gargoyle, but there always seemed to be more 'not good' energy around it - and finally I 'called it a day'.

That night I was absolutely 'frozen' in bed, and had to call on great help from 'Upstairs'. When I went to use my computer in the morning, it would not work, just showing a green face - this was before coloured screens were known. So I made an appointment to have it repaired, carried it to my car, and found that a tube for the heating system had broken, spewing green anti-freeze all around the foot area. Hardly a coincidence - I considered this to be a demonstration of 'not good' powers being used against me, for whatever reason.

Further Clearing

There are some other 'things' that need to be cleared. Bill Askin has discovered that curses exist on land that were created in the time of Dinosaurs !

To remove curses you must ground and protect yourself, then locate the land in your mind, use a map, or go there physically.

Dowse if any curses have been placed on the land - and on any adjoining land (sometimes to clear one area you may have to cover a much greater area) and ask permission to proceed (*"Can I ?, May I ?, Should I ?"*).

If this is given, then ask the help of 'The System' to lift all the curses and take all the energies involved 'into the Light or heal them in the way that is Highest and Best for All Creation' as described above. Remember to thank all who helped

Gleanings - The Protection Files

We teach the 'ninja technique of invisibility'. The egg is actually the shape of the subtle bodies as far as the outline or border of the 'emotional' body. The invisibility is an energetic thing, not actual. For protection, (flat tire in a scary part of town), we envision that the 'shell' of the 'egg' is two inches of body armour - no negative intent or person can focus on you.

However, all positive energies pass through (friends, etc, the good hearted). I have travelled all over the world including war zones in the Middle East with no harm. You can practice with panhandlers etc. - they don't 'see' you.

Also for those who seem to drain our energies, we have a volume control in the Heart Centre - Anahata. When you begin to feel any draining, 'pump up' the volume. Sometimes the energy you send out causes the person to step back a step.

Thank you so much for your very specific explanation. I've been trying for six months to get something this concrete that I can try. I've tried the more abbreviated explanations of surrounding with protective white light and found that I got dizzy and nauseated after about an hour. Perhaps being specific about allowing all positive energies to pass through is the difference.   SS

MF said: *"My pretty little car was rear-ended by someone in a hurry and since then I have felt under siege by aggressive shoppers".*

Hey ! All Dowsers should wise up on self-protection, vehicle protection and property protection. They're almost the only people who can make sure they have it right - via Dowsing.

I tell my car not even to get scratched in car parks. But it's taken some years to get it right.

I had set up driving protection, but after years of having no 'agro' from other drivers or any shocks or damage, met a lady driver on the wrong side of a blind corner 8 years ago.

Dowsing it afterwards, she had a towering need for self-punishment running and I hadn't 'written in' wholly crazy people !

It probably needs the help of other people, maybe even some enabling things like numbers or patterns. Worth research, anyway.
Dan Wilson

I have dowsed that Silver light is more powerful than white light, by a factor of 10, when used for clearing and protection. Metals themselves don't enter into it, just the colour Silver. Why silver I have no idea. Would have thought golden light to be more powerful than white, but no - golden light represents the Spirit World, apparently.

Mediums, when asking for the name of a person they 'see' will get the name in Gold if the person is in spirit, or Silver if the person is still living. GS

We have found that gold is now the colour used for protection.

When you ask for protection, that is what you want: Protection. What you don't want is Attraction.

What does White do ? White attracts the dark. You don't want to purposefully attract the dark. Gold has a higher harmonic.

In the past few years 'new' colours have come in. Not necessarily new to our eyes, not necessarily new with regard to wave lengths, but 'new' with regard to purpose, and perhaps slightly different than they were before. Gold, and the use of gold, is one of them.

And Silver does have its use too, perhaps for some things, silver would be used for protection. Perhaps, in some circumstances for protecting the body. Silver contains Blue. Blue attracts Oxygen.

Perhaps to protect oneself from a physical deterioration, such as a cancer, which is anaerobic, one might use Silver which means Blue, which attracts oxygen and which is anti cancer.

We used to ask for the White Light of Protection, now I ask for Gold. M

To Understand just 'How We Be'
Our Hidden Energies we must 'See'

Our Energy Body

So far I have not been able to see auras, except for the energy that is immediately around the body and can be seen emanating from the tips of fingers. So what follows is an assembly of reports from those people who have described their viewings and other discoveries, so that you can put these together to get a better understanding for yourself.

William Wilks' Experiments

The first report is the most unusual of all. The late William Wilks of Mayne Island, BC, had not been trained as a Dowser - he used the 'angle wires' and a tape, as developed by Francis Nixon in her Vivaxis studies. He calls Vivaxis the 'Vital Centre'.

The 'angle wires' that he used are actually 'L' rods. The 'tape' is described as 'a piece of strapping/binding used to cartons/boxes together' about 30 inches long, which 'should be vibrant, alive, and springy'; this corresponds to a Bobber, except that sideways and rotational movement would be restricted.

Wilks later abandoned the strapping in favour of using a roll-up carpenter's tape measure, the extended length being varied according to the flexibility of the tape measure.

In recent experimentation, I have encountered and detected at least eight upright vertically placed bands of energies within the body's field or aura.

These bands or segments are quite easy to detect and to evaluate within a limited way, limited because I have recognized in my testing that these bands seem to have a shifting or changing position in relation to the body; in other words, they are not precisely fixed, but are probably undulating in characteristics.

To study the aura, I took the two angle wires in my hands and stood with my back to my own Vital Centre, endeavouring to have the wires detect the first layer or band that lies very close to the surface or edge of the body, with elbows placed well back and the wires held nearly touching my chest; both wires then become activated and respond by pointing crosswise to my chest, this band being about one inch in width.

The next band is about seven inches in width, in this band the wires will point outwards or away from the body, both wires pointing parallel.

Extending your arms outwards, the next band is about one and a half inches in width, the wires within this area will point parallel to the body.

The next band encountered is about four inches in width and the wires in this area pointed outwards or away.

Then the next band or layer was about one and three quarters inches in width, pointing parallel to the body, followed by the next band of about 5 inches that pointed the wires outward or away, then another band of about two inches that turned the wires parallel to the body, crosswise.

Beyond this I ran out of arm and was unable to determine what control or condition extended beyond a fringe of two or three inches, however the point of direction at the edge was outwards or away.

The indications are that this alternating of wide and narrow bands with the wires in the narrow bands pointing crosswise and the wider bands pointing outwards could extend or continue to the full extent of the aura or field. My measuring of the aura indicates a width of approximately nine feet.

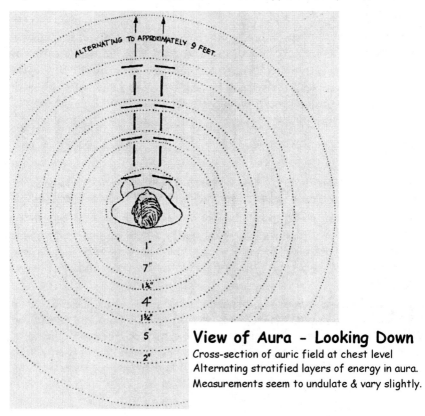

ALTERNATING TO APPROXIMATELY 9 FEET.

1"
7"
1½"
4"
1½"
5"
2"

View of Aura - Looking Down
Cross-section of auric field at chest level
Alternating stratified layers of energy in aura.
Measurements seem to undulate & vary slightly.

Some further testing of these bands with the angle wires revealed that when standing or facing from any position (i.e. irrespective of one's position relative to one's Vivaxis) the recording or results were the same. The narrow bands running crosswise totalled four, those facing outwards numbered four, for a total of eight alternating flows or bands of energy.

Perhaps there are more, as I indicated, but this was as far as my arms could reach.

Now, to look at another newly found part of Man's aura - this is an energy that flows and functions compatibly with the vertical form we have just examined, but one that flows horizontally and one that complements the vertical bands just discussed.

From the drawings it will be apparent that the human body is 'boxed in' within a force or energy mantle, and is surrounded by an energy sophistication that flows vertically and horizontally to enclose the

Horizontal

Energy Bands

These bands are identified with the angle wire. The wire will spin with alternative directions depending which band is being tested.

The wider section, as shown, is the only reliable area to find or receive your vital Centre's direction.

Other bands are shown, are not found to be linked.

These sections are part of the sophistication of the field or aura and no doubt affinitive and compatible to the vertical bands shown elsewhere.

To test hold the angle wire within any of the bands far enough from the body to allow the wire to pass and then observe the various bands spinning either clock-wise or anti-clockwise.

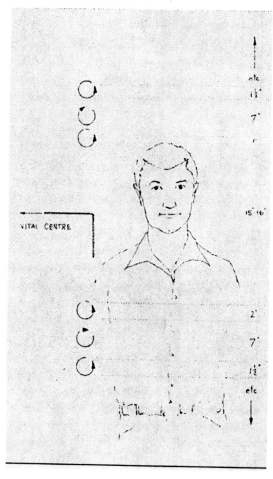

elemental human body, together with its accompanying bio-electro-magnetic sophistication, within its common environment. This new fact I uncovered just recently and reveal for the first time.

These two energies are perhaps similar, but distinct and separate, though perhaps identical in structure, and co-ordinate their functions to create a vertical and horizontal screen of alternating flow of energies that compose possibly the major parts of the field or aura.

In the horizontal stratification there is a difference or exception in the structure, form or sophistication of the layers, and that is found in the area of the body from the top or tip of the head downwards to a position just below the arms, perhaps to the area of the Thymus gland in the upper centre of the chest.

It is confined to this particular area of the body. Here we are able to use the angle wires successfully to find and locate the Vital Centre and its energy flow, an important fact to remember when using the angle wires to locate your 'line'.

Keep your hands and wires well within the confines of this vital area, as this is the only reliable area where personal energies can be detected when they are flowing into the body.

This whole area of investigation is becoming more and more complex and I will do my best to explain at least some of the rules and order. The angle wire when held within this band or area - the band is about 15 or 16 inches in width - will point towards your Vital Centre.

If held above or below this area, the angle wires can come under the influence of the horizontal alternating layers of energy. This influence is from the top of the head upwards and from that position in the chest area just described, downwards, to the ground.

The influence of these alternating energy bands' waves are detected by the angle wires spinning, either in a clockwise or anti-clockwise direction, depending on the layer or band in which the angle wire is placed or held.

The functioning of the energy flows described above are valid only if the body is free or freed from the induced energies derived from the eating or consuming of living foods, or acquired by a direct contact with other living entities.

These foods' Vital Centre energies will take over and assume partial command of your personal circuitry, and this will obviously create rearrangements in the relays and circuits within you.

A very little of this has been charted, but much more will be. It is most important in these experiments first to clear the body of all outside energies and influence by using the ramrod military stance.

This you do by simply standing or facing into your own personal Vital Centre's direction - this stance or position you hold and maintain for just an instant of time.   Having completed this, you are now 'clear' and can enter into the next phase.

Take your angle wire in hand and stand erect.   Hold it so that the wire's horizontal arm will just pass over the tip of your head; holding it as close as possible, allowing the arm of the wire to just pass by when it becomes activated and begins to swing, circling over the head.

In this position the wire encounters that layer of force which is one inch in width immediately above the head.   In this first and narrow band, the angle wire will turn anti-clockwise, circling.

Raise the arm and the wire upwards: you will encounter the second horizontal band above the head.   This band is about seven inches in width, and will turn the wire clockwise, again in a circular or spinning motion.

The next band upwards is again narrow, about two inches, and the spinning will once again change direction and spin in an anti-clockwise motion.

If you study the drawings you will be struck by the similarity of the structure of the layers of the alternating bands of energies.

I am quite convinced that they are quite the same in design, with one exception, and that is within and between the area of the top of the head downwards to a position just below the arms and just above the centre of the chest, as described above.

The remaining portions of the body downwards are divided into further alternating flows of energy or force until the ground is reached.

It is difficult to measure and test the lower alternating bands, due to the shortcomings of the arm and the wire.   It is quite difficult to manipulate the arms and the wire with any degree of exact success. Perhaps this can be done with the help of another person.

I believe some modification or special apparatus will have to be designed to gauge these bands.   However, you should be able to achieve enough checking in this area to establish that the lower bands do exist, and do alternate, and are in layers, and that they are similar to the bands as found above the head.

The structure and the mechanics of these energies indicate that the human body is surrounded and boxed within these flows.

In my attempt to measure the width of the aura or field of another person I use my trusty tape. First I touch the person with the tape, thus charging the tape with the person's wave length or vibrations; then, beginning close to the person, point the tape downwards towards the ground, watching the tape activate and vibrate with its own particular motion.

I walk slowly with the tape outwards until the tape ceases to vibrate, measuring the distance from the person to the place where the tape stopped its pendulum-like motion, which will give an accurate measurement of the width of the aura.

This is a simple and accurate method to accomplish this task.

Information derived from other sources indicates that the aura's measurements could be undulating and therefore likely to be variable and unstable. Constant monitoring will prove or disprove this. Be sure to 'ground yourself' before and after making this test, using the ramrod method.

The result given here is quite admittedly subject to variations. I believe that many reasons could be given to explain the undulations of the human field or aura; despite all this, I believe the basic structuring as I described it will hold up.

There is no doubt in my mind that much of the sophistication of these esoteric forces, and particularly of their functions, will soon be revealed. Note that the measurement of these bands simply reveals their reaction as forces; this testing reveals nothing of the shades of colour as attested to by others.

Levels of Auric Bodies

In her book 'Hands of Light' (Bantam) Barbara tells how she sees the human energy field having seven levels, each penetrating through inner levels (of lower 'frequency') and the body.

The odd-numbered levels are seen as structured fields of standing, scintillating light beams, while the even-numbered levels are filled with bioplasma - formless substance/energy: second level being gaseous, the fourth fluid-like, and the sixth like the diffuse light around a candle flame.

This bioplasma is of various colors, density, and intensity, and flows along the lines of the structured levels. Your human experience varies with its strength and wellness - correlating directly with your emotions.

Life exists in each level, differing according to the makeup of energy-consciousness in that level. By changing one's tuning to different auric vibrational levels, different levels of the auric field can be more clearly defined - and easier to work directly with them.

First Level - Etheric Body

Feeling of all physical sensations, painful and pleasurable. Numbness correlates to no flow of energy along the lines of the first level of the field. When a healer works to start a flow of energy there, the feeling sensation returns.

The first level seems to be about ¼" to 2" from the physical body, of fine, thin, energy lines 'like a sparkling web of light beams' in constant motion, pulsating at about 15-20 cycles per minute; sparks of bluish white light move along these energy lines.

The colour of the etheric body is of a light aqua-blue colour for quiet, sensitive people, thicker, coarser, and a darker blue-gray for strong, robust people. Athletes and dancers tend to have more lines of energy - thicker, more elastic, and bright blue.

The etheric body seems to be a matrix into which cells grow; in a seedling it has been found to give the shape of the completed plant.

Second Level - Emotional Body

The second level, shaped to the outline of the physical body, indicates your feelings or emotions about yourself. It appears to be like more clouds of fluidic fine substance in constant motion.

It has bright colours of cloudlike energy with positive feelings; darker, dirtier shades if negative feelings. All colours can be seen and these flow along the structured lines of the first field level.

If you allow the feelings about yourself to flow (both negative and positive) the aura keeps itself balanced - the negativity is released and transformed. Otherwise the energies become stagnant, with dark, dirty clouds of various colors, which clog up the system and disrupt healthy functioning, and cause stagnation in the first and third levels of the field, which are adjacent to it.

Third Level - Mental Body

The lines in this level are very delicate, like the finest thin veil, light lemon-yellow coloured pulsating at a very high rate, extending to about 3" - 8" from the physical body.

When this level is balanced and healthy, the rational and intuitive mind work together in harmony as one - we experience clarity, balance, and a sense of appropriateness. When our thoughts are negative, the pulsations are slower, the lines dark and distorted.

'Thought Forms' are seen here, of various shapes, colours, and sizes; they are sometimes activated by colours emanating from the emotional level - such as negative thought processes, often squeezed into action by stagnated emotions from the second and fourth levels.

The natural state of energy is constant movement; when the movement of energy is stopped in the second and fourth levels, some of that momentum is transferred into the third level - distorted because it is not free to move naturally.

Fourth Level - Astral Body

Our whole world of relationships, all our feelings about each other. The energy of the fourth level is thicker than that of the second, even though it is at a higher vibrational level, more like coloured fluid; it extends 6" - 12" from the physical body

If of low vibrations, this energy will be experienced as dark, thick, heavy fluid, just like the mucus you accumulate in your body when you have a cold, having a very strong negative effect on your health.

When two people interact great streams of coloured fluid-like bioplasma reach out from each to touch the other, the nature corresponding with the energy-consciousness involved.

Love shows a lot of sweet rose energy in soft waves; with passion the rose will have a lot of orange, and the waves will be faster, with higher peaks. Envy will be dark, gray-green, slimy and sticky. Anger shows as harsh, sharp, pointed, penetrating, invasive, and dark red.

Barbara Ann Brennan explains that the first three levels of the aura indicate our physical, emotional, and mental experience in the physical body; the fourth level acts as a bridge between the physical and spiritual domains; the higher three levels represent our physical, emotional, and mental experience in our spiritual world, and are the templates for the three lower levels.

Fifth Level - Etheric Template Body

Viewing this level is a bit confusing, since everything appears to be reversed, like a blueprint. What you normally experience as empty space is cobalt-blue light, and what you normally experience as solid objects are composed of empty or clear lines of energy.

There is an empty slot or groove in the fifth level into which each blue line of light of the first level fits. This egg-shaped body extends 18" - 24" from the physical body. It is observed that at this level 'sound creates matter'.

It contains not only the form for your body but the form of all other life - the unfolding evolutionary pattern of life that manifests into form. It is described as the level of Divine will, divine intent manifested into pattern and form - subject to your free will. It is a world of precision and of precise tones - the level of symbols.

<u>Sixth Level - Celestial Body</u>

The emotional body of the Spiritual plane - Divine love; seen as beautiful streamers of light radiating out in all directions, extending about 24" - 33" from the physical body. It contains all the colours of the rainbow in opalescent tones and pastel shades, having a gold-silver sheen. It is unstructured and is of very high frequency.

When this level is unhealthy, it is dark, thin, and undercharged and its beams of light sag. This is usually a result of lack of Spiritual nourishment, such as a trauma of some other personal nature that results in the person's rejection of God; sometimes a gap exists between the adjacent levels, and the normal communication channels between the levels are closed.

<u>Seventh Level - Causal Body</u>

Divine mind - the mental body of the Spiritual plane, called the 'Ketheric Template'; it is egg-shaped, extends 30" - 42" from the physical body, made of tiny threads of gold-silver light, and containing a golden grid structure holding the other auric bodies; the outer edge being thicker and stronger, like an eggshell. It contains all the associations of a person's incarnation.

When healthy, it is composed of beautiful, extremely strong golden lines of energy that scintillate at a very high frequency, which are interwoven to form all the physical components of your physical body, knitting everything together, whether they be the cells of an organ, a body, a group of people, or the whole world - the universal divine mind field.

If the seventh level of the field is not healthy, the golden lines will be dull and weak, will not hold their form, and may be thin in some places - even torn open, allowing energy to leak out of the system.

The Chakras

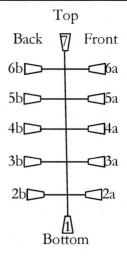

Schematic Power Grid

Chakras look like vortices, or funnels, of energy. They exist on each of the seven levels of the field, and chakras two through six appear on both the front and the back of the body. Their major opening is about 6 inches diameter, about 1 inch from the body.

Most descriptions of Chakras tell that they have 'petals' (like a flower) of various sizes and colours that spin. Barbara Brennan sees these petals as being rather like individual ice-cream cones contained in a larger cone for each Chakra.

The internal connection is near the major nerve plexuses (which are understood to connect to the glands), to a major 'power line' (probably interspaced with the spine) running from chakras below the body to others above the head.

The vertical power line is about one inch wide in most people; in Healers who have a high altered state of consciousness, it can become as large as six inches in diameter. Each colour is woven together, somewhat like a rope made of beautiful pulsating light of all colors.

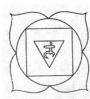

1. Muladhara - Root Chakra

The first or Muladhara / Root Chakra is located between the legs. Its fine tip seats right into the sacral-coccyx joint. It is associated with the senses of body position, of body movement, and tactile/touch, and to our will to live - supplying the body with physical vitality, and energy to the spinal column, the adrenals, and the kidneys.

2. Svashisthana - Seat of Life

The second Svashisthana / Seat of Life Chakra is located just above the pubic bone. Its tip seats directly into the center of the sacrum, through which we sense emotions. It is related to sensuality and sexuality, and supplies our sexual organs and our immune system with lots of energy.

**3. Manipura
- Power Chakra**

The third - <u>Manipura /Power Chakra</u> - is located in the solar plexus area, with its fine tip seating into the diaphragmatic hinge, between thoracic vertebra twelve (T-12) and lumbar vertebra one (L-1). It supplies the stomach, liver, gall bladder, pancreas, spleen, and nervous system with energy, and is associated with our Intuition, who we are in the universe, how we connect to others, and how we take care of ourselves.

**4. Anahata
- Heart Chakra**

The <u>Anahata / Heart Chakra</u>, in the middle position, has the front aspect is related to love, the rear aspect to will. Its fine tip seats into T-5. It brings energy to our heart, circulatory system, thymus, vagus nerve, and upper back.

**5. Visuddha
- Throat Chakra**

In fifth position is the <u>Visuddha / Throat Chakra</u>, associated with the senses of hearing, tasting, and smelling. Its fine tip seats into cervical vertebra three (C-3). It supplies energy to the thyroid, the bronchi, lungs, and alimentary canal, and is related to giving and receiving and speaking our truth.

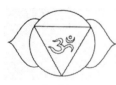

**6. Ajna
- Third Eye Chakra**

The sixth <u>Ajna / Third Eye Chakra</u> is located on the forehead and the back of the head, with its tip seating into the centre of the head. It supplies energy to our pituitary, lower brain, left eye, ears, nose, and nervous system. The front part of the chakra deals with conceptual understanding, the back to carrying out our ideas in a step-by-step process.

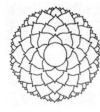

**7. Sahasrara
- Crown Chakra**

The seventh major chakra, the <u>Sahasrara or Crown Chakra</u>, is located at the top of the head, with its fine tip seating into the middle of the top of the head. This is described as the 'thousand petal' chakra, and may comprise one chakra of gold within a many petalled chakra of violet.

The Crown Chakra supplies energy to our upper brain and our right eye, and is associated with direct knowing and the integration of personality with spirituality.

In general, the front aspects of the chakras correlate to our emotional functioning, the back to our will, and the head chakras to our reason.

Barbara Marciniak identifies additional chakras above the head - connecting to our Solar System, galaxy, and universe. Perhaps the highest is our connection to the Godhead, to 'All That Is'.

The Chakra - Power System shown here is normally recognized as the 'Kundalini System'. Full opening, including to higher levels, can give enlightenment - and this seems to be a prime aim of Yoga; forcing this, however, can cause major health problems.

Unfortunately most practitioners of Western Medicine are not conversant with these problems - usually leading to incorrect diagnoses, which then make such problems worse.

Others have described minor chakras at each and every joint - including Ankle Chakras of silver and green that may be anchoring our bodies together. Working with these Ankle Chakras has been advised to facilitate leaving one's body.

The Hara Line

The Haric level has been defined as 'the foundation upon which the aura rests'. While the aura is related to your personality, the Haric level is understood to be related to your intentions, and corresponds to your life task or your deeper spiritual / incarnational purpose.

The Haric level is said to consist of points along a laser-like line that is on the center line of our body, at the emotional/astral level. This line is about one-third of an inch wide and consists of 12 strands - perhaps it is a misunderstanding of this that has led some of the 'New Age' gurus to talk about a '12 strand DNA'. It extends from a point about three and one-half feet above our head, to down deep into the core of the earth.

The first point is a clear-coloured (all colours, no colour) centre above the head that looks like an inverted funnel, called the transpersonal point. Its wide end pointing down is only about one-third of an inch wide, and may represent our first individuation out of the godhead and our reason to incarnate.

The second point is a beautiful diffused aqua or aquamarine light in our upper chest area, between the heart and throat, called the Thymus Chakra, connecting the Hara Line and emotional body to the Kundalini Line and etheric double; it corresponds to our emotion, our spiritual longing that leads us through our life. It is very specific to our life task.

Ch'i Hung (aka Qigong) identifies this chakra as the acupuncture meridian Conception Vessel 17, also called the 'grief point', located between and about three inches above the nipples, on the breastbone. When you find it, you will know immediately; it is painful and sensitive to pressure. By doing so, one experiences compassion.

The Hara Chakra itself, called the Tan Tien, or Sea of Ch'i, is the will centre from which all martial artists move when they perform. It appears to be a ball of power about one and one-half inches in diameter, having a strong membrane around it (so it looks a bit like a rubber ball) and may be gold in colour; it is located about two and one-half inches below the navel.

This is a will center. It is your will to live in the physical body. It contains the 'one note' that holds the physical body in physical manifestation.

The Hara Line, when correctly grounded, extends down into the molten core of the earth; so grounded, Healers can gather great power known to Ch'i Hung as Earthly Hi, or the life force one draws from the centre of the Earth.

When so used, the Tan Tien can turn very bright red and become very hot, and Healers may feel intense heat all over their body.

Other Chakras

These, perhaps of lesser importance, have been identified in Ch'i Hung (Qigong) as on the Hara Line. Three Hara centres are placed between the primary chakras above, and another three outside them.

The Causal Body Chakra is located between the transpersonal point and the Thymus, in the base of the skull where the neck meets the head at the back; it looks like crimson yarn wrapped around a golden core.

Some see this centre as blue; it must be activated and balanced to achieve its purpose of bringing mental commitment to one's life purpose. Is it this activation into life force that changes the colour ?

This centre is also a major transformer of non-physical information into consciousness as in channelling, automatic writing, and working with spirit guides for psychic healing.

The Diaphragm Centre between the Thymus and the Hara chakra, at the level of the physical diaphragm muscle, approximately just above the solar plexus, of colour lime green, also known as the Triple Warmer-11 (T-11) acupuncture point, the adrenal gland centre.

Some see a membrane dome of energy at this location, which they name by the seed sound of mumin (moo-mm).

The dome is a filter, separating spiritual from material energies and allowing only what is finer-tuned to pass through. Activation of this centre may provide a clearing and detoxification of any obstructions to the fulfillment of one's life purpose - cleansing the entire Hara Line. Thus it has been called the 'garbage chakra' or 'vomit chakra'.

The Perineum Chakra of deep ruby or maroon colour, found between the Hara Line and the centres in the knees.

Reiki students know it as the Hui Yin position; in Indian meditation / yoga as the 'moolband' or 'root lock'; it is known in acupuncture and Ch'i Hung as the 'gateway of life and death' (Conception Vessel 1).

It is the place of activating and anchoring one's life intention and purpose into physical plane reality.

Three smaller chakras pairs complete the Hara Line.

A pair of silver vision chakras behind the eyes, paving the way to using the eyes as lasers in Healing.

A pair of forest green or tan movement chakras behind the knees, to direct movement forward on one's life path.

A pair of brown grounding chakras in the soles of the feet to root the Hara Line into Earth Hi - and root one's purpose into physical direction and manifestation.

There may be two Earth chakras; one is about six inches below the feet, seen by Diane Stein as shiny black. This seems to be our grounding link to the earth's surface. In my Healing work I find yet another Chakra further below - perhaps our connection to the molten core of Gaia, as described by Barbara Brennan.

Interaction between Auras and Chakras

Genevieve Paulson, in her book 'Kundalini and the Chakras', gives detailed descriptions of many more chakras.

Perhaps some could be identified as communication points between our meridian system and our 'Light Bodies' or auras, since many correspond to the points described and used in acupuncture and associated modalities.

The Core Star Level

Barbara Ann Brennan sees a 'core star level' - a quantum leap deeper into who we are than the Haric level, and related to our Divine essence. It is located one and one-half inches above the navel on the centre line of the body.

On the level of the core star, everyone looks like a beautiful star, each star being different, the internal source of life within, and radiates out infinitely permeating all the other stars.

In this inner place, we are the centre of the universe, beyond the limitations of time, space, and belief. It is the individual aspect of the Divine - we are wise, loving, and full of courage, an inner essence that has not changed with time.

Our reactions to negative experiences may have shrouded it to some extent, but they have never really changed it - it is our most basic nature.

Assemblage Point

The Assemblage Point / Beam system is not reported by Diane Stein, Barbara Ann Brennan, or most clairvoyant Healers.

The first reference that I could find to it is in Abbé Mermet's book; Carlos Castenada also mentions it, but neither of these authors gives much information to its location, form, or purpose.

The first person to publicize the Assemblage Point is Dr Jonathan Whale - in his excellent books 'The Catalyst of Power' and 'Naked Spirit - The Supernatural Odyssey'. Jon has also made enormous strides in developing laser-type crystal therapies for Healing.

Much of this section is based on the website of Dr Whale: www.whalemedical.com/ap1.html - see this for more information - or better still, buy his books !

Robert A. Monroe's book: 'Journeys Out Of The Body' contains graphic diary accounts of supernatural experiences of others; it makes a number of significant disclosures that are relative to the Assemblage Point.

Monroe found himself leaving his physical body to travel via a 'second body' to other locales far removed from our conscious physical and spiritual realities. He conducted a series of experiments that conclusively affirmed the existence of a 'second body' that could be projected from his physical body.

Using disciplined mental techniques, he could shift his conscious awareness into his 'second body' and travel to distant locales while his physical body remained behind in a trance state.

While on one of his frequent out of the body excursions, he discovered that his second body was attached to his physical body via a cord consisting of hundreds of tendon-like strands packed neatly together.

This cord was attached to the centre of his back and the hundreds of strands or filaments spread and fanned out to form his second body. This suggests that his projected 'second body' had an Assemblage Point entering at the centre of the shoulder blades.

Another intriguing disclosure of his was that when he occupied his second body, his body image was reversed, his left leg and left arm was on his right side and vice versa - a 'mirror image' effect. Monroe assumes that he is not unique and that every human retains the possibility to project or possess a 'second body'.

Dr. Carlos Castaneda undertook specific shamanic instructions to gain mastery over his dreaming double or 'second body'. The Assemblage Point is intrinsic in the shamanic teachings of Don Juan Matus as recorded in Castaneda's books both in relation to the physical body and the second body or dreaming double.

Don Juan discusses the importance of the Assemblage Point of the physical body with regard to health and disease.

Assemblage Point information presented here is entirely to do with the Assemblage Point of our physical body - not the Assemblage Point of the 'second body' or dreaming double.

Although Don Juan used powerful hallucinogenic plants to shift Castaneda's Assemblage Point, he gave Castaneda stern warnings of the dangers of uninformed use of drugs and other adverse incidents that can cause an involuntary shift.

Throughout his book Castaneda records Don Juan's intimations that an involuntary or unconscious shift of the Assemblage Point causes serious physical and mental problems, even life threatening.

The Human Assemblage Point

The epicentre of the human energy field is called the Assemblage Point. The location and entry angle of the Assemblage Point with respect to the physical body dictates the shape and distribution of the human energy field.

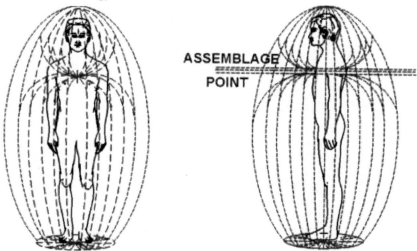

The biological activity of the organs and glands determines the position of the Assemblage Point, and thus the shape and distribution of biological energy throughout the physical body.

The location and entry angle of the Assemblage Point regulates how we feel and behave. Disease also dictates the Assemblage Point location and entry angle. Any type of severe trauma can cause an involuntary shift of the Assemblage Point to a dangerous location.

An unstable and displaced Assemblage Point may occur if we had a consistently negative home relationship. Genetic reasons or disease can similarly produce abnormal and unstable Assemblage Points.

Sufferers of an involuntary Assemblage Point shift downwards experience that 'something' deep inside them has changed. Although they can remember how they behaved and felt before the incident, returning to their former energetic and happy self is impossible for them.

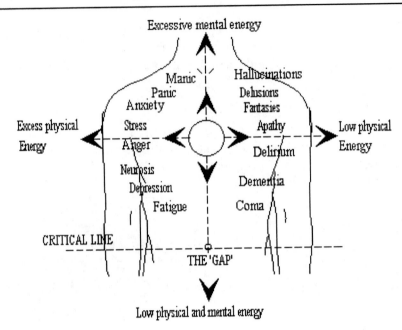

That indescribable 'something' deep inside all of us that can suddenly shift following an adversity, changing our whole perception of reality and our physical health, is the location and entry angle of our Assemblage Point.

If the Assemblage Point drops beyond a certain distance it is very difficult for the individual to recover their former health and state of being.

Raising the Assemblage Point location and angle upwards, closer to the centre of the chest, is an essential consideration in such cases.

Unfortunately, accepted orthodox medical diagnostic and management procedures do not take the patient's Assemblage Point location into consideration, although gross misalignment of the Assemblage Point location is present in many diseases.

Extreme locations to the right side of the chest with an acute angle are associated with extrovert psychotic behaviour such as violence, bullying, rape, stalking, murder, terrorism or fanaticism.

Extreme locations to the left side of the chest are associated with introvert psychotic behaviour such as hallucinations, autism and downs syndrome.

High locations are accompanied by symptoms of hyperactivity, anxiety, panic, insomnia and so on, along with hyper liver/adrenal

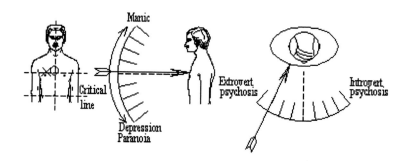

activity.   Attention deficit hyper-activity disorder (ADHD) in children is now very common and is an example of this.

Low locations are accompanied with hypo-activity, the depressive illness spectrum and hypo liver/adrenal/thyroid activity.

The bipolar disorder spectrum or manic depression is accompanied by an oscillating Assemblage Point location which switches between a high manic location to a low depressive position on the right side of the chest.

With the autistic spectrum the Assemblage Point will almost certainly be found on the left.

A good stable physical location near the centre of the chest is essential for good mental and physical health.

The location for an average healthy woman is slightly higher than that of an average healthy man.

If, for whatever reason, the Assemblage Point shifts outside the central location, distressing physical and mental symptoms can and do frequently occur.

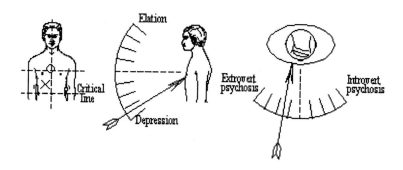

Hunger, thirst, shock, trauma, drugs, alcohol, accidents, violence, intimidation can and do cause the Assemblage Point to drop to a dangerously low location.

Ironically the drugs and therapies used in treatments for many diseases often depress the patient's Assemblage Point location even further down towards the critical line.

Death results when the Assemblage Point crosses the umbilical region. In the case of comatose patients on life support systems, regardless of any electroencephalogram tests, the patient will not be brain-dead until their Assemblage Point has traversed the umbilical region.

With all serious diseases in their chronic phase, the patient's Assemblage Point will be found in a low location perhaps as much as 20 centimetres or more below that of a healthy person.

For those patients that have a serious physical or mental disease it is imperative for their recovery to adjust the location of their Assemblage Point back up to a location of that of a normal healthy person.

This simple action will greatly help the patient's restoration of normal levels that are essential for good health. Not only are the Assemblage Point diagnostics and correction principals applicable to mental and physical disease but, for a normal healthy person, regular correction to the central location can dramatically improve mental and physical efficiency.

With most people the Assemblage Point will be found entering on the right side of the chest's central meridian line; this is due to the excessive left brain activity resulting in physical and mental activity, which is demanded by today's stressful life style.

Drugs, toxins, illness, accidents and emotional trauma are the most common causes of serious misalignment.

Once misalignment has occurred it is very difficult, if not impossible, to re-establish the original position by one's own efforts or by orthodox medical therapies.

Serge King in 'Kahuna Healing' says that the main source of 'Mana' or 'Life Force' is from the 'Higher Self'; he sees *"a 'white hole' in the centre of our Being through which energy come streaming from another universe."* He does not call this the 'Assemblage Point' but it seems to fit the description. I suggest that it is not 'another universe', but a source beyond, a 'cosmic' source.

Dowsing and the Assemblage Point

Since we know that a Dowser can change the flow of a deep water vein that is a great distance away, it can be expected that this skill can be effective in correcting the location and direction of an Assemblage Point - and the total grid system which it controls.

Kristina Nielsen has taken courses on the Assemblage Point; as a brilliant clairvoyant Healer she was able to see it - and experiment with the use of Pendulums to make corrections. See her site www.clearyourpath.ca for further information.

Kristina has had some wonderful results; one young boy was most unstable, causing intense frustrations at his home and was suicidal; after just a single session with Kristina, he changed completely - to become a caring, responsive young man.

Meridian System

Donna Eden, in her wonderful book 'Energy Medicine', gives clear pictures of this system, excellent explanations of its purpose, and clearly defined exercises to both locate and clear the meridians.

There are 14 of these meridians within the body; they are very fine, tubes of 0.5 - 1.5 microns diameter - so tiny that western medicine has only recently been able to see that they do exist; they show on infra-red photographs, in the locations described by Oriental Healers.

Two of these, the 'Governing Channel' (from the tailbone, straight up the spine, over the top of the head, to the upper lip), and the 'Central Channel' (from the lower lip and down the front of the body to the bottom of the pelvic bone) seem to be of great importance to all the other meridians.

The channels are connected by placing the tongue on the roof of the mouth and contracting the perineum. Movement of energy through this circuit involves circulating Ch'i (life force) through the connected channels and the Hara Line chakras.

This is called the Microcosmic Orbit, or Large and Small Heavenly Cycle, and is the basis of the Qigong / Ch'i Hung discipline.

The remaining 12 meridians are subject to 'tidal flows' - each having a 2 hour high tide, and 12 hours later a 2 hour low tide. This tidal flow is upset by long distance jet travel, and so the organs fed develop problems.

Peak Tides for Meridians - Based on 24 Hour Clock

Liver 1-3	Lung 3-5	Large Intestine 5-7
Stomach 7-9	Spleen 9-11	Heart 11-13
Small Intestine 13-15	Bladder 15-17	Kidney 17-19
Circulation-Sex 19-21	Triple Warmer 21-23	Gall Bladder 23-1

The points used in Acupuncture (this term is used here to include associated systems such as Acupressure) seem to act as amplifier stations, similar to those used in telephone systems.

The meridians supply energy to every system in our body; their flow is as critical as the flow of blood - if a meridian is obstructed or the flow unregulated, the systems that it feeds are jeopardized.

There are 'alarm points', 'strengthening points', and 'sedating points' along each meridian. These can be used to check the meridian and take appropriate action.

It seems that each organ and each gland has associated meridians - when health problems exist remedial action on the meridians concerned may well enable a return to good health.

Kirlian photography and sensitive electric instruments have indicated that there is a higher electric potential at the skin where these points surface.

The recognized 'end points' of the meridians are numerous - in the feet, hands, ears, teeth, eyes, and the head area. It may be that these 'end points' are in fact 'linkage points' to a meridian (or similar) system in the auric bodies. Perhaps this is also true for the nervous and other systems.

In the chapter on Vivaxis we will read Mike's Story - how Francis Nixon found 'receptors' - that seem to correlate with Acupuncture points, and their connections outside the physical body.

Lymph System

Lymphocytes are specialized white blood cells (about 25% of the total) seen as clear liquid when coming out of a cut. They are produced in the many lymph nodes in the body, and carry proteins, hormones, and fats to cells; they also eliminate dead tissue and other waste products, and are a key part of your immune system.

This system, unlike most others, seems to lack a pump ! This is why tapping your 'lymph points' to ease congestion is so effective, and perhaps a main reason why so many people go to massage therapists.

Donna Eden gives many guidelines for identifying problems in your meridians and lymph systems, and exercises for improving your health - and that of others with whom you can so co-operate.

My best advice is to buy, read, and understand her book 'Energy Medicine' - definitely a 'Best Buy' !   And then to actually do the exercises that she suggests !

Gnomes

Once when I was working on a problem with my left hip I 'saw' a Gnome - or at least the upper part of one; he had a smiling face, looked at me, and winked; he was wearing a floppy sort of top hat that was coloured red.   Have you heard of 'genomes' in medical science ?

I asked *"was this Gnome in charge of my hip ?"* and was told YES.   It seems as if Gnomes are 'in charge' of all our major organs and joints, being responsible for obeying orders received and maintaining the health of what is in their care - unless ordered to cause or allow a problem of some description.

I spoke to the Gnome, and asked if he needed anything - and was told 'Manganese'.   So I purchased manganese tablets, Dowsing for which brand was best for me.

It seems that the colour of the hat represents their place in the Gnome hierarchy - the colour order may be similar to that of the major Chakras.   Dowse to see if this is correct, and if you are clairvoyant, look at the Gnomes in your Being.

Your Heart Gnome (or Dwarf ?) is your major link to 'Upstairs', and should be working harmoniously with the 'Head Quarters Gnome' (in charge of your head) and the Gnomes in charge of the various parts of your brain - who give instructions to the other Gnomes, and receive feedback concerning any problems.

In considering our 'Ship of Being' these Gnomes would be the officers and petty officers who do the work, perhaps assisted by other elemental Beings - even Elves, Pixies, and Fairies looking after muscles, bones, and cells !

My impression is that they work as a team with our life, immune, and Healing systems - but I have not delved into the details of their operation.

My understanding is that Gnomes function in this way in all animalistic and insect life forms - and are in Souls, Angels, Archangels, and other 'High Energy' life forms, perhaps as the 'Essence' of Gnomes - their Mental or Spiritual form.

They are elementals - but a very special type. Like all elementals, they are assigned a task and will carry out that task as ordered - but seem to have a limited ability for reasoning. It is as if they run programs in response to a stimulus. So an important way of getting a more satisfactory operation is to re-program - or adjust and amend the programs that they run.

The key point here is that we can communicate with the Gnomes within our own Being - and of others who we help as Healers.

'Food for Thought': Could organ transplants be more successful if the co-operation of the Gnomes involved be obtained ? Would they adjust blood types, etc, to match ? Is the transfer of the Heart Gnome (or Dwarf ?) the reason for memories and personal choices of the donor surfacing in the recipient ?

If there is an invasive life form, perhaps the 'Gnome Medics' could be asked to come and remove the Gnomes in that life form and take them to their rightful place to be Healed.

Gleanings - The Aura Files

On one of my lectures about Dowsing for a group of doctors, I had offered to carry out the following experiment: the patient stood at the centre of an audience, and some doctors with L-rods measured the borders of his biofield.

Previously, I explained to the patient that he/she should:
  1) Think of something extraneous,
  2) Mentally to abuse all by the most bad words,
  3) To pray.

Using L-rods, the doctors measured the borders of the biological field of the patient three times. Result of the first measurement: 1 metre; second: about 30 centimetres; third - 3 metres. The doctors were surprised at the results.   O

I am glad that Russian doctors are sufficiently open to even try the L rods; I think we would have to get Australian doctors drunk on Vodka before they would even consider using Dowsing.

I have been involved with similar experiments, but with some variations, particularly in teaching people how to voluntarily adjust the strength and depth of their bio-energy fields to suit particularly difficult to handle situations.

This technique is particularly useful when working in areas where contagious diseases are prevalent.

Again, the experiments and effectiveness of a person to learn to do this can be checked using Dowsing instruments.

The world that exists beyond traditional scientific acceptance is simply wonderful.   B

When I map Dowse, I suppose that I do imagine myself walking around the target site, 'being there' as it were. I have great problems thinking of myself 'split' - a bit here at home, and a bit somewhere else, possibly 200 miles away.

However, I have to admit that at the very least, I do imagine myself on the scene. Maybe we do have some form of 'contact' with a distant site.   J

Hinmm, to Dowse your own aura ? Yes there is a way, but it is kinda far out, but bear with me on this one.

Set a kitchen chair in the middle of the room. Just ask your aura to sit in the chair. Are you still there ? Now to measure an aura just use a pendulum or some other instrument.

Back away from the chair about 8ft with your pendulum in search motion; now as you walk forward toward the chair that your aura is sitting in you will find the edge of it about 5 - 6 ft out from the chair.

But unless you can teach some one else to find aura it would be almost impossible to check your aura while you are doing map Dowsing. The minute some one says any thing to you your aura comes back to you.

Don't forget to call your aura back when you are done. We do this in my classes.

We have some good looking gal come up to the front and stand near one corner of the room. Then 6 or 7 Dowsers come up and find the edge of her aura in a semicircle.

Once they find the edge I get her to ask her aura to go to the other corner. It is a very funny look on the Dowsers face when they can't find her aura any more. Then couple of them will go over to the other corner and there it is ! Nobody over there, but the aura is. Then she calls it back. Lots of laughs.

I got to thinking about that one night so when I got up the next morning I went into the den and ask my aura to 'go over there' and measured my aura, called my wife in there and she measured it also.

Thought I was nuts but she did find it. Surely you can find one more Dowser in the neighbourhood.

J's question of what would happen if you forgot to call your aura back to you made me do an experiment with my own aura.

I asked my aura to stay right here in my chair while I went to town to play cards this afternoon. Marta checked my aura before I left the chair and after I got in the other room. My aura was still in the office. I was gone for 2½ hrs and Marta checked the office when she got home before I did and my aura was still in the chair area.

She checked me when I got home and only the living aura was still with me.

We both came in the office and found my aura still right there in the area of my chair. It hadn't moved at bit. I sat down and Dowsed what would happen if I didn't call it back.

Pendulum says that it will return on it's own in less than 7 hours. I could feel no difference with or with out the extra aura. My card playing wasn't very good today. I don't think the lack of part of my aura was to blame.   Joe

About four weeks ago, my yoga teacher broke both ankle/foot on each leg falling off the LAST step of the studio stairs. Some people freaked out and thought she was 'pushed' (she was alone) and that negative thought forms and entities were responsible.

I Dowsed to ask if I needed protection, and got the answer NO. There were indeed residues of fear and pain in the stairwell 'resulting from the accident', but nothing that I needed protection from, and they needed simply to be cleared.

An interesting question - in an accident like this, could a person, in fear, shock and pain, leave part of their aura fractured off, for a brief time, that other people could feel ?   S

The earth is multi-dimensional, multi-levelled, so is nature, and so are we. I have been out of body and looked back at my body sleeping in bed. Well, let me re-phrase this, as it is actually a 'dual' state of consciousness.

I was aware of being in my body, feeling my heartbeat and my breathing, and I was 'also' consciously floating beside my body 'trying' to see it, (two of me) but I couldn't see it real well because of some flames of white fire that was surrounding it, about 2 feet out and going all around.

So I look around. I see someone floating beside me. Looks like a blobbly misshapen sphere or egg, mostly dark colours, ah, my brother is sleeping and wandering around unconscious. My younger sister comes into the room in her 'etheric' body, I can tell it's her because it looks like her and she's a soft grey-blue mist.

She was attracted to the room because of the bright blue living beam of conscious slanting blue light that was in the room, it 'woke her up'. So my brother is floating around in his astral body, my sister is 'walking' around in her etheric body, and I'm there in my whatever body, probably astral.

There's also mental body (and finer), but the world can't be seen real well from the mental body, it's all light and colour, very bright.

Each of these bodies extends from the physical within it's own level of dimensionality. If you have etheric vision, or sensitivity (we all do), then you will sense or see the etheric body. If you have astral vision capability (we all do, but not aware of it usually), then you will see the astral aura (body), etc.

Each of these bodies (auras) extends relatively further the more refined it is. For instance, the causal aura extends up to 30 feet or more in some people. It can actually extend huge distances in highly evolved people.

Since people usually are focused into a singular consciousness (there is also non-selfconscious consciousness !) they must go to sleep to enter another state (body) of consciousness, but the physical nervous system is usually not refined enough to register the finer realms so they are not 'aware' of it.

Projecting the consciousness 'out' of the body is the shifting/raising of awareness to a different 'body', (related to the 'raising of the Kundalini', as most 'out-of-body' experiences are the reflection upon nature of a naturally active Kundalini, and the resulting stimulation of the higher chakras/bodies.

The long and short of it is, each of these auras is the counterpart (body) of us in the corresponding level of nature.

Each of these bodies (auras) has it own way of perceiving and interacting with nature, and mostly very unfamiliar to us.

Imagine a baby trying to reach for the light on the ceiling and not understanding why he/she can't reach it.

That's what it's like, we have to learn these refined senses and interactions.   We can be conscious in one or more level simultaneously, and be in more than one location at once, but not on the same plane usually !

I didn't read this stuff - I 'woke up' when I was about 6 and spent most nights (and some days) 'touring' the world and beyond. This caused my family some real trauma so I learned to hide it. This kind of perception is not supported in society at large, it's generally considered as 'psychosis'.

After spending a lifetime of wondering how to 'evolve' people so they would 'wake up', I came to the conclusion that I can't. Each person has his/her own path and history, and karma. So I just figured out we should simply be kind to each other, and that's a mouthful. Let us all practice compassion.   J

Think of it in terms of Dowsing. There are those who use it to receive information only; and there are those who eventually learn how to turn it around and consciously broadcast with it.

Of course, we need to also realize that these processes both occur unconsciously, as well, albeit at a different level, and that we receive intuitive hits without actually having to Dowse for them, and that we are also able to send good thoughts to others though our very nature, again, without having to consciously pray for someone.

As energy beings, we are constantly acting as two-way radios; receiving and broadcasting. If one looks at this in terms of signal reception, as in Signal-to-Noise-Ratio (SNR), there are a lot of interesting parallels.   F

I have contended that the act of considering our self to be 'defensive, unavailable, and unreachable', involves the subconscious creation of an astral wall, or block, so to speak.

Not sure that I am correctly using the terms presented by J - I have never distinguished the difference between the finer bodies and tend to call them all astral.

I, too have done out of the body travelling while awake and by intent. I was not aware of my physical body and when I returned, I kind of slammed into my physical body again not really knowing what happened for a moment.

You ask: *"In an accident like this, could a person, in fear, shock and pain, leave part of their aura fractured off, for a brief time, that other people could feel?"*

My feeling is YES; we can leave some part of our energy in a place because of trauma, and site the group who travels into other realms to recover these lost part of yourself.

The other way people can feel that event is by being aware of the Akashic records which leaves us a vibrational record of the events that have occurred at a specific place.   E

In cases of any severe shock, such as an accident or learning of an unanticipated death of someone close, it is my belief a very real part of us gets left behind, perhaps to catch up to us at a later time. But in that interim period, I would think it is very necessary to call in extra energy to make up for the loss.   LN

My friend and I started a business, and studied and learned on our own, by reading, way beyond Dowsing reading and into Remote Viewing, quantum physics, etc.

Our observations are: We imprint everything we do; depending on our depth of emotion, etc, the deeper the imprint. Some imprints can last a very long time, even centuries.

Try checking an original oil painting, or oriental rug, for this imprint. You may find the imprint of the creator of the item, as well as of one or more owners that may have been deeply attached to it. This imprint can be 'tracked' by a Dowser that knows how to focus on it (by making the properly stated request).

People 'project' their thoughts all the time, especially someone planning to do something big in their life. Dowse the location of a friend planning the big 'getaway vacation' of the year/life, and you'll get their location at the vacation spot !

Our extensive reading has helped us to understand that all of seeable creation is really frequency based wave lengths, some of denser or looser density.

That includes us, our bodies and auras. In the frequency soup that we really are a part of, we are all one picture, one being, just each of us as a hair, toe, etc of the One.

Therefore, we are all connected to this frequency of life, and therefore we are able to access any part of it.

It is like tuning in a radio. As a Dowser we are learning to 'fine tune' our observations.

Part of this frequency of life is the unseen world, and if any of you have experienced sporadic Dowsing especially using rods, you need to be aware that with the magnetic field of the planet dropping, the 'film' between realms is becoming very thin indeed. You may be 'intercepted' by beings that are at a frequency that we can't see, but the rod can find. Some of these are positive, and some aren't.

Put your protections around any Dowsing area, room, etc, that you want your results to be as accurate as possible in.   LJ

I've noticed something when driving. I'll be driving along and suddenly experience a small shock of adrenaline, my heart speeds up and I am prompted to suddenly brake, grab the steering wheel more tightly and swerve to avoid something. A few feet further on I'll see a deer lying on the side of the road.

On other occasions I also experience somewhat the same reactions then further up the road I'll see someone pulled over being issued a speeding ticket.

This has happened so many times, I've developed a theory.

I believe a thought form has been left at the site and I am experiencing it as I drive through it. The strong emotions projected by the person who sees the deer or red flashing lights in his mirror is somehow leaving an imprint or an actual charge in a specific geographic location.

That thought form or charge dissipates fairly rapidly, maybe in two or three days there's nothing left.   I don't understand the mechanism. Maybe someone here does ?

Once I went into a house a friend of mine had just rented. It was a big old manor. I walked in the front door and felt the impression of a piano. It felt good. I walked toward where I felt the piano should be, wanting to see it, maybe play it.

I walked into a room, then into the other side of the room, then turned toward the source of the feeling. There was a blank wall, actually a small piano size alcove. I could feel the wall vibrating to the presence of the piano harp.

I turned to tell me wife that I thought a piano might have been in this location once, and then saw that in the side of the alcove there was a small open closet literally filled with music books and sheets for piano. That was enough validation for me !

It's a whole 'new' frontier for science, the word 'science' taken in it's most pure etymological basis, i.e., 'to know'.   J

I think J has hit the nail on the head - everyone projects a message of some sort, be it fear, love, anger, compassion or sorrow.

Whatever state of condition our soul is in, is in our aura. We as Dowsers have learned to gauge the depths and strength of that aura. Everyone has the ability to do that, but it is a gift that has been lost through generations of being taught and convinced that it is an evil talent.   A

This past week I took my daughter to a Dowser for a healing. In a nut shell it was determined there were 9 entities bound into her aura all of which were removed rather easily except for the last few.

The results were visible in that my daughter know something was really going on and became flushed when this happened.

The beginning dimensions of the aura were measured and noted.

The final dimension were also documented and showed a very symmetrical aura envelope. The long and short of it is that she is well now ! There were 9 entities that were removed in all.

No wonder why she had an elongated and displaced aura !

I found the process extremely interesting and very satisfying - and yet another example of how Dowsing can supplement the established medical system.

Believe me we have been through a tough few years dealing with a BAD addiction and all of the associated problems. Conventional medicine did not help heal my daughter at all but only put her to sleep.

Dowsing and Healing are a wonderful combination and for all of you who do these activities may I say it is appreciated.   BM

I found that Leadbeater has written some excellent books on Thought Forms, the Astral Plane, and the higher Devachanic Plane.

Some other interesting booklets were written by Swami Panchadasi in 1912 on the Human Aura and on the Astral World - these have been published by the Yoga Publication Society.

You may be able to download these as ebooks from:

http://www.gutenberg.org

- their catalogue of free downloads is absolutely unbeatable !

John Living

When other Life Forms come to Stay
It's Hard to Make them Go Away !

Influences of Entities

Let us now examine the effects that other life forms have upon a human being when they invade the various bodies.

Many people find that there are rather peculiar pains that seem to move around in their body - or within a certain group of their body parts, such as hip, thigh, knee, leg, ankle and foot.

Such pains are typical results of invasion by 'other dimensional life forms' of some description that have penetrated auric protection, invaded the patient, and taken residence in his body, often hiding in the muscle tissues. This may have happened when such auric protection was weak or damaged - as happens in surgery, or a serious accident.

Physicians find themselves unable to cure these pains, only giving medicines as pain killers or telling the patient that 'it is all in the mind' or just imagination.

I have suffered from such pains. One instance occurred around 1993, when I fell heavily on the ski-out at Sunshine, near Banff in Alberta - and I was a pretty good skier, accustomed to far more difficult ski slopes. I could not lift my right arm even to shave for over a year - and normally my physical problems heal very quickly.

Conversing with the life form involved, using my 'Message Chart', I understand that it was the soul of a baby girl that had been aborted, and had now found a good home (for her, not me !). It took 12 years for me to be free of her influence.

Over the years I have tried many different ways of overcoming these intrusions - some with considerable (but not complete) success. It also seems that it is easier for an invader to gain access than to leave ! They need help to get out again.

'Remarkable Healings'

In her book of the above name, Dr Shakuntala Modi, MD, tells of her experiences as a psychiatrist using hypnotherapy, giving examples of the way her clients described problems and how these were overcome.

Her background is that of structured western medicine, her approach being that all problems exist in the physical body - but she extends her investigations into the Soul.

She does not pretend to be clairvoyant, and it seems that she has no understanding of auras and thought forms. At one point she mentions auras, but in a somewhat disparaging way. The recurring theme in possession and interference is that of 'Satan and his Demons'.

Heaven Divided

Some of her reports that include regression to the start of Soul life tell how 'God' and Lucifer parted company - that there was a rebellion in Heaven, and Lucifer left to control his own domain, taking many angels with him.

She reports that many good angels were tricked into becoming under the control of Lucifer, and how these were then tortured in various ways under the direction of a 'black cloaked and masked being' that was called Satan.

These tortured angels were given bad jobs, in hurting and interfering with Humans and Souls, and warned that if they did not do so or failed in their allotted tasks they would be returned to Satan and given more torture. From this point on, the possessing entities did not mention Lucifer, but Satan.

This is a common belief in many religions - that Lucifer and Satan are different names for the same Being. This belief seems to be false; in fact Satan is also called Isis using the Egyptian terminology, and has the repute of being a great loving and healing Being.

It is possible that the black cloaked figure was Lucifer or one of his cohorts - and that the use of Satan's name was to deter the Angels and Souls from going direct to Isis/Satan and being Healed.

Additionally all really bad stuff has been blamed on Satan/Isis in most religions. This is similar to the way that Hitler blamed all problems on the Jews !

Some years ago I thought to take battle against Satan, who I perceived as the leader of the 'satanic forces'. I found, to my amazement, that Satan was a female, a Goddess, full of genuine Love. The so-called 'satanic forces' were the dark forces controlled by Lucifer and his cohorts.

'I Am' and 'I Not'

Humans have a memory of a 'Good God' called 'I Am' - 'the Holy Creator of All That Is, in All Times, in All Dimensions'. I have been finding that there was also 'I Not' - a destructive influence, that infested Lucifer (who seems to have been in charge of 'All Light') and caused a rebellion against 'I Am'.

It is my understanding that after the rebellion in Heaven, the 'I Not' / Lucifer crowd tricked 'I Am' and engineered that he be killed, so that Lucifer has been in command since that time - ruling a 'bad god system' that has caused pain and suffering to all life forms, especially to and by humans.

It may be that when 'I Am' was killed various elementals saved parts of him, and that the rest of his body fragmented. Perhaps this fragmentation was similar to the fragmentation of Soul parts as observed by Shamans, occurring under extreme trauma.

It is possible that these fragments became the 'Higher Selves' of humans, and that further fragmentation of these 'Higher Selves' formed Souls - this conforms to the observation 'As Above, So Below'. If this is so, then human beings are fragments of 'I Am'.

Even if this is not the case, the energy of 'The Creator' is in all human beings - and in all other life forms. I believe that this energy is the energy of 'True Holy Love, Namaste'.

The Holographic Universe

If the universe is holographic, whereby each part has a 'picture' of the whole, then the 'God Energy' or 'God Essence' in each human contains the overall picture of 'I Am'.

When a coherent laser-like light passes through the pieces a three dimensional image appears. The more small holographic pieces that are combined in illumination, the greater definition of the picture.

There is a problem, however - so many of these pieces in Souls have become infested by the dark forces that the overall picture is not clear and is often distorted.

This may be the reason for various religious groups trying to do their best, but fighting other groups that have slightly differing viewpoints - and many of these are differences in moralistic applications, procedures, and the labeling of higher level Beings.

Problems in Heaven

Other reports from the Soul level tell of many problems in Heaven. The clearing of memories of past life in a Soul is but one result; misuse of Karma and of Soul Contracts has been having a most traumatic effect on Souls and Human Beings.

It seems that a group of God Beings and Angels remained who are committed to fight against Lucifer and his cohorts - they have been operating similar to the French resistance movement against the Nazi occupation, and have given help as best they could to those who called for their assistance.

The 'bad god system' may be the reason that Angelic help has to be requested - that the Angels have been prevented from acting on their own initiative to give help, the excuse being that they cannot interfere with the 'free will' of humans.

This rule does not seem to apply to the dark forces, who exercise their own free will to interfere with humans and cause trouble !

Results of Hypnotherapy

Dr Shakuntala Modi regresses her clients using hypnosis to identify the causes of problems. She reports that her clients see 'black blobs' at places of their body associated with problems, and that most are coming from traumatic experiences in both present and past lives.

These 'black blobs' are further identified as 'Soul Fragments' - whereby a portion of the Soul split away due to the intense trauma, often to safeguard the rest of the Soul. They are still 'of light' but have become covered with a 'not good' gooey/sticky substance.

Communication is established with the fragment, its identity and the nature of the trauma are determined, and then Angelic help is requested to remove all the dark gooey muck (the 'Demons'), Heal the fragment, and return it to its rightful place.

Sometimes re-assurance is needed to help the fragment return - this is especially so with fragmentation that occurred during the present life, and is similar to the reports from Shamans who use 'Soul Retrieval' techniques.

Most of the traumatic experiences from past lives occurred at death. In discussion with these fragments, they tell that they await the return of the Soul in a reincarnation, and attach themselves to it.

Such fragments seem to have little memory other than of the situation leading to death, and of death itself.

The case histories presented in Dr Modi's book tell that Healing of both emotional and physical problems occur - yet again indicating that the causes of many illnesses in the physical body have non-physical causes.

Samskara

This is the term used by Samuel Sagan, M.D., of the Clairvision School in Australia (www.clairvision.org) for 'Soul Fragments' that invade humans - not always at the level of possession, but still causing problems.

Dr Sagan, MD, has explained these very well in his book 'Entity Possession' published by Destiny Books, ISBN 0-89281-612-0. It has an alternative title 'Entities: Parasites of the Body of Energy'.

Dr Sagan took a considerable time working with patients to discover their problems when he started his work, but was able to achieve substantial Healing in his patients in only a few sessions using a non-standard technique that he developed.

In his work, patients are taken in meditation to view the life form involved - and most are able to do this, but it takes some time. It helps if the person working with the patient, a 'connector', who is best a clairvoyant, can give hints as to what can be seen. This is especially so if the patient lacks any clairvoyance - or this Soul sense has been blocked.

The 'connector', not necessarily medically trained, helps the patient relax and concentrate on their body, to 'feel' any problems. The connector then guides the patient by asking questions to help the patient fully understand the cause of the problem, by 'feeling' emotions attached.

This 'feeling' is the outcome of placing one's awareness on the problem - without any hypnosis or drugs, being solely guided by non-leading questions asked by the connector.

In many cases 'black blobs' are described similar to those reported by Dr Modi's patients. There is one difference, however - Dr Sagan is clairvoyant, can see these entities in detail, and is fully aware of the metaphysical world in which they operate.

Dr Sagan's book 'Awakening the Third Eye' (published by Clairvision, ISBN 0-9586700-5-6) is probably the best introduction to 'Soul Sight' that has ever been written. The ability to see clairvoyantly is critical to being an accomplished 'connector' - to be able to 'see' the entities involved.

Although trained in the western medical system, Dr Sagan pays great heed to the knowledge of Chinese and Indian Healers - which is based on experience extending over thousands of years.

Problems at Death

Dr Sagan describes the human being as having physical, etheric, astral, and Spiritual bodies. During sleep, the astral-Spiritual bodies go wandering in the higher dimensions, linked to the physical-etheric bodies by a silver cord - as described by many other mystics.

He uses these simple linkages in describing his methods, without going into the demarcation of the astral-Spiritual bodies into those of the higher dimensions.

Dr Sagan tells that when death occurs, the silver cord breaks. The conscious human being is in the astral-Spiritual body, and may not be aware of death - and usually stays around the physical-etheric body for a few days.

The etheric body, now without its silver cord 'life-link', starts to decompose and return to the etheric layers of the earth, while the physical body starts to rot as it loses the protection of the etheric body.

If death was traumatic, then a fragment of the astral-Spiritual body could be split off. The rest of the astral-Spiritual body seems to go through the astral world, shedding more fragments, until the 'core essence' of the Soul reaches Heaven, probably after passage through worlds above the astral. Dr Sagan calls these fragments 'Samskaras'.

In some cases the Soul, residing in its astral-Spiritual body, remains earth-bound for various reasons - good and not so good. Both Modi and Sagan consider that it may contain its own set of fragments accumulated from immediate and previous past lives.

It so seems that such Souls and fragments of Souls attach themselves to family members and/or other people - especially those who have similar likes and dislikes. These Samskara may well take refuge in a person attending the funeral (small children are very vulnerable) or in a relative - especially if they feel a close connection.

A point is made that black clothes worn at funerals seem to attract Samskara; this is a western practice, unlike eastern cultures where white garments are worn.

Sometimes this may include an attempt to impose their will on the relative to teach a lesson - this may be tied into religion, where the relative is perceived as needing 'encouragement' to follow the beliefs of the Samskara.

The fragments may frequent places where they can meet suitable people, such as at bars and hospitals; hospitals in particular can be most dangerous places. When a person has low vitality, and especially when drugs and anesthetics cause the Soul to leave the physical-etheric body, it is easy for another life form, such as a fragment, to gain entry. And deaths that occur in hospitals do leave many Souls and fragments seeking another home.

Even if such a fragment or Soul is not malicious, even if having beneficial intent, they do drain your life-force and energy, and usually imprint their own desires and behaviour on the host - which may be contrary to those of the host.

A special case is that of miscarriages and abortions; although the physical body may leave the mother, the etheric (and perhaps the astral-Spiritual body or even the complete Soul) may remain - and if so, cause major problems for the mother.

When a further baby is conceived, there may well be conflict between the previous and incoming Soul - and if there is also a gender difference, the result may be a baby that grows to be 'gay'.

Thus such mixed gender may well occur 'naturally' to a person - and any effort to remove such a fragment or Soul may lead to far greater problems than are intended to be solved. Note that this potential cause of mixed gender is not mentioned by Sagan or by Modi.

Dr Sagan advises that all operating rooms should be 'cleared of bad energies' and that special energetic clearing of the mother should be undertaken whenever a baby is conceived but not born alive.

Nature of Fragments

In the many case studies that Drs Sagan and Modi present, it is apparent that all the various fragments seek recognition. For example, a fragment from a traumatic death seeks to rejoin the rest of the Soul, cannot get into Heaven (for whatever reason), and awaits return of the Soul in reincarnation.

When it finds its reincarnating Soul, it attaches itself; but all its awareness is of the trauma that occurred. So it endeavours to replay the traumatic experience in the hope that the Soul will recognize it, give it Healing, and help it to rejoin.

The problem here is that the conscious Soul has little or no memory of any past life - any such memory that does exist lies in the domain of the sub-conscious, and it seems that various impediments have been placed (by the 'bad god system' of the 'dark forces') to prevent such Healing, since the dark forces seem to thrive on unhealthy emotions - and do all that they can to create more.

Dr Sagan points out that when a fragment is seeking its reincarnating Soul it is comparing vibrational patterns. If Souls are themselves fragments of a 'Higher Self' then other Soul fragments of the Higher Self may have the same vibrational pattern.

So it may be that the past life expressed by the fragment was not experienced by the host Soul, but by another Soul in the same group or family. This can explain the instances when a person recalls more than one life during the same time period.

Do not assume that the traumatic circumstances were experienced by the particular Soul; the intent is to Heal the fragment (or other form of life) so that it can have a good life in its correct place - and also, perchance, to be free of its attention and accompanying hurts !

The 'Demons'

The Healing intent should also apply to the 'Demons'. In all my work I have found that each and every life form wants to have a good life. The life forms in a demon were all originally good, but as Dr Modi explains, often have been tricked by the dark forces.

In my discussions with them, they were forced to do a bad job by threats against themselves, their friends, or their families. In many cases control devices were implanted or given as gifts, badges, and reward tokens - and these also need to be removed and Healed.

Dr Modi has found a most effective way to implement such Healing - call on the help of the Angelic Forces. It may be best to also ask the help of 'The System' - which has the knowledge of which specialists should be giving the Healing, and has the ability to call these guys into action.

Misuse in the Black Arts

Since other life forms in the physical world also have a Soul (or similar energy level) in the astral plane, these may seek a home in another physical life form (including human) or even be directed there with malevolent intent by a person using 'black arts'.

In such cases, the sender will usually lie to these Samskara, pretending that they are being given a job having 'good intent' - when the opposite is true. This may be the basis of some strong 'spells' that operate at a different level than thought forms - although having some similar characteristics.

When a high level 'not good' entity is involved, or even the Spirit of an animal mis-used by a 'medicine man', constraints may have been placed on the smaller life forms within the invader to enforce negativity; if so, then these constraints must be removed so that all life forms can be Healed.

In many cases an effigy is used, such as a wax model, a photograph, or a stuffed toy. Part of the remedy includes Healing all included in such an effigy, and the placement of protection around it to prevent future mis-use - and this may have to be repeated from time to time, in case the mis-user tries to interfere with such protection. Paper Radionics machine may be most helpful in this work.

I had a problem with a Cree Indian Medicine Man - who, unknown to me, had a history of using 'bad medicine'. In a 'Clairvision' meditation I was able to see him making a doll (teddy bear ?) to represent me, putting a pipe that I had given to him in the mouth of the teddy bear, and casting various spells.

It seems that he used 'shape shifting' techniques to persuade the teddy bear that he was me, and that I was him - the intent being that if I sent any hurting thought forms back to him, they would instead come to me !

He also mis-used animal Spirits, by torturing and then killing animals, pretending that he was me, and getting the help of the animal Spirits to obtain revenge against me. All very complicated again, and done with great ceremony.

I discovered 3 instances of deceased family members who had invaded my body - not always with good intent.

The 'Real Nasties'

Unfortunately real 'bad guys' do exist. The key to dealing with them is to know that each and every Being is made of smaller teams and families of even smaller Beings, until you get to the smallest of all, the 'Lights'.

All these smaller groups all want to have a good life - and to help all others like them to have a good life, with plenty of Love, but they are ruled by the leader of the Being - in the same way that a dictator rules. They believe that they are 'tied' to that Being, and must accept such ruling.

I have found that the most effective way of dealing with 'the nasties' is to get these small guys to leave them and come into 'The Light', to join the 'Force for Good'.

I send them THLN, tell them I love them - but do not like their behaviour; this is the way that good parents handle mischievous children. In a parent-child situation it helps further to ask them *"What is the best way that you could behave in these circumstances ?"* so that they themselves gain confidence in making their own decisions.

So I then speak to all the Lights, and tell them that the Love sent to them has freed them, and that they are now able to leave the 'not so good' being, and ask them to go and be Healed.

I then send more THLN to all who remain, ask *"Do you like to hurt others, or Love to have a good life ?"*, and tell them *"Judge yourselves now"*. The overall result is that the 'Force for Good' gains extra recruits, and 'the nasties' lose their power.

Other 'Entities'

Sagan reports instances of life forms that have no known correspondence in the physical world. Shamanic wisdom is that although the shape may look terrible to you, so that you tend to have fear, when you show your recognition of it as a fellow life form and send it your Love, your perception of the shape may change so that it appears beautiful - you overcome the tendency to be afraid.

Perhaps the perception is generated in your own mind - and your mind may not have a full understanding of the life form encountered.

Some people have a great fear of bacteria - not realizing that their bodies (and especially their digestive system) relies on friendly bacteria. Yes, some bacteria can be damaging - usually because they are in the wrong place; certain bacteria do a great job in digesting a garbage pile - but these same bacteria can cause problems with your health if they enter your own system.

Viruses are life forms that may have been formed as Healers - to engineer re-growth of damaged body parts. It is possible that their assigned job was changed by a 'bad god system' to cause illness and disease.

Background of the Thought World

In most metaphysical understanding, thoughts are real in the level that they exist. If an energy, a team, or a family of Lights is told that something has happened, then this 'Is So' - a form of hypnotism.

Hence if the teams forming constraints are told that they are 'stuck' in that position due to something, then they belief it to be so - and it 'Is So'. It could also be that in some cases the belief of a constraint is effective, even if no such actual constraint exists.

It also follows that any constraints that have been imposed are also made of Lights, operating at a lower 'family / team' level than those that they constrain.

Since (in my understanding) 'All that Is' is made of 'Lights' doing forming families and teams to make various dances at different speeds, we can communicate with them - we are 'All the Same'.

This is the key to working with Samskara: communicating with them to find who they are, their purpose, if they were sent by others (if so, full details about the senders), and asking about their shape, and their colour. Show interest, develop rapport.

Ask what do they really want for themselves - because helping them to achieve their desire will certainly be most important in sending them 'on their way'. Show you care about them - even if you have suffered from them !

Negotiations

The key to all negotiations is to have respect for others involved, to be aware of their needs, and to be prepared to put all your effort into finding a win-win solution - and to make contact so that negotiations can be started.

This can be achieved by concentrating one's awareness on the hurting that is felt - especially to 'feel' the hurt with as many senses as possible. Even if one lacks clairvoyant sight, one can place one's awareness on the pain - since that is how one recognizes that the pain exists.

It is important that one's attitude is one of calm, sympathetic inquiry without any antagonism - which would immediately raise another barrier to successful negotiation.

Have respect for another life form - even if it is causing you trouble ! Your intent is to help it to be Healed and sent to its rightful place.

Although you may not be aware of the life form that is causing the problem, be assured that the life form is fully aware of your intent and attitudes ! Your intent to be helpful and Heal is known - and if your intent differs, negotiations may be blocked.

It seems that it is necessary to deal with one particular cause of hurt at any one time - give recognition; open negotiation; ask if those in the cause would like to have a good life, to be with their friends and those that they love; and then ask them to be taken away to be Healed and sent to their rightful place.

'Blanket Healing' does not seem to be effective in many cases - perhaps because each individual involved wants recognition, and must agree to be Healed. Without such agreement the Angelic Forces may not be able to act.

Dr Sagan's approach seems ideal - but in fact a minimum amount of guided visualization is used. So much emphasis is placed on 'seeing the cause' that if a patient is blocked from such sight, extra guidance is needed to steer the patient to the problem. This 'zero-ing in' helps the patient to be better able to 'feel' the cause of the problem - and feeling may be better than sight in the negotiations.

Hypnosis may be a good method of overcoming such blockages; perhaps it is a matter of labeling - since in all cases the connector/ hypnotist is acting as an assistant to help the patient to enter a relaxed state of mind, to be aware of the life forms involved in the problem, to ask the needed questions to open negotiations, to find what the life form truly seeks, and help it to participate in a win-win solution.

'Let the Search Begin !'

Dr Sagan's suggestions are similar to those propounded by Vernon Woolf in his book 'Holodynamics' (published by Harbinger House, ISBN 0-943173-33-7) which deals with Thought Forms - a composite structure from the writings of both experts is:

1. Relax

Be completely relaxed - as in meditation; go to your 'special place' if you have one, or imagine that you are in surroundings that are totally serene and safe.

This may be the time to ask assistance from your Angels and Guides, to help you to be physically and mentally prepared for the work in hand, and to help you in that work.

Remember that your attitude must be to make friends with all involved in the problem, with the intent of helping them to have a better life - to operate for the benefit of all.

It is possible that the Guides that you now have are not sufficiently advanced to help you as needed - so it is best to ask 'The System' to assign to you special Guides and Angelic Beings who are experienced with similar problems and competent with such work.

- Do you have a Guide who will help you with your problems ?
- Is this Guide 'In the Light' ?
- Is this Guide willing to help for the benefit of all ?
- Are you now co-operating with your Guide to seek a win-win solution to your problems ?

2. Focus on the Problem

Place your awareness on the problem, be it a pain, a habit, or a set of circumstances. Concentrate on being 'one with the problem', getting the deepest possible connection.

If the problem is not active at this moment, go in your memory to when it was operating.

Let your awareness wander where it wants to go, seeking the cause - not being confined to the effects. Do not try to have any control - that would be coming from your rational mind, and all this work must be done by your intuitive mind for success. Your Heart is the key to having Intuition and Compassion, and in linking with your Guides.

- What is the problem ? . . . What is your part of the problem ?
- Are you prepared to put all your effort into solving your part ?

3. Use your Sense of Feeling

Without trying to visualize anything at the start, just use your awareness to feel for the cause of the problem.

Can you smell, taste, or feel the cause ?
* Can you describe the smell . . . taste ?
* Does it feel large or small ? ... heavy or light ?
* Does it feel old or young ?
* Does it have any shape ? . . . any colour ?

Such neutral questions help you to 'get in touch' with the cause - and may find that you 'know' much more about it, even becoming aware of the traumatic circumstances in which it was formed.

Questions about country or time of occurrence, or even gender at that time, should be avoided at the start of negotiations - but may be asked when a rapport has been established.

<u>4. Establish a Friendly Relationship</u>

Acknowledge that all involved in the problem are life forms, that they are doing their best in the job assigned to them, and thank them for all their work, and for the help that you have received.

Remember that these guys are operating in or around your mind - they know you better than you know them, so if you lie to them or are not honest with them, negotiations are unlikely to lead to a satisfactory outcome.

Their ability for intelligent thought may be very low - probably at the level of a very young child - so keep things simple !
* Do you accept my gratitude for the help that you give me ?
* Will you now communicate with me as your friend ?
* What is the true intent of your actions ?
* What do you want for yourself ?
* If you continue with your actions what will you finally get ?
* What would it feel like to have what you really want ?

Sometimes the answer may not seem very friendly - *"I Hate You !", I want to kill you !"* or similar. Remember that this may be based on misunderstandings or even untruths.

Further delving will eventually uncover a positive/beneficial intent - so keep at the questioning until this is found. Often the intent may be very good, but the way of achieving this be very immature.

"So, if you hate me so much and want to kill me, what will you <u>finally</u> get from that ?" - "Peace !".

5. The Best Win-Win Solution

a. Thought Forms: unless there is some sort of pain that moves the cause may be a thought form - so handle it with Love and find an alternative job for it, as already described in the 'Healing Overview'.

If we classify 'entities' as life forms that are not intrinsic to the host, then we include thoughts that are sent by one being to another; if these are reinforced by multiple similar thoughts, a 'thought form' may be made.

A person can create his or her own thought forms, but usually thoughts sent by others are more effective in creating a thought form - coming from others it seems to have 'more weight'. The conscious remembering of such thoughts, and of the feelings and emotions so generated, gives extra weight to them.

The stronger the attached emotion the greater the power attached to the thought form; whether the emotion is good or not so good does not matter, only its strength is important in establishing power.

They have the intent to be helpful, but the mode of action may be outdated (as when formed from instructions given to a baby by its parent), may be mistaken (as when you created them due to misunderstandings of what you perceived), or may be erroneous (as when sent by another with intent to hurt - but disguised as intent 'to teach a lesson').

These thought forms have an effect on all your thinking actions (and automatic re-actions) which have any similarity to themselves. Finding them is relatively easy, since all you have to do is generate a similar thought so they become operative.

b. Other Life Forms: You may have recollections of an incident that started the problem - something you did, or a past-live happening (which may not be yours !). This is part of the acknowledgement that is often sought by life forms that are involved in such problems..

The cause may be deeper, such as a curse on you or on occupiers of the land, or interference from other dimensional Beings or from dark forces.

Ceremony to Free Invading Life Forms

I asked for advice and help from 'The System'; I opened dialogue using my 'Message Chart' and was given instructions on how to proceed - which follow. It is written for yourself - but you can change the context to be effective for another person; if so, endeavour to get them to join in all Blessing and giving of Thanks, Gratitude, and Love.

It is most important that your attitude is one of love to all who cause problems - like a parent: you love your children, but do not like their behaviour; you seek to help them have a good life in the future.

In all this ceremony use your Pendulum spinning clockwise over your 'other' hand (as your 'Handy Chart') to manifest the current part of the ceremony; it may make a number of circuits to deal with various aspects; wait until it stops completely before proceeding.

You can, if you wish, check with your 'Handy Chart' the percentage effectiveness of any stage involved.

"I open in 'True Holy Love, Namaste' (THLN), with that Love of Truth, and with Good Intent."

"I Bless with THLN, Blessing 995, and Healing 997 'The System' and all Life Forms who help in this ceremony."

"I ask 'The System' for help to free all Life forms that are within [your] being and causing interference - including pains, hurts, suffering, disease, and ill health."

"I ask 'The System' are you able to so help ?", if YES, *"I ask 'The System' are you willing to so help now ?"* - if either is NO, ask 'The System' for advice as to further action (which may involve overcoming anger, greed, etc., or the need to forgive). If YES to both:

Tune into the invader (by thinking of it - and the interference caused); *"I send THLN to all Life Forms in your Being; this ceremony will not hurt any of you; it will set you free so that you will have a good life in the future."*

Next dialogue with the invader (by clairaudience, your Message Chart, or other means) to discover the identity of the invader, what job it has been given, the reason for the job (its purpose), who gave that job - and was it given in THLN, in Truth, and with Good Intent ?

Usually the invader will not have checked this last aspect - so tell the invader that you will do this check now on behalf of the invader.

"I ask 'The System' to link me to the sender; I send THLN to the sender, and ask if the interference was sent with True Holy Love, Namaste, with Truth, and with Good Intent ?"

The usual answer is NO !

"I Bless with THLN, Blessing 995, and Healing 997 all Life Forms that are within the total Being of [myself] and others who are sending, causing, or giving this interference.   As in all Heavens you are now free of all hypnosis".

"Light dissolvers are now sent to each and every part of your Beings to dissolve all devices, all bindings and all constraints so that you are now free; you will now open your heads, open your mouths, release all hooks, release all cords, and be free; Angelic Beings will now take you to be Healed, and be in the Light" - repeat this twice more.

"I request 'The System' to scramble the vibrational patterns and energies of all that have failed to obey this instruction or fail to be so dissolved and to transmute them to be beneficial in all aspects".

"We now go back in time to before any such interference was sent to [me]".

"I Bless with THLN, Blessing 995, and Healing 997 all Life Forms that have sent interference or are in any way involved with such sending to [me] in all or any 'nows' or 'times' and ask that they now be Healed with THLN."

"I Bless with THLN, Blessing 995, and Healing 997 all Life Forms who are involved in Healing the Life Forms that have sent interference to [me]."

"I request 'The System' to take all needed action to restore [my] Health to the level that existed before such interference was manifest or better, so that my Health will now be perfectly good in all ways and in all aspects, including to eliminate all cellular and other memory of hurts and pains."

"I Bless with THLN, Blessing 995, and Healing 997 all Life Forms who are involved in Healing [me] Good in all Good Ways, and send you the Light, Energy, and Blessing of my Heart with my Thanks, Gratitude, and Love."

"I request 'The System' to place all needed protection to prevent these or any other forms of interference from being sent, penetrating my being, or causing hurts, pains, or suffering to [me], to be effective in all ways, in all aspects, in all planes of existence, in all dimensions, in all domains, in all times, and in all nows."

"I Bless with THLN, Blessing 995, and Healing 997 all Life Forms who are involved in protecting and guarding [me], and send you the Light, Energy, and Blessing of my Heart with my Thanks, Gratitude, and Love."

You may care to check if this has now been manifested, the degree of effectiveness, any time needed for completion, and if any further ceremony or work is needed.

Remember that you may have dialogued with but one of perhaps a number of Life Forms - you may need to work with others that have invaded the Being.

You may find this effective in overcoming possession, as an exorcism ceremony - it seems to deal with a deeper level of energy than most other ceremonies.

Sometimes attacks are made on possessions such as our car or computer - this may also be used to negate such attacks and prevent their re-occurrence. But it is not meant to be used for normal problems or lack of care - and you must ask permission first!

Vivaxis: Life Links to Birth Places

Vivaxis was the name given in the 1960's by Frances Nixon and Bessie O'Connor, of British Columbia, to an energy they discovered. The name is a conjunction of 'viva' meaning life and 'axis' to describe the place where things join together. They found that when a person was born, a seed sprouted, or even a line was drawn, an energy link was created to the place where this happened. They believed that it was a 'magnetic effect'.

'Magnetism' has been applied to many things - such as animal magnetism and Mesmerism (now called hypnosis). This stems from the past, when magnetism and electricity (1840 definition: 'the energy of the Goddess Electra') were not well understood.

However Turenne, investigating unknown (or 'occult', meaning 'hidden or not understood') forces for the French Military in the 1890's, did discover that there is a metaphysical magnetic effect. It is at a right angle to the physical magnetic field and can be found by Dowsing on metallic magnets, as well as on 'non-magnetic' items.

Bessie and Frances, during their experiments, unknowingly confirmed the previous discoveries made by Turenne.

One major problem with their approach, and with Judy Jacka's continuation of their efforts, is that almost everything that they found they linked to Vivaxis, like horses wearing blinkers !

So in reading their books be most careful to understand that many of their discoveries of non-physical methods and effects, although valid and interesting, have zilch to do with Vivaxis.

How Thoughts Travel

Perhaps it is easier to understand Vivaxis by considering the movements of thoughts; they travel at many times the speed of physical light, and go where you send them by thinking of a person, plant, or place; since people move around, the thoughts have to find the present location of a person.

So a possible explanation for Vivaxis is that it is the location of records of the person or other life form; when you meet a person you store their ID code, including their Vivaxis - at a place near where they were born.

When you think about a life form, you send a thought to their Vivaxis, retrieve their current location, and the thought then goes to the life form. Further communication is then direct.

Since all matter is understood to have life and intelligence, when we link to something we can also determine its place of birth.

This was confirmed by a series of experiments conducted independently by William Wilks of Mayne Island, BC, after studying the works of Frances and Bessie. He was able to find where a carrot was grown, and the place where certain rocks were formed before being displaced by earth movements.

All of these experimenters had not been trained as Dowsers, but developed their own Dowsing tools - and used them in ways similar to most other people trained as Dowsers. And they all found out other new facts !

They showed that the line of communication taken by a thought to go to its destination depended on whether you were above the destination (go directly) or below (go in the opposite direction, travelling right around the earth, taking the long route).

They tell how the thought travels horizontally from the vicinity of the pineal gland until it is directly over its destination, and then drops vertically - this if traveling direct.

If below, it is possible that the thought rises first before starting its journey. They also showed that a block of salt, when put in the path, blocked such travel. These experiments were done locally - perhaps if a mountain range was in the way they would rise above the peaks.

Cellular Alignment

The alignment of cells in our body seems to be in harmony with our Vivaxis. The sub-atomic particles in cells spin about an axis - including to have a wobble like our earth. It seems this axis of rotation is aligned to (or works in sympathy with) that of our place of birth.

This spinning may be in harmony with intergalactic influences - which would also affect the planets in our solar system. If so, this would help explain how astrology (which uses our time and place of birth) can predict our progress in life.

X-rays, when given to a part of a body, 'overwrite' the Vivaxis of that part, so it is not now in harmony with the rest of the body.

Any other strong energy system may well have similar effects - such as is found with Electro-Magnetic Forces (EMF) and the radiations of energies from the earth due to water veins and the Curry Grid.

Bessie and Francis developed a complicated system of locating the genuine Vivaxis of the person, walking in a 'military manner' towards and away from that point, and hitting the affected part to cause re-alignment.

They quote many instances of how people were cured of very serious diseases, including multiple schlerosis and damage caused to a child by a mother being X-rayed while pregnant.

There is no doubt that they had found a most important link between X-rays and future health, and that the methods used were effective in curing the cause of the problem.

It is certain that X-rays have an effect on those cells in the body that are X-rayed. But what, exactly, is this effect ? How does it work ?

Being an Engineer I like to get to understand the mechanics involved, so that I am better able to suggest possible solutions, consider improvements to existing techniques, and find new ways to use the information obtained. And I was stuck !

Can Astrological Influences be Validated ?

Then I heard a talk by Sira Beaumayne at the Canadian Society of Dowsers Annual Convention 2000; she was talking about 'Astrological Psychology', in which I have very little interest.

But her approach was different ! She likened all the activity in our cells to that of the solar system, and suggested that we were affected by the places of planets, etc., in relation to us - because it had an effect on the rotation within the cells, on the alignment of the axes of rotation of the parts within the cells, just as if they were planets.

This new concept not only helped me to give more respect to astrology, but gave a clue to the X-ray problem.

Perhaps when a cell was given an X-ray, or subjected to any similar intense energy, the axis of rotation would be changed.

And Frances had mentioned in her book that one lady, born in Winnipeg, had her main Vivaxis directed to that city, and the X-rayed part to a completely different place where the X-ray was given.

Dowsing and Vivaxis

Now we know that not only had the ladies not been trained as Dowsers, but also that the Dowsers of that day did not have all the knowledge that we have - the Internet helps spread knowledge and ideas, many more books have been published, and Dowsing societies are more active, with some excellent teachers.

In Frances Nixon's book 'Born to be Magnetic' Vol 1 she mentions one of her first young instructors, Brian Cole. After attending the Canadian Society of Questers (CSQ) convention in 100 Mile House, BC, I visited Brian and his wife, Wenda, in their home on the Sunshine Coast, and picked their brains.

I had not realized before that Brian and Wenda had both been involved with 'Therapeutic Touch' and Radionics - and that Brian had been one of the instigators in getting the first Dowsing society formed in Canada - the CSQ.

Since talking with Brian and Wenda Cole I have used the technique that they recommend - with outstanding results. At the recent workshops in Red Deer and in The Pas the participants reported improved vitality - some were able to see auras for the first time.

King Cole's Technique

You can ask your Bobber (in 'Find' mode) to locate your Vivaxis, use your Pendulum (remembering to ask if the 'to' or 'fro' swing is the needed direction), or an 'L' rod.

If you use an 'L' rod. be sure to complete a full circle in 'Find' mode, since initially it may point to one of the 90° sub-directions; when your 'L' rod 'sticks' to one direction after a complete circle, it will probably be your Vivaxis.

You should stand upright - head held high, like a soldier on parade - facing into your Vivaxis, and take two to four deep breaths.

Then turn 90° clockwise and repeat; another turn and repeat; and yet again.

Now turn again (back into your Vivaxis) and repeat this whole procedure - but turning anti-clockwise until you return into your Vivaxis.

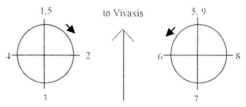

Order of movement when doing Vivaxis 'ceremony'
Face into the direction indicated.

Your hands are energy transmitters, so when you complete the Vivaxis turns, coming back to the starting point, then hold your hands about a foot away from your ears and send 'True Holy Love' to all parts of your Being

Can Dowsing make Corrections ?

Bessie and Francis probably knew that Dowsers could locate water veins and site wells. But did they know that a Dowser, by 'banging a stake' or just using the 'Power of Thought', could move a water vein into a well ?

I thought, *"If I can move a water vein that is not part of me and is often quite distant, then surely I can get all the cells in my own body to re-align themselves - to make sure that their axes of rotation were all in harmony with that of the 'master cell', probably in my pineal gland !"* And my Dowsing indicated that this was so - except, of course, that I was not doing the moving, but just asking that the 'Force for Good' for their help in getting it moved.

More Meridians

Bessie and Francis discovered much about our bodies, even about 'brain receptors' and paths taken by 'pseudo-meridians' outside our physical bodies.

In the understanding of Chinese Healing the various meridians start and end at certain places, and have treatment points along the meridians.

Perhaps they do not 'end' - but connect to similar meridians in our auric bodies. The 'brain receptors' that they located are in similar positions to the points known in Acupuncture.

Mike's Story

Mike was only five years old at the time when a bullet from a .38 caliber pistol. held in the hands of a six-year-old boy, pierced through his upper torso and through his upheld left hand.

For many gruelling months the small boy balanced between life and death but as time went on life began to return to his paralyzed arms.

However, from the waist down Mike remained paralyzed and at the age of fourteen years he had neither movement nor feeling in either leg.

A huge burn extended about six inches down his left leg, angry and red with little sign of healing although it had happened a month before.

His merry eyes twinkled as he related the story of how it happened.

My cousin had me strapped behind him on his motorcycle. It was real keen ! We were playing chicken with this other guy, in a field near the river. We came charging at this guy and he swerved his bike and jumped just before it hit a tree.

My cousin's bike skidded and he yelled. "*Jump !*" - but I couldn't, I was strapped on ! The bike fell against my leg and the exhaust pipe started my pant leg burning. My cousin cut me free from the bike and carried me to the edge of the river. It was real weird how my leg all steamed as he held it in the water.

On another occasion he broke the leg bone above the knee. At the time he was participating with a group of children in a yogic exercise.   Mike was sitting on the floor and with his hands was attempting to pull the lifeless leg towards the opposite shoulder.

He described the result: **Suddenly there was a loud crack like a firecracker. It startled the kids and they asked "*What was that ?*" - I replied "*I think I broke my leg*", and sure enough I had.**

An even worse fate threatened him, for the doctors said his spine was collapsed and repeatedly they had been pressuring his mother to grant her permission to have it fused with animal bone. Mike would lose his ability to bend his spine for the remainder of his life.

Mike went to Francis Nixon for Vivaxis treatment; at each session groups of disturbed code receptors were reinstated with their correct energies and each correction brought more movement into his limbs.

Speculating why Mike had the complete use of both arms but was paralyzed in the legs led to a significant discovery.

The bullet perforated Mike's left hand, but his mother felt it was of little consequence compared to his other wounds since it merely pierced the flesh between the left thumb and forefinger and he had soon regained its full use.

On a hunch Francis tested the part of the hand between the thumb and forefinger on her husband's left hand; she found that as he sent a message to move his leg the communication was received by receptors located in this section, and that the stimulation ceased when the message terminated.

Testing showed the corresponding section between the big (first) and second toes of the left foot was also a vital communication centre - and with Mike these and associated receptors on the head exhibited distress signals.

About six hours after the correction by Vivaxis techniques improvements became apparent and Mike now had much greater ability to lift his knees.   Additionally, bladder problems requiring a leg bag were overcome.

The changes had taken place immediately after the communication area between the left index finger and thumb had been stimulated.

Healers Need Protection

From discussions with people who worked with Frances and Bessie I have discovered that they both suffered in health - although they were helping others.

In the books that they wrote I did not find any mention of them 'grounding' themselves or placing any protection against being hurt as empaths.

Brian and Wenda Cole confirmed that most Vivaxis healers did not take precautions before doing their Healing, and this was probably the cause of so many suffering in later times.

Using your Knowledge of Vivaxis

It seems that they considered their Vivaxis discovery to be the 'beginning and end' of healing; due to their determination to pursue their investigations and healing work we have gained new knowledge.

But it is important to recognize the other factors involved with health as well ! Treat Vivaxis as another very important tool in your 'Healing Kit'.

The subject of Vivaxis was been raised from an unexpected source - in preparing her workshop on 'Energy Healing' based on Donna Eden's work, Kristina Nielsen reported that *"Spirit has told me that linking with your Vivaxis before Dowsing or Healing improves your abilities - so I am incorporating it in my workshop".*

Mineral Prospecting

Prospectors can use this knowledge - it would be useful to gold prospectors, etc. who are seeking the 'Mother Lode'. Its Vivaxis is where a stone or mineral became solidified - if it is melted afterwards it gets a new Vivaxis.

If you have found a nugget, you can hold it in your hand as a 'witness' and ask to be shown the direction of its Vivaxis, where it was formed, and follow the trail - or use your 'Map Dowsing' skills.

Practice: Dowse whether you have any of your cells mis-aligned due to X-rays or other influences. If so, Dowse to ask if they can now be re-aligned to the correct Vivaxis for all your body - to be in alignment with your 'Master Cell'.

If so, ask that it now be done - and then check if it has been done, or if time is needed for it to be done.

Also send Love to all your cells, and ask them to re-establish communication with the 'Wisdom of your Being' and obey all instructions that they so receive.

Take some locally grown produce, hold it in your hand as a 'witness', and locate where it was grown on a map.

Think of the Unemployment that would Ensue
If All Health were Perfect - What would we Do ?

Illness

Let us define illness as any condition of our Being that results in a dis-ease effect on our physical body - since that is when we know that something is wrong.

Dis-ease is just that - not 'at ease', the vibrational patterns of some parts of us are stressed beyond limits, our body cannot cope with what is happening, signals to us that there is a major problem, and that action is needed to deal with this stress.

Most of the Western medical concepts are primarily concerned with overcoming the symptoms - cancelling the signals that are given and manifest in the physical body.

Most of the modern day pharmaceutical medicines have been derived from plants - the same plants that were used by ancient 'medicine men' (and often women) and are now used by homeopaths and herbalists.

There is great opposition from the pharmaceutical companies against those who use the natural medicines in their original state; 'purity' of manufacture is claimed, yet these man-made medicines have been shown to have many side effects that do not occur with the plants when used naturally by those who understand them.

Perhaps this is due to the pharmaceutical companies dealing with medicines as just a chemical soup - they deal with the 'dead' chemical constituents, ignoring the Life Force that is in the natural plant. Anyway, they can sell more medicines to deal with the side effects - more profit !

Most medical doctors choose that career because they wish to be Healers; at medical school they learn about the physical body and how to recognize symptoms of illness. Then they are taught only which pharmaceutical medicines to prescribe !

Let us recognize that the pharmaceutical companies have a massive influence on western medicine - they have their profits to maintain !

They give grants to medical schools, free samples to doctors, advertising revenue to professional journals, and funding to the medical associations.

Governmental staff, who are supposed to safeguard the national health, are often 'guided' by the drug companies - and the senior people later may be found lucratively employed by these same drug companies.

Research that is submitted to obtain permission to sell drugs is usually done by university researchers, the cost of research being subsidized by the pharmaceutical companies.

If the result is not beneficial to the pharmaceutical companies, it usually is not submitted to the authorities - and the research establishments involved may suffer a reduction in funding.

There are instances when cures are determined, yet tests cannot be funded - money is not made available for a simple reason: the treatment cannot be patented, so profits will not accrue to the drug companies.

Yes, there are many researchers who want to do a good job - but research is expensive, and they have families to house, feed and clothe.   But the corporate mentality that is prevalent nowadays, including in universities, is geared to money. A change would be beneficial to all !

We have seen that the Human Being is far more than just a physical body - yet these other aspects are mostly ignored in western medical practice.

For good health, all aspects need to be considered.

Injury

The one form of illness that is primarily physical is injury - breaking a limb, or damaging flesh and skin by tearing, burning, or other similar calamities.

Let us be thankful for the skills of the surgeons who work on these problems, and for the advances in their knowledge.

In past times it was the barber who cut off a damaged limb, perhaps with the help of the blacksmith to sear the cut end. This was not always successful, since germs were not acknowledged, and there was not any attempt to maintain a clean environment.

Ridicule was poured on those who first realized that germs existed - they were vindicated only when microscopes were invented and germs could be seen.

Germs

The smallest of these are viruses - like sub-sections of DNA that infiltrate a cell, change its DNA, and replicate. These are indeed life forms ! They have the intelligence and knowledge to do their job - even after centuries of freezing in space.

Some even establish miniature factories within a cell, each one making a component - when ready, these are assembled and put into action.

Originally they may have been intended to repair and replace damaged cells - to re-grow a damaged part; this may be a source of some uncontrolled growths, such as some cancers.

The present purpose of a virus seems to be to effect change. Perhaps they have played a key role in evolution of our species. But generally our bodies do not like change, so the result is usually harmful to us.

Bacteria are far larger than viruses - many within us are beneficial to us; they are needed to help consume food and recycle unwanted cells, such as those that have been injured or died a natural death.

There are quite a few that are not so beneficial - or are doing their job in the wrong place or in an incorrect way.

Bacteria are needed to purify rivers - many of these consume oxygen, just like us. Generally bacteria that consume oxygen are beneficial, while those that do not have to consume oxygen do their work in different ways.

This can be observed in a rubbish pile - if it has plenty of air, then we do not smell bad fumes. Without such ventilation, it stinks.

The one thing that is common to both viruses and non-beneficial bacteria is that they like to multiply in a poor environment. If a person is in excellent health, then they are less likely to be the subject of a successful attack.

This can be described in another way - if your Life Force is strong, action is not needed by viruses or bacteria to correct the situation.

There are some viruses which will attack anyway - perhaps they are nature's assistants in keeping the human population within limits acceptable to the rest of nature; to prevent any human population explosion that results in a plague of humans - that devours all the resources of nature, to the detriment of other life forms.

This, of course, leads to the NIMBY syndrome - 'Not In My Back Yard', meaning take somebody else, not me, or my family (except, of course, my mother-in-law !).

The best defence is to keep healthy - which includes having a healthy diet.

To put this in perspective, statistics show that the world's population has grown by about 2,500 million since 1950 from 5,000 million to 7,500 million - a 50% increase.

By 2050 it may well reach 10,000 million, most of this increase coming in the lesser developed countries.

'We Are What We Eat'

- And drink, such as 'Diet Drinks' using aspartame which have been shown to have poisonous effects (to humans, not the bottom line of the drink makers).

The Ecologist reports that aspartame was listed by the Pentagon as a biochemical warfare agent. Today it's an integral part of the modern diet. Sold commercially under names like NutraSweet and Canderel, aspartame can be found in more than 5,000 foods.

Independent scientists say aspartame can produce a range of disturbing adverse effects in humans, including headaches, memory loss, mood swings, seizures, multiple sclerosis and Parkinson's-like symptoms, tumours and even death.

It may be the prime cause of Attention Deficiency, for which so many tranquilizer drugs are prescribed, causing further problems in children 'down the road'. Aspartame now accounts for the majority (75 per cent) of all the complaints in the US adverse-reaction monitoring system.

A report on the Internet (source identity lost) :

In October of 2001 my sister started getting very sick. She had stomach spasms and was having a hard time getting around. Walking was a major chore. It took everything she had just to get out of bed; she was in so much pain.

By March 2002, she had undergone several tissue and muscle biopsies and was on 24 various prescription medications. The doctors could not determine what was wrong with her. She was in so much pain, and so sick ... she just knew she was dying. She put her house, bank accounts, life insurance, etc., in her oldest daughter's name, and made sure that her younger children were to be taken care of.

She also wanted her last hooray, so she planned a trip to Florida (basically in a wheelchair) for March 22nd.   On March 19th I called her to ask how her most recent tests went, and she said they didn't find anything on the test, but they believe she had MS.

I recalled an article a friend of mine, a lawyer, had emailed to me and I asked my sister if she drank diet soda ? She told me that she did - as a matter of fact, she was getting ready to crack one open that moment. I told her not to open it, and to stop drinking the diet soda ! I emailed her the article.

My sister called me within 32 hours after our phone conversation and told me she had stopped drinking the diet soda AND she could walk !

The muscle spasms went away. She said she didn't feel 100% but she sure felt a lot better. She told me she was going to her doctor with this article and would call me when she got home.

Well, she called me, and said her doctor was amazed ! He is going to call all of his MS patients to find out if they consumed artificial sweeteners of any kind.

In a nutshell, she was being poisoned by the Aspartame in the diet soda - and dying a slow and miserable death.

When she got to Florida in March 22nd, all she had to take was one pill - and that was a pill for the Aspartame poisoning ! She is well on her way to a complete recovery. She is walking ! No wheelchair !

Environmental Conference

At a conference, the keynote address by the EPA announced that in the United States in 2001 there is an epidemic of multiple sclerosis and systemic lupus. It was difficult to determine exactly what toxin was causing this to be rampant.

I stood up and said that I was there to lecture on exactly that subject.

When the temperature of Aspartame, marketed as 'NutraSweet', 'Equal', and 'Spoonful', exceeds 86 degrees F, the wood alcohol in converts to formaldehyde and then to formic acid, which in turn causes metabolic acidosis.

Formic acid is the poison found in the sting of fire ants. The methanol toxicity mimics, among other conditions, multiple sclerosis and systemic lupus.

Many people were being diagnosed in error. Although multiple sclerosis is not a death sentence - methanol toxicity is !

Systemic lupus has become almost as rampant as multiple sclerosis, especially with Diet Coke and Diet Pepsi drinkers. The victim usually does not know that the Aspartame is the culprit. He or she continues its use; irritating the lupus to such a degree that it may become a life-threatening condition. We have seen patients with systemic lupus become asymptotic, once taken off diet sodas.

In cases of those diagnosed with Multiple Sclerosis, (when in reality, the disease is methanol toxicity), most of the symptoms disappear. We've seen many cases where vision loss returned and hearing loss improved markedly. This also applies to cases of tinnitus and fibromyalgia.

If you are suffering from fibromyalgia symptoms, spasms shooting, pains, numbness in your legs, cramps, vertigo, dizziness, headaches, tinnitus, joint pain, unexplainable depression, anxiety attacks, slurred speech, blurred vision, or memory loss - you probably have Aspartame poisoning !

Dr. Espart remarked that so many people seem to be symptomatic for MS and during his recent visit to a hospice, a nurse stated that six of her friends, who were heavy Diet Coke addicts, had all been diagnosed with MS. This is beyond coincidence !

Diet soda is NOT a diet product ! It is a chemically altered, multiple sodium (salt) and Aspartame containing product that actually makes you crave carbohydrates. It is far more likely to make you gain weight !

These products also contain formaldehyde, which stores in the fat cells, particularly in the hips and thighs. Formaldehyde is an absolute toxin and is used primarily to preserve 'tissue specimens'.

Many products we use every day contain this chemical but we SHOULD NOT store it IN our body !

Dr. H. J. Roberts stated in his lectures that once free of the 'diet products' and with no significant increase in exercise his patients lost an average of 19 pounds over a trial period.

Aspartame is especially dangerous for diabetics. We found that some physicians, who believed that they had a patient with retinopathy, in fact had symptoms caused by Aspartame.

Documentation and observation also reveal that thousands of children diagnosed with ADD and AHD have had complete turnarounds in their behavior when these chemicals have been removed from their diet. So called 'behavior modification prescription drugs' (Ritalin and others) are no longer needed.

Truth be told, they were never needed in the first place !

Most of these children were being 'poisoned' on a daily basis with the very foods that were 'better for them than sugar'.

Dr. Roberts warns that it can cause birth defects, i.e., mental retardation, if taken at the time of conception and during early pregnancy. Children are especially at risk for neurological disorders and should never be given artificial sweeteners.

Stevia, which is a sweet herb, helps in the metabolism of sugar, which would be ideal for diabetics. It has now been approved as a dietary supplement by the FDA.

It is known that for many years the FDA outlawed this true sweet food, 'due to their loyalty to MONSANTO Chemical Company'.

According to the Conference of the American College of Physicians, *"We are talking about a plague of neurological diseases directly caused by the use of this deadly poison"*.

Preservative and other Additives

So many foods on grocery shelves have additives to prolong shelf life - and this is especially so when it is a manufactured food.

These are not natural - and our bodies have been designed to consume natural foods. Even raw foods have often been poisoned by the pesticides and herbicides used by farmers - including farming corporations.

Fast Food outlets get a lot of disparagement; some of this is deserved, since many of the animals that are 'used' are stuffed with anti-biotics, maltreated during their life, and killed without dignity.

This also applies to most meat products in shops, however.

Traces of these pesticides, herbicides, and anti-biotics accumulate in our bodies - and can prove very troublesome as this accumulation grows.

Suppose we become vegetarians - would this help ? Many believe so, but studies have shown that humans need some vitamins, etc., that can only come from consuming animal matter.

It has also been accepted that the types of humans differ - some need a strong meat diet, whilst others can thrive on lesser amounts.

Our bodies need many nutriments for good health - especially vitamins and trace minerals. A food product may look attractive on the store shelves, but be of little or no nutritional value.

Mark Purdey has investigated 'Mad Cow' disease. He has found this to be quite widespread among wild deer and other animals in areas where there has been little human contact.

These animals have not been fed any recycled animal foods, which have been accepted by most governmental authorities as being the cause of 'Mad Cow' disease.

But there is one common denominator - high manganese and low copper content of the soils; this means that the grasses that grow, though they look fine to the animals, do not give them all the needed minerals. There are many trace minerals that we need for good health. See Nexus Magazine: Vol 10 nos 3 & 4.

There is a very strong case for consuming 'organic' produce - food that is not subjected to chemicals, but uses natural fertilizers from plants recycled by Mother Nature; by eating meat and eggs from animals and chickens that roam free, not penned in tiny cages or filled with anti-biotics.

Unfortunately the pesticides and herbicides that are used by many farmers kill many of the bacteria and enzymes within the soil, so reducing its ability to regenerate.

Insects that are killed are then eaten by other insects and by birds, and they lose their own good health. In 2007 there are reports that the bee population in parts of Europe and the USA are not surviving - which may prevent pollination of plants and so cause a great shortage of vegetables and fruit.

These poisons are washed into streams, ponds, rivers, lakes, seas and oceans.

Warnings have been issued about restricting the amount of salmon consumed - they range the oceans and they have been found to be contaminated by the poisons (including industrial wastes) dumped by people in 'civilized' countries.

Perhaps one of the best ways to ensure that you have good food is to grow as much as you can yourself. In England, during the 1939-45 war, dollars and shipping could not be spared to import food - and much was sunk by U-boat action.

So people grew food in their own gardens, or they obtained 'allotments' (small pieces of land where they could grow their own plants) if they lacked gardens. This helped the Brits to survive - and maintain good health. It gave them extra food over and above their rations.

This system still exists, and is common in many parts of Europe. Sometimes the quality of soil may be very poor, not normally able to grow much, as was the case with Findhorn in Scotland.

By making a concentrated effort to work with nature, showing respect to the land and giving love to the plants, good crops were grown both at Findhorn (a desert-like barren spot) and at Perelandra in the USA. Do an internet search to find more information.

From Siberia comes the wonderful story of Mind working with nature to help the Russian people to grow good food on small lots - and this has succeeded to the extent that a considerable portion of the Russian food requirements is now grown in 'Dachniks' (miniature Dachas) - and is of excellent quality.

This story is told in a series of books about the 'Ringing Cedars of Russia' - the website www.RingingCedars.com has more details.

Life Force in Food

It may be that Love is the real 'Life Force' throughout nature; and when we give Love to plants they respond by doing their best to help us.

But it is so easy to kill this life force by overcooking - raw food is usually best for us, although digestion may not always be so easy !

One of the most sure ways to kill this life force is by 'microwaving' food. Microwaves work by moving the cellular parts of a food extremely quickly, similar but far more intense than the increased speed of cells resulting from heating them.

Independent research by Dr Hans Hertel in Switzerland first identified and quantified this problem - the corporations went to extreme lengths to stop the publication of the results.

Do a Google search for 'Hertel Microwaves' to see more details.

Microwaving Your Food Isn't Safe

by Larry Cook (Reprinted from Natural Life News & Directory)

If you have ever wondered whether or not microwaved food is safe, here's an experiment you can do at home. Plant seeds in two pots. Water one pot with water that has been microwaved, the other with regular tap.

The seeds that received microwaved water won't sprout ! If microwaved water can stop plants from growing, think of what microwaved food can do to your health !

In 1989, Swiss biologist and food scientist Dr. Hans Hertel studied the effects of microwaved food. Eight people participated in the study. For eight weeks, they lived in a controlled environment and intermittently ate raw foods, conventionally cooked foods and microwaved foods. Blood samples were tested after each meal.

They discovered that eating microwaved food, over time, causes significant changes in blood chemistry:

(1) A decrease in hemoglobin and cholesterol values, in the HDL (good cholesterol) versus LDL (bad cholesterol) ratio and in white blood cells, weakening the immune system, and an increase in leukocyte levels, which tends to indicate poisoning and cell damage. The study suggested that eating microwaved foods can cause degenerative diseases and/or cancer.

(2) *"The measurable effects on man through the ingestion of microwaved food, unlike untreated food, are blood alterations, that can also be found at the beginning of a pathological condition, also indicative of a beginning cancerous process"*, wrote Dr. Bernard Blanc, who assisted in the study.

(3) Microwave ovens 'cook' food by forcing the atoms, molecules and cells within the food to reverse polarity billions of times per second, causing friction - the more the friction, the more the heat. This oscillation tears and deforms the molecular structure of food. New compounds are formed, called radiolytic compounds, which are not found in nature.

Interestingly, microwaves are actually used in gene-altering technology to deliberately break cells and neutralize their 'life-force' so they can be manipulated. Microwaves destroy the life-force that gives food its vitality and nourishment. When this life-force dissipates, micro-organisms start breaking food down and it begins to rot.

In early 1991, a lawsuit was filed against an Oklahoma hospital because a patient died from receiving a microwaved blood transfusion. Hospitals routinely heat blood for transfusion, but not in a microwave.

The effects of microwaving breast milk have also been researched. John Kerner, M.D. and Richard Quin, M.D. from Stanford University said that: *"Microwaving human milk, even at a low setting, can destroy some of its important disease-fighting capabilities"*.

(4) After more research, Kerner wrote in the April 1992 issue of Pediatrics that: *"Microwaving itself may in fact cause some injury to the milk above and beyond the heating"*. And a radio announcement at the University of Minnesota said that, *"Microwaves are not recommended for heating a baby's bottle. Heating the bottle in a microwave can cause slight changes in the milk. In infant formulas, there may be a loss of some vitamins. In expressed milk, some protective properties may be destroyed"*.

(5) Another study in Vienna warned that microwaving breast milk 'can lead to structural, functional and immunological changes', and that microwaves transform the amino acid L-proline into D-proline, a proven toxin to the nervous system, liver and kidneys.

(6) In Russia, microwave ovens were banned in 1976 because of their negative health consequences and many studies were conducted on their use.

Here are some of their findings on microwaving food:

1. Microwaved foods lose 60% - 90% of the vital-energy field, and microwaving accelerates the structural disintegration of foods.
2. Microwaving creates cancer-causing agents within milk and cereals.
3. Microwaving alters elemental food-substances, causing digestive disorders.
4. Microwaving alters food chemistry which can lead to malfunctions in the lymphatic system and degeneration of the body's ability to protect itself against cancerous growths.
5. Microwaved foods lead to a higher percentage of cancerous cells in the bloodstream.
6. Microwaving altered the breakdown of elemental substances when raw, cooked, or frozen vegetables were exposed for even a very short time - and free radicals were formed.
7. Microwaved foods caused stomach and intestinal cancerous growths, a general degeneration of peripheral cellular tissues, and a gradual breakdown of the digestive and excretive systems in a statistically high percentage of people.
8. Microwaved foods lowered the body's ability of the body to utilize B-complex vitamins, Vitamin C, Vitamin E, essential minerals and lipotropics.
9. The microwave field next to a microwave oven caused a slew of health problems as well. Aside from these studies, many people find that microwaving their food doesn't help them feel good.

Stephanie Relfe, Kinesiologist, found herself feeling 'grey and rather low' one day and discovered that she had inadvertently eaten microwaved food at a restaurant.

In her practice, she found that all of her patients gave body signals of having allergic reactions to microwaved foods. Another Kinesiologist, David Bridgeman, said *"Of all the people I test for allergies, 99.9% so far show severe sensitivity to any microwaved food".*

In conclusion then, the safest way to heat your food is to use your stove top and throw away your microwave !

Improving Food Value

I was brought up in a strict religion where food was always Blessed. I rebelled against the narrow-mindedness of this group, and so also abandoned their procedures - including the Blessing of food.

When I learnt how to locate auras, I experimented on the food that I ate. With blessing, the aura of food doubles in size ! Since this indicates an increased life force having more love, I now Bless all that I consume.

Use your Pendulum to check the size of the aura of your food before Blessing it - and then check again afterwards.

Then as a further experiment, Bless your food with 'Blessing 995' and 'Healing 997' and check the size again !

Pains that Move

Many people find that there are rather peculiar pains that seem to move around in their body - or within a certain group of their body parts, such as hip, thigh, knee, leg, ankle and foot.

Physicians find themselves unable to cure these pains, only giving medicines as pain killers or telling the patient that 'it is all in the mind' or just imagination.

Those who studied science at school may remember one of the major differences between solids and liquids and gases.

With both solids and liquids, if you place one into another by immersion or mixing, the volume to hold these is the same as before such mixing. Put a stone into a jar of water, and the level of water rises to accommodate the volume of the stone.

But you can have a container full of one gas and then pour the same volume of a different gas into the same container without spillage - the molecules of one gas fit into the spaces between the molecules of the other gas.

In such a way 'other dimensional life forms' of some description may have penetrated auric protection, invaded the patient, and taken residence in his body aura, hiding in the auras and tissues of muscle.

Although they are 'other dimensional', they have an effect on the muscles themselves - which suffer interference due to invasion.

This may be the cause of muscle cramps; when I treat them as invasive 'other dimensional life forms' I get success in their removal - and relief from the cramps.

German New Medicine

Dr Ryke Geerd Hamer has made a most interesting discovery - that when there is any illness in the body, a CAT scan of the brain shows distinctive patterns at spots corresponding to the site of the illness, and these patterns change with variations of the stage of the illness.

He questioned patients who were suffering from serious diseases, and ascertained that in almost every case the patient had been traumatized to some extent just before the onset of the disease.

Dr Hamer postulates that these are connected - similar to the 'fight or flight' reaction that is well recognized, but being of a far longer time span.

He suggests that the sub-conscious takes what it understands (perhaps incorrectly !) to be the needed corrective action - and that this is recognized by us as an illness.

He explains that if the trauma is overcome, then this reaction moves to a healing mode. Failing this, an even more serious illness or death may occur. The longer that the trauma remains active, the more difficult is recovery to good health.

This makes sense ! It is an excellent reason for a person to take precautions against being traumatized - and if this does occur, to take action to negate the effects.

This means that the events causing trauma must be recognized as potential threats to our own good health. Trauma is essentially emotional, and taking action such as the 'Emotional Freedom Techniques' (EFT) can be a great help in releasing such causes of future illness. Typical traumatic experiences include:

- Loss of a friend, relative, associate, or pet.
- Relationship problems at home or at work.
- Loss of employment or failure to be promoted.
- Injury to a person that you love or feel responsibility.
- Recognizing that you hurt another in some way.
- Anger at behavior of others.
- Worries about ourselves or others.

In many cases like these the traumatic event has already happened - there is nothing that we can do to change the event, but we can change our own re-action to the event.

Recognition of a trauma, and that it can cause ill-health to our own self is sometimes difficult - we lose a close relation, and are so upset that we do not realize that we are hurting ourselves !

Would it not be better to just be thankful for the experience that you have had with the deceased, wish them well in their next existence, and get on with your own life ?

You may have been left in a financial mess in this way, or find problems in 'carrying on'. Do not worry about these - just know that the situation could be far worse, that other people have gone through similar times and survived, and that somehow or other things will be fine in the end.

Do your best, and remember that you can always ask the help of 'Upstairs' !

Dr Hamer further proposes that most of what the medical profession sees as illness is, in fact, part of the Healing process. His propositions can only be described as turning medical practice 'upside down' - and so the medical authorities are rather incensed !

If Dr Hamer is correct, then the medicines produced by the drug companies would not be needed - and the potential loss of these profits is certainly stirring action to ridicule his findings.

This, of course, is the typical reaction of 'the Establishment' to any new thought that threatens those that are now 'in Power'.

Historically the medical profession is a prime example - witness the reaction to the theory that sterilization of surgical tools would reduce sickness, the battle waged against Radionics, and the persecution of Dr Rife.

If you would like more information on Dr Hamer's work, see www.GermanNewMedicine.ca - it is not easy reading, but is worthwhile !

The **key point** is that we must recognize traumatic events as potentially disease causing to our own selves, and take action to protect ourselves - including to use EFT, which costs nothing except our own time and effort, cannot cause any harm, and has a proven track record.

Prison Regulations - Hygiene is Important !

Each day all prisoners will change their socks.

Prisoners will line up in numerical order, take off their socks, and pass them to the prisoner on their right.

There are Those that Love 'Being Ill'
To get Compassion, Control Others Will !

Simple Healing

We are all Energy Beings - and since we are 'All the Same' we can help each other. Some things are easy for us to do - and some almost impossible (for us !).

But these 'almost impossible' things may be quite easy for those 'Upstairs' to do, using 'God Level' resources that we may lack. And the converse is true - we may have abilities in the physical plane that are not directly available to 'Upstairs'.

When we work together as a team, all things may be possible !

If our ego is in control, then teamwork may be very difficult; with our Heart in command, co-operation becomes relatively easy.

This is, perhaps, the biggest and most important skill in Healing - to know (and accept) that we do not give Healing ourselves, but act (like a conduit) as a link for the 'Healing Energies' from 'Upstairs' to go and help another Being.

These Healing Energies are attracted when you have the intent to help another - not for reward, but because it is 'the best way to Be', to want to assist others for good purposes.

This does not mean that a professional Healer should not charge for their own time - they have to feed, clothe, and house their families, and perhaps pay rent, staff and travel expenses.

The problem comes when their fees are excessive, when they are charging for the help given by 'Upstairs', not just for their own expenses.

In this discussion, you will be the 'Healer', and the other person who is being Healed we will call the 'Healee'.

Protection

There are many reports of people who do Healing getting hurt themselves.

Before doing any Healing work, always clear and protect yourself. Ask 'Upstairs' or 'The System' to protect you.

A simple way is:

> *"I ask The System to clear from me all negativity*
> *And to protect me in this Healing work,*
> *To enclose both myself and the Healee in Light and Love.*
> *Let nothing that is not mine come to me;*
> *Let nothing that is not their own go to the Healee;*
> *Except the Light, Love, and Healing from 'Upstairs'.*
> *As I work to Heal others, let myself be Healed as well.*
> *All Healing to be without harm to others.*
> *I send you my gratitude and my Love"*

"Once More, Dear Friends !"

Another aspect which, unfortunately, is not generally recognized is that there are many energies, other dimensional life forms, that have themselves been hurt, perhaps by being given bad jobs that they do not like - such as being involved in anger or hate.

These energies that have been hurt seek Healing for themselves; when they find a Healer who is actively working to Heal others, they may come for Healing themselves.

The Healer in many cases does not understand this, feeling the effect of these energies as being detrimental, and telling them *"Go to the ends of the universe and never trouble any Being again".*

This is like you going to a doctor and being told to 'F… Off' !

It is so simple to help them, and it costs you nothing. Just ask the 'Force for Good' to come and take them to be Healed, so that they can again be 'In the Light' and in their rightful place.

When you do this, you may be extremely surprised at how the atmosphere around you improves - do it often !

Grounding

We stand upright between the earth and the sky; and there is a voltage difference (perhaps small) with change of height. This is measurable in the physical dimension - and also effects the other dimensions. They need to be 'Grounded' as well !

It is well known that if a person keeps his 'Head in the Air' without being 'Down to Earth' problems arise in many ways. These may include energy patterns in and around our body, and may contribute to poor health.

As explained before, thoughts are perceived as 'Real Things' in the other dimensions; these (and other energy patterns) can find release if you are 'Grounded'.

How do you do this ? Just imagine that you have roots that extend from your body down into the earth - just like a tree ! Sound ridiculous, perhaps - but it works !

So imagine that you have roots growing from your feet and the base of your spine, and that these move with you - to connect you to 'Mother Earth'.

Being 'imaginary' these roots go straight through carpets, floors, concrete foundations, and all things that would prevent or disrupt connections in the physical world.

Washing Machine

This is a very simple method that does not require any medical knowledge, just good intent and lots of Love.

It was developed by Joe and Marta Smith, a farming couple from Nebraska, and has been used by them (and by many others) with great success.

This is how Joe tells about this wonderful system:

Hands-on Healing is a good way to help others. I'll take you through the method I like to use when possible.

To do this you should have 2 people and practice on each other. You will be the 'Healer', and the other person the 'Healee'.

For the Healee, get your partner or a close friend that you always drink coffee with and doesn't think you're completely nuts but will humour you.

Step 1: Set the Healee in a chair right in front of you. During all this exercise both you and the Healee should breathe in through your nose and exhale out of your mouth. It also helps if you both take 3 'Pranic Breaths' to start - feeling the energy at the top of your nose as you inhale.

Step 2: You take a step back and say something nice to the Angels who you are going to work with you and send through you the Healing Energies that are needed.

God has all these Angels up there that love to help you do this Healing if you just call on them - so get serious, look up to the Heavens, and tell them how grateful you are for them being able and willing to help you.

Don't kid your self into believing that you alone are doing this. This power comes from somewhere else !

Step 3: Now ask the Angels to send the Healing Energies down into a spot right in front of you and just behind the Healee. As they do this, step into this spot with your elbows at your side and your hands ahead of you, the palms turned up to receive this energy. Feel the warmth and love coming into your whole body.

Step 4: Ask the Healee if it is alright if you touch him - or her, as the case may be. Walk up behind them and place your hands on their shoulders, sending God's love into his/her body.

Stand there for a while feeling the power flow through your hands into the Healee.

Ask the Healee to visualize that his/her body is a washing machine and you are sending God's love in the form of a warm cleansing soap to cleanse their body of all the hurts and pains of their life.

(You may find that sending 'Blessing 995' and 'Healing 997' with God's Love help it to work better - these have been found to work well, for some undetermined reason. Like additives to detergents ?)

"To cleanse all the fears, all the disappointments, all the 'shoulds' and 'should nots', animosities for others, and add forgiveness for those who have animosity toward you."

Throw anything else in there as you are guided - things that come to your mind that need clearing. You know this work is using Intuition, so add to or take off what you want, as your Intuition guides you to do.

Now back to the washing machine; take your index finger and apply light pressure to the front of the Healee's body just below the collar bone. This is where you send Healing Power to the Heart.

Do this for several minutes, or until you get the signal that the job is done. You will know !

Then using your thumbs, press slightly on their back 2 inches above the shoulder blade and 2 inches from each side of the spine - these are 'release points'.

As you do this, tell the Healee "spin out all this stuff that has been bothering you for years. Spin it out just like a giant washing machine."

As you are talking about all their problems you may feel them tighten up, and as they spin it out, they seem to just let it all loose and relax. If they are still a little tight ask them to spin it again - that you don't think they got it all out the first time.

If they need it, do the process again and send in more of God's warm love. Sometimes it takes several sessions to get the relief that the subject needs.

Step 5: You now fluff their aura just like you would a pillow - only don't hit the Healee; this is like putting the clothes in the dryer ! As you try this, you may feel the aura push back so very gently and lightly.

When you fluff their aura, you disperse any old, unwanted energy that is hanging around, just like the breeze taking away dampness on clothes hung on a line to dry.

Step 6: Often clothes look better when they are ironed; to do this put your hands in front of you, and with your palms facing each other bring them almost together several times - the air between your hands seems to get thicker, more 'bouncy'.

So do this motion, standing sideways to the Healee, bouncing the aura all the way down on one side, then the body itself, then go the other side and bounce that side.

You can stand in front and back, too, to bounce the aura from side to side, doing it in front, around the body, and the back.

Step 7: Another thing you can do is to 'fold the clothes' - move your hands over their body noticing any area that feels either hot or cold. This works best if they are on a massage table.

As you move across the area of an injury, or a diseased area, it will give off heat into the palm of your hand. It will feel like a warm breath of air, very subtle.

Ask the Angels to change any 'not good' energies in these places with Love so that all the energies in these places are beneficial.

Step 8:   Most important - ask the Healee to join with you in sending Thanks, Gratitude, and Love to 'All who helped in this Healing'.

Even Angels get excited when their help is appreciated - and they may queue up to help you when needed !

Joe tells more:

"An example of heavenly help happened to me in Georgia one night. A lady came over to the place where we were staying and wanted me to work on her - using 'hands on' Healing.

She had a real bad case of shingles in the face - her face was badly swollen, especially the left side. So I took her to one of the bedrooms, sat her on a dressing stool, and did the Healing work.

After I got through I let her sit there for a while and 'come back to earth'.

As it turned out I wasn't kidding. She said that she had an 'out of body' experience while I was doing the healing.

As she was floating in the ceiling she looked down and saw herself being worked on by an angel, a big white angel - I wasn't even there ! These were her words, not mine. "

Healing in General

It is necessary that you have the permission and co-operation of any person that you may help with Healing. The Washing Machine is a good example - you are asking the Healee to release 'not good' energies themselves, to release their own problems.

If they hang onto their anger, hate, etc. and refuse to release it, then they will not get the full benefit of Healing. Yet these 'negative emotions' seem to be the cause of much illness.

The Angelic Forces will not over-ride the 'Free Will' of people - if a person decides that they will not release it, there is not much that any Healer can do.

Cases where you may not be able to get the conscious permission of a Being that needs Healing include babies and small children, those who are unconscious for any reason, animals and plants.

In this case you can still ask the Angelic Forces for their help, but ensure that you ask that it 'be in the highest and best good' of the Healee.

Note that the term 'Angelic Forces' may be better than 'Angels', since these are labels that we apply, and the Healing may need help from Beings who may be different from Angels - but still members of the 'Force for Good'.

Even the most knowledgeable medical practitioners and Healers may not know exactly the best type of Healing that is needed; they may have a good idea, but use general terminology - perhaps the Angelic Forces know more than we do !

Let them choose how to give their Healing - accept that you are just a conduit for their energies, a willing tool that they use.

Ego may not like this, but Heart understands.

In cases of very severe illness with much suffering, it may not be possible (or in the Healee's best interest) for a physical healing to occur - the suffering may be mitigated by the Angelic Forces, however, until death occurs and the Soul moves on.

If you cannot obtain permission for a Healing, or the Being is far away, then you can always send them your Love and ask the Angelic Forces to send Healing Energies to them, always to be used in the 'highest and best good' of the Being.

More 'Map Dowsing'

Body Dowsing has two meanings - to use your body for giving a Dowsing signal, and to consider your body as the subject of Dowsing.   Here we have a map of a body - and we will now Dowse that map.

Get a piece of paper, and sketch on it your body, similar to the sketch shown here.   Using your Pendulum, locate your heart, your liver, your kidneys, and your adrenaline glands, and mark them with a pencil.

Front   drawing by Joe Smith, Digital Dowsers   Back

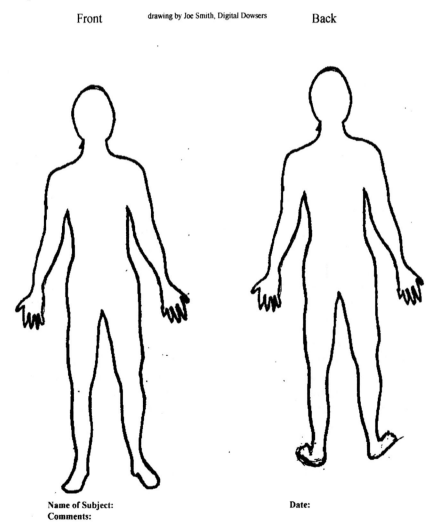

Name of Subject: **Date:**
Comments:

Now use your Bobber, Pendulum, or L-rod to ask *"Do I have any problem with my [heart, etc] ?"*, and if so, then take the very first thought that 'pops' into your mind and ask *"Is ... the problem ?"*.

It is important to listen to that very first thought - often the logical part of us says *"Nonsense, I don't believe it ! It must be something else"* and so the Intuitive thought is discarded. But that Intuitive thought is probably the truth.

Check your overall health, as a percentage of the maximum good health (100%) that you could enjoy, by using your counting ability. If you use your 'other' hand as an indicator, you could change the meaning of the fingers - let your middle finger indicate normal (the average person), the next finger be plus (or minus) 20 %, with your little finger / thumb representing plus (or minus) 40 %.

Now ask permission from your partner to check for problems, and if agreed then do this same exercise - using another similar sketch as a map of your partner's body.

First check that the organs are in the same place (does s/he have a heart ? - perhaps a kidney has been donated !) and then check the overall health.

Discuss the results, see how you both agree, but remember that you are not qualified to diagnose unless you have a medical doctorate. You can only say *"My Intuition indicates that you may have a problem - I suggest that you have your . . . . checked by a professional in the . . . . Field"*.

Remember that if you find a problem 'in the heart' this could indeed be a physical problem, but it may be a 'broken heart' or 'love problem' instead !

Aura Dowsing is exactly the same ! Make other sketches of your partner's body, this time both a front view and a side view. Now Dowse where to draw their aura around the body on each sketch: locate a start point, and then let your pencil be guided to draw the outlines - be open to the 'feelings' that you get.

Notice if their aura is lopsided, or is closer to the front than the back of your body.

If so, ask (by Dowsing) if their aura needs to be balanced - and if YES then ask to have it balanced, and that it now be balanced; check *"has it now been balanced ?"*

Next use your 'Map Dowsing' skills to see if there is any hole or weak spot in their aura. If so, get permission and (if granted) ask that the damage be repaired with True Holy Love.

You can Dowse for colours in your aura and their location, and then 'intuit' their meanings - note the first explanation that comes to mind for each colour.

You can use your map Dowsing skills to find any thought forms that are causing major problems, and ask in the same way that the thought forms be Healed so that they do not cause problems in the future.

Advanced Healing Overview

There are as many ways to help with Healing as there are stars in the sky. Not any single method is perfect - but some may be better than others in any particular circumstance.

It is important to recognize that our own method may not always work - that the method of another Healer may be more suitable for a person. We all have strengths and weaknesses - and it is when we work together in a team that more can be accomplished.

If you wish to improve your Healing abilities, you can read about the different modalities in general, select those that you think will suit you best for more study, read more in depth about these, and then work with Healers having experience in these - you will learn in practice much more than from study, but study provides a good foundation.

If you keep an open mind, you can ask 'The System' to help you to become proficient in a healing modality - you may receive hints that are not generally known, even by the experienced Teachers, and tell others so that they can improve.

A brief overview of some modalities follows.

<u>Healing Touch, etc.</u>

'Energy Medicine' by Donna Eden, is one of the most important Healing books. In it she uses Kinesiology, a form of Intuitive signaling.

The book has a magnificent explanation of meridians and points, plus Chakras and Auras, combined with the use of hands to move energies to Heal - with practical demonstrations which have been tested and work well. Videos for instruction are available.

Reiki

Reiki formulates the rituals used in Healing by using symbols. Diane Stein's book 'Essential Reiki' enables people to understand the techniques and use its Healing Power without paying enormous amounts of money for the privilege.

Rituals help you to remember the correct way to do something - a program loaded in your mind; when done by many people all over the world, the patterns are 'set in stone' - and so easily called for use by all practitioners

Flower Essences

Particular diseases are associated with emotional problems, such as heart problems being associated with anger. The emotional problems may be alleviated by herbal essences, such as Bach Flower Remedies - but the deeper reasons for allowing hate, greed, anger, etc., to be in the person in the first place must be overcome.

It may be advantageous to use these essences to identify the problem, and then use other methods to eliminate the causes.

Reflexology

Based on the Chinese understanding of meridians, which all have terminal or connector points at many places such as the eyes, ears, teeth, hands, and feet of a person.

The feet are excellent places to work with the meridians - they are more spaciously placed, located without undue effort, and you can work on them easily.

Reflexology practitioners can often extract 'other dimensional life forms' (such as having a pain which moves around) and give great relief; many of these take up residence (like squatters) in the meridians and the muscles of the body.

Acupuncture / Acupressure

The ancient Chinese knowledge is that there are subtle energy channels that run throughout our body, coming to the surface at certain places, and probably having connections between these places within our auric bodies.

These channels are known to surface in our feet, our hands, our ears, and our eyes. Iridology is based on examining the eyes - where indications of diseases can be recognized, even before the disease becomes apparent in the body itself.

When these channels become blocked, illness occurs; by applying pressure or lancing into the channels (especially where these channels have major points) the blockages are released, and health improved.

Shamanic Healing

This is a far deeper aspect of Healing which is beyond the scope of many.   But the books 'Urban Shaman' and 'Kahuna Healing' by Serge Kahili King are well worth reading.

One simple Shamanic method is to attach all of a particular worry to a piece of paper - writing down the problem, putting all your feelings into the writing, visualizing all aspects of the problem being removed from your own Being and put into the paper; and then burning the paper.

I was with one Shaman when he cleared the 'not good' energies from a house; after working within the house, he chose a small pine tree in the garden, stripped a section of bark from around its trunk, and tied tinsel and other bright objects to the tree.

He then gave instruction to the people in the house to cut the tree down in about a week and then burn it. He explained that the tinsel and bright objects would attract 'not good' energies to the tree, and then they would be changed in form when burnt.

This may be the origin of a Christmas Tree - to clear away 'not good' energies at the end of a year, so that the New Year would start free of past negativity. Perhaps the original intent was not understood when the Christian religion included Christmas Trees as part of the Pagan Festival that they renamed Christmas !

What is the effect of hanging an effigy of an Angel on such a tree ?

Power Animals

One of the key abilities of Shamanic practice is working with Power Animals - working with them to do work, getting their help to visit places both 'Above' and 'Below' and to overcome problems and obstacles, and so do Healing in whatever way is needed.

'Power Animals' in this context includes the Spiritual Essence of animals, birds, fish, reptiles, plants, trees, insects, and all other life forms, although the co-operation of animals and birds are used in most reported cases.

When doing Healing work, do not be surprised if such a Power Animal comes to assist ! Give thanks - we need all the help we can get !

Soul Retrieval

One of the main ways that Shamans heal is by 'Soul Retrieval'; when a person has an intensively traumatic experience, some part of them, such as a 'Soul Piece', seems to disconnect from them.

Soul Retrieval includes identifying the trauma, locating the missing Soul Piece, persuading it that is now safe to return, assuring it that is will be welcomed and loved, and bringing it back to the rest of the Soul.

It may be that when a person dies, the chances of any missing Soul Piece being reconnected disappear; perhaps they try to have a separate existence in the 'Astral Plane'.

Perhaps other aspects of a person, that are 'not good', also separate from a Soul when it departs a human body at death. Eastern wisdom tells that these are the main inhabitants of the Astral Plane, and that they will try and get back into a living human being - usually causing unwelcome effects if successful.

For example, if such a part has been used to drug use or heavy drinking, they may hang around places where this occurs, seeking to find a human who has such a tendency, and then endeavouring to join.

Such cases are examples of the saying 'Like seeks Like'.

"The Pattern of Health"   by Aubrey Westlake, M.D.,

It may sound surprising, in these days when specialization starts at about 11 years of age, that I left school at eighteen without any definite idea of what I wanted to do, beyond a rather vague notion that I wanted to study Health.

This at first seemed promising, but on going into it I soon found that to study Health, it seemed, one had just to study Disease, which seemed a contradiction in terms.

Dr Bach and his Flower Remedies

My first firm contact with the new fields of medicine I was destined to explore came about in the following way. A woman told me her son had been cured of meningitis by a remarkable doctor - a Dr Bach - who had only used remedies which he himself had found and prepared in a special way from wild flowers.

This intrigued inc very much, as from my then medical knowledge I could not imagine how flower preparations could possibly influence (let alone cure) such a serious pathological condition as a meningitis, and so I asked her to tell me more.

It happened that she had worked with the doctor and had had instruction from him in the preparation of his remedies, and had subsequently used them herself in treatment with the greatest success.

Dr Edward Bach was a well-known Harley Street bacteriologist and a brilliant research worker. Suddenly for no apparent reason he threw up all his work and his lucrative practice and retired to the wilds of Wales, there to hunt intuitively for the flowers and trees which had special vital healing force.

These flowers, prepared in a special way either by strong sunlight or boiling, could deal effectively, so he claimed, with the disharmonies of the personality and with all the emotional states lying behind the physical, and thus restore peace and inner happiness to the sick and distressed. thereby curing all diseases in a simple but fundamental way.

For example, if you suffered from known fears, you took Mixnulus; if you had had a shock of any sort, the remedy was Star of Bethlehem; indecision was treated with Scleranthus; lack of faith with Gentian; obsessional thoughts with White Chestnut; and panic or any urgency with Rock Rose.

As with all pioneers. his path was by no means easy. His medical colleagues thought he was slightly mad, and his friends were filled with regrets for what they felt was a sheer waste of his brilliant talents.

But Dr Bach had no doubts and no regrets. He knew he was on the right path. He finally found thirty-eight remedies in all, chiefly from the common flowers or trees of the hedgerows.

But the obtaining of any given remedy was a very severe strain, as previous to finding the flower which gave it, he experienced in toto both the physical and emotional states of which it was the antidote.

Dr Bach's claim that treatment of the emotional state or states is all that is necessary to cure the patient, or, in his own words, *"only through tranquility of mind and soul can a human being reach bodily health"* seemed too far-fetched, and at first I was frankly skeptical.

So I proceeded to try the remedies. To make the test as conclusive as possible I eliminated all other therapeutic factors so that with only one factor operating - the Bach remedy; if anything happened it would presumably be due to the remedy and to nothing else.

I treated a variety of conditions in this way, and much to my surprise I became completely convinced that the remedies acted as Dr Bach had claimed, even in acute conditions. I obtained remarkable and dramatic results.

In these early cases the remedies were chosen as suggested by Dr Bach by an assessment of the emotional state or condition. I found, especially in complicated and chronic conditions, that it was very difficult to assess the emotional state of the patient.

I found that I could get over this difficulty by using myself as an indicator.

I took the patient's left hand in my right and then, after a short interval to get 'attuned', working blindly I took up each remedy in turn in my left hand, running through the whole thirty-eight.

On some I got a reaction. i.e. a sort of tingling sensation which started at the back of my scalp, and, if strong, would go all over me.

If and when I got this reaction on a bottle, I put it aside. At the end I looked to see which bottles I had put on one side. and I took it that these were what the patient needed. The numbers chosen might vary from one to six, seldom more.

I was not sure how accurate this method was, but it seemed to work, judging from the fact that one could work from the remedies obtained into diagnosing the emotional state of the patient - and this diagnosing was strangely accurate. This so to speak. was proof in reverse, as the indicated Bach remedies gave me an insight into the patient's emotional make-up.

One of the most spectacular cases in which this method worked was a child aged about six, who was brought to me because she was 'a queer little thing', according to her parents. She seemed retarded both mentally and physically, though she was certainly not mentally deficient. I 'bached' her, as I called it. and got a terrific reaction on Clematis.

This was given to her, and from that time she began to become normal in every way, and never looked back. It was the turning point in the child's life.

I am not convinced that they will cure a patient by themselves - direct treatment of the physical may be needed as well.

"I don't Mind,
You don't Matter"
Defining Mind and Matter

It is a Matter of Form

It is my understanding that 'All that Is' is made of the same 'Baby Energies' or 'Lights' doing different three (or more) dimensional 'dances' at various speeds to form everything, and doing so in families, teams, teams of families, and families of teams - the complexity of the dances growing with the size of the numbers of dancers involved.

Physicists know that atoms are made of sub-atomic particles of various form, and that electrons are there, then not there - then somewhere else an electron appears, perhaps a replacement.

It seems that they are moving in and out of the physical dimension - and so into a different dimension, perhaps operating at a different speed, if this is the difference between dimensions.

Not only are these dances performed to form matter, but also to form thoughts and auric patterns, and doing this in all levels of existence, in all dimensions.

'As Above, So Below' implies that this is the 'substance' of 'Energy Beings' at all levels, including Angels, Elementals, Spirits, etc.

Sub-atomic Particles

When examining the way that sub-atomic particles operate, physicists find that different particles can be recognized by their attributes: the form of the dance that they make, and the effect of that dance upon others - such dances being consistent for any particular form of particle.

Patterns can be described as mathematical rules and formulae - intelligence must be involved in making these, to define the basic steps, and the ways that these are joined to form more complicated equations.

This has been recognized by mystics as the basis of 'Sacred Geometry', and demonstrated by computer users experimenting with Mandelbrot pattern growth.

The Dancers

If the idea is correct that everything is made of these dancers, then they must intrinsically 'know' what to do, or that they follow a 'Dance Leader' - who must know what is required for a dance.

In either case this implies that all who are involved in such dances have the ability to think (what do I do next ?), to act (I do the dance), to feel (does the dance feel correct ?), and perhaps to Love (I Love to do a dance which is beneficial to others !).

If so, then each Light and Baby Energy is a Being in its own right ! Even more important (for us) is the understanding that 'We are All the Same' - and so can communicate with others like us. Not just other human beings, but with 'All that Is' - 'Above' as well as 'Below'.

How can we use this ability ?

Vibrational Patterns

These are the dances made - the vibrational patterns being the small movement of a microscopic (or even far smaller) dance.

Any thought that we have is itself a vibrational pattern - and wave studies have shown that when waves meet, their patterns are affected, the new patterns embodying the contributory patterns.

This is the basis of holography, which proceeds to 'untangle' the combinations to obtain copies of the original contributory patterns, using the knowledge that each tiny part of the combination has its own picture of the whole - including the original patterns.

Therefore it follows that whenever we send a thought, we have an effect on the recipients - whether or not the recipients are those that we intended.

The more precisely that we direct our thoughts, the higher the concentration of the thought that can be expected to be received by the intended recipient.

Improving the Environment

By propagating good thoughts, we will improve our immediate environment - at home, work, or play. The more people who do this, the stronger will be the effect.

Emoto and Backster have demonstrated that water and plants are responsive (and we know this is true for animals) so we know that our thoughts can be expected to have an effect on the total environment - even throughout the world.

Unfortunately there are a lot of people having 'not good' thoughts of various types, so we may have to work very hard to make any substantive change on a large scale - but every little effort helps !

Home First !

We can expect to get the best results when we work on a small scale - on ourselves, our family, our working environment, and our community.

We ourselves are influenced by the thoughts and actions of others - and especially how we respond !

It is our response which activates reaction within our own Being, so the less negative emotion that we attach to the thoughts and actions of others, the less we are affected.

Love is the strongest force, the greatest power - so when something happens that could be detrimental to us, just send thoughts of Love to those involved, to help them be healed of their problems.

Energy Healing

We do not like being hurt. If 'As Above, So Below' is correct, then this applies to all life forms, which are all made of energies.

Often it is those who have been hurt in some way who 'take it out' on others. It may be that the energies in those who are causing problems have been hurt, and that they need to be Healed.

This can apply to the energies within ourselves - who may be the cause or effect of hurts. So sending Love and Healing to yourself, and to all the energies in your total Being, can effect Healing of yourself - and your problems and illnesses.

By sending this Love and Healing you are changing the vibrational pattern of your components such as your cells and organs - changing them for better, and helping them to Heal.

By blessing your food, you increase its 'Life Force', its 'Love Energy' - when you eat it, it is more beneficial for you !

Making Water into Medicine

Dr Emoto has shown that water is responsive to thought, even changing its physical structure according to the thoughts applied.

Since water is the major component of our body cells, any beneficial vibrational pattern that we apply to the water that is in these cells will itself be beneficial to ourselves.

This also applies to the water that we drink, which will go to these cells; this can be used as a method of changing normal water into a medicine !

The late Malcolm Rae set out in the 1960s to find a method of copying the healing potential of known therapeutic substances into a neutral medium (such as water). Before he began this work, Rae was fully aware that the possibility of 'geometric healing', as this work was sometimes called, had been repeatedly discussed in the philosophical and medical literature of the Western culture since the writings of Plato. Many people have sought the secret to geometric healing, and thought that it lay hidden in the esoteric field known as Sacred Geometry.

Rae established that three elements must be present around any healing substance: the substance itself; the invisible but all-pervasive magnetic field of the Earth; and the invisible but radiesthetically detectable 'field signature' of the substance under study.

Rae hypothesized that somehow a substance and the Earth's magnetic field interacted to form the unique field signature of that substance, one must have two elements: the presence of the Earth's magnetic field, and a representation of the field signature of the substance one wanted to recreate.

This line of thinking represented a radical departure from the traditional operations of Sacred Geometry, and opened up the possibility of new discoveries. Although it de-emphasized the role of geometry in the solution to the problem, it introduced magnetism into the equation, thereby providing a powerful new force for the development of a remedy's energy pattern.

Rae's experiments demonstrated that his observations and reasoning were correct. If he placed a geometric representation of the signature of a healing substance into the Earth's magnetic field, the healing properties of that substance could be duplicated into a neutral medium, such as water.

Radiesthetic researchers commonly measure the boundaries of the field signatures of various substances from the centre of the substance to the edge of the field.

Through trial and error Rae discovered that eight measurements were sufficient to uniquely represent any substance. If he took eight measurements, each locating one portion of a field's edge, he would obtain a unique representation for that healing substance.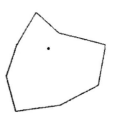

Malcolm Rae continued his research for more than 15 years, eventually developing a clinically-precise system for reproducing the healing potential of various remedies from printed patterns. Each magnetic pattern is a series of concentric circles. They differ from one another only in the number and location of the partial radii within each pattern.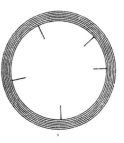

By working closely with a number of doctors, Rae was able to test his results clinically at each stage of the work; he thoroughly verified each step of the process.

Some years ago some symbols similar to Rae's 8-measurement diagrams were published in a book called 'The Paper Doctor' by Don Gerrard in the USA - but intense legal action by the US drug companies and medical associations forced it to be banned - and copies were even burnt, signifying that it was really important !

These symbols were noted by Don as requiring a magnet to be placed precisely below the dot, and the glass of water (only 1/8th inch depth of water) also had to be centred over the dot. A total of 58 remedies were given in the book.

We can consider two dimensional symbols as 'maps' of the three dimensional dances - not the 'real thing', but a representation. Notwithstanding this, they are effective - they work !

The Sanjeevini Symbols

These were developed in India, and bear a remarkable resemblance to the circular symbols which were Rae's ultimate choice.

Luckily, these Sanjeevini symbols are outside the jurisdiction of the authorities in the USA. They have been placed on the Internet - to download them without charge, with full instructions for their use, visit: **www.saisanjeevini.org**

This diagram is a 'Sanjeevini Card'. You can download these cards for the Healing of 60 different body parts and 186 diseases !

One way to use these Sanjeevini symbols is to select the needed symbol, and place it under a glass of water for 15 seconds - very simple !

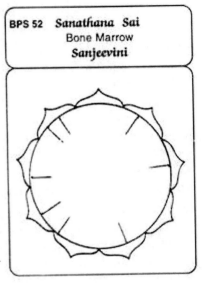

BPS 52   **Sanathana Sai**
Bone Marrow
Sanjeevini

The symbol puts the needed vibrational pattern for Healing into the water - an analysis of the water would not show this, since the vibrational pattern is 'too subtle' to be ascertained by physical examination. This is just like any Homeopathic remedy.

It appears that the Sanjeevini symbols are more powerful than the 'Paper Doctor' symbols - and more Healing patterns are available.

It is also similar to the way that my Pendulum moves when doing a major Healing - going back and forth in various diameters.

The web page includes a manual which explains other methods of use, including how more than one symbol can be combined, and the use of carriers other than water; there are pages of just the symbols.

If you print the downloaded symbols then you can cut them to business card size and laminate them. I have a laminator, and found it worked well when I placed the cut symbol between kitchen sealing plastic (also cut to size), put them in the lamination holders, and ran them through the laminator - cheap and effective.

It is probably best to use Bill Askin's technique (which follows) to remove unwanted vibrational patterns from the water before imprinting it with the Sanjeevini pattern.

I also suggest using your Pendulum, rotating clockwise, to imprint the 'essence, vibrational pattern, and energy' of the Sanjeevini symbol.

Making your own Medicine

Bill Askin is a trapper from northern Alberta, highly skilled in the Silva Mind Method and in Dowsing - he introduced Raymon Grace, a leading Silva teacher and internationally known Shaman, to Dowsing.

Bill has developed a very simple method of demonstrating the use of one's Power of Thought with a Pendulum:

1. Take a glass of water, and taste it - remember the taste.
2. Use your Pendulum to make anti-clockwise rotations over the glass of water, asking that *"All things not good for me be removed from this water"*.
3. Taste the water again - it probably has a better taste.
4. Use your Pendulum to make clockwise rotations over the glass of water, asking that *"All things needed for my good health be installed into this water"* or *"that the vibrational pattern, essence, and energy of all medicine needed to cure the causes and effects [of a problem - Health or otherwise] be put in this water"*.
5. Taste the water again - it probably has an even better taste, and is now medicine designed just for you ! Drink it all.

Remember to express your gratitude to all involved in so helping you to have such good water !

Do not expect to be completely Healed at the first sip that you take - like most medicines, time is needed to be fully effective, and further doses may be needed. See p.172 for help with toxins, etc.

People who have done this experiment are amazed at the way the taste changes, even without noticing any immediate medicinal effects. Experiment yourself - unlike most man-made medicines, there will not be any side-effects, so you cannot be hurt.

You do not have to know the name of the medicine that is needed; you can just ask 'The King of All Plants' to decide which plant essences would be best, and to install their vibrational patterns and energies, in the quantity needed.

If you want the very best medicine, say when installing with a clockwise rotation:*"I Bless this water with 'True Holy Love, Namaste', with 'Blessing 995', and with 'Healing 997'. I send my personal thanks, my personal gratitude, and my personal Love, to all who help in this ceremony"*.

Remember to be sincere when doing any of this work !

This last blessing can be used with all that you eat or drink - better still, Bless 'All that is Consumed' for a greater effect.

It might be a good idea to make a glass of water-medicine for yourself first thing in the morning and last thing at night - asking 'The System' that 'the water be charged with all the essences, vibrational patterns, and energies that you need for perfect good health'.

Protect One Self !

Have you found that when you are with certain people, they really seem to enjoy your company - but afterwards you feel drained ? Some people do suck energy from others !

To overcome this, visualize a protective shell around you that prevents your energy from being sucked or drained by other life forms (not by only humans) - doing this as a safety precaution.

Do not make it so that it stops all energy, since then you would not get the incoming good energy that you need.

You do not have to specify the shape or colours of the shield - ask your Guardian Angel (or other Spiritual Helpers) to make it and place it in position.

Often 'Upstairs' may need you to put some physical energy into anything that you do in other dimensions. They may not use it as it is, but transform it into something else - physical energy is quite strong, and using the energy provided helps 'Upstairs' to do more.

A simple clapping of your hands may be all that is needed; perhaps it is meant to help you understand that you must help yourself, not just rely on others. <u>Remember to thank all who so help you !</u>

You will probably find that the energy sucking people do not relish your company so much - they cannot steal your energy, perhaps the main reason for being friendly with you !

You can take similar steps to prevent or reduce harassment or other such problems at your home or workplace.

Mind over Matter

These experiments will probably have helped you to realize that you have great 'Mind Power' - all humans have this, even if they are not so aware.

As described in the film 'The Secret', there are many 'energies' in Creation that are waiting for a good job - a job that is beneficial, that gives them a chance to help others.

The Human Mind has the ability to call on these resources, and to work with other levels of 'Being-ness' to improve life for all - not just other humans !

Our thoughts can identify what is needed, visualize the completed design, and take steps to 'make it so' - not only in the physical dimension, but as we have seen, also in the dimension of thought.

When we 'plant a thought' it will grow according to the nutrients supplied - including the comparable thoughts of others.

The more people who think in the same way, the greater the likelihood that the thought will flourish.

The greatest of all nutrients is Love; as with the light from the sun, this is needed for growth - and lots of Love will enable good, strong growth.   There is little difference between 'Love' and 'Life' - as written, or in reality.

Viciousness, violence, greed, selfishness, and similar negativity are all like herbicides that have a detrimental effect - perhaps even killing the plant.

Orgone Energy Generator

You can make a very simple, cheap, and effective Orgone Energy Generator using household aluminium foil and corrugated plastic sheeting - as used for election signs in many political campaigns; it comes in many colours, being about 1/4 inch thick: these normally come in 4ft * 8ft sheets; you will need a 4 feet by 2 feet section, which you cut it into 6 pieces - each 16 inches long by 12 inches wide, the width of the aluminium foil.

One sheet is enough for four of these generators.

Section of Plastic Sheeting

Now make three identical units by laying the aluminium foil over one 12" by 16" piece, then covering it with another piece, and using sticky tape bind these together to form a sandwich, and make a mark on the sandwich to show which foil side is uppermost and the direction in which the foil was placed - this is needed since the finished sandwiches must always be placed in a special way.

When not in use, stack the three sandwiches with all the directional arrows pointing in the same way.

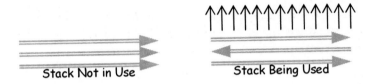

Orgone Energy

Stack Not in Use

Stack Being Used

To use, turn the middle sandwich so that its arrow goes in the reverse direction - then stand on the stack in your bare feet, or place the stack under an injured area of your body. Most people will feel a boost of energy.

It seems that a cone of energy is projected from the generator, gradually widening as it rises.

When I stand on my Orgone Generator I hear excited yells:

The Parade is coming !

The Parade is coming !

The Parade is coming !

These are just as if the 'energies' (perhaps in the spaces in the plastic sheets) were spectators at the sort of parade that is held in large cities on major occasions !

Standing on them (in the grand-stand ?) I certainly feel their excited energy !

All about LuLu

Lulu is a skeleton form of the human body encased in plastic and about 18 inches long, and comes with an unsharpened wooden pencil - you place its eraser end on LuLu where a joint is to be adjusted, and tap it to make the correction

You write the person's name on the plastic, or have it clearly in your mind - either one will work. It is best if you have 'witness' attached (or by the side) such as a photograph or piece of hair - the more evidence that you have to ensure a correct connection the better.

Now start with your Pendulum on all the person's joints and spine. When you find a vertebrae out, Dowse which side should you tap, and the number of taps needed to put it back in place.

Then use another pencil or your finger as a 'mallet' to make the taps on the pencil, holding the eraser end on the vertebra.

You can use this procedure for other types of Healing as well - and for more detail you can use a book that has detailed descriptions of the body instead of the plastic model skeleton.

You may find that some Health problems can be Healed with your Pendulum by itself - tapping an organ may not be the best way to proceed.

Note that working with Lulu - and other 'direct' Healing on the hurts and pains is relieving the symptoms; the causes of such problems need to be addresses as well.

Remember that so many illnesses seem to be caused by 'things' in our auras, in our 'Light Bodies'. Treatment is needed at these levels.

Gleanings - The Lulu Files

Does LuLu work ? Yes it does. I had a friend from Kansas City call with a problem. She had been working on a lady that had serious back problems but hadn't done much good so she called me.

I told her I would work on it and I did so two different times over the next two days. Today I got a check in the mail saying her back was feeling fine, no more pain.

I didn't tell her that I found she might be starting a stomach ulcer. I'll tell her later.

The check wasn't asked for, she just sent it. I have even used this system on myself and my wife.   JS

I also have LuLu.   In Qi-gong healing, we use a model with numbers on the spinal column.

An acupuncture needle is inserted on a spot on the spinal column that corresponds to certain dates for the time frame that you are doing the healing.

A laser pen is put directed at the point where the needle is inserted in the spinal column of the model after Dowsing for the correct length of time to keep the needle inserted.

I have incorporated colour healing with this, using Dinshah's colour zones, colour filters, and the laser light. Then I say the Qi-gong mantra over the person - I do not touch them.   JZ

After getting the original LuLu I found the side with the muscles difficult to read because the numbers were blacked out.

So I first bought a anatomy colouring book and was able to see where all the muscle groups were on LuLu and, of course, a lot more. I also started to LuLu the anatomy book.

All this seemed to be working very well as feedback has been universally positive. I have been very hard on people I have worked on to be truthful about how they are feeling, not just tell me they are doing better because they do not want to hurt my feelings/ego.

Anyway, I have now picked up a book of 37 different anatomical charts and have been working on my wife and friends with what appears to be great success.

I had just been doing the normal pulled/tense muscles/tendons or bone injuries to these parts of the body. But with the new book I have access to the entire body.

My wife had an echocardiogram done last year showing the beginning of heart disease. Before her last test I did a check and found something going on with a pulmonary valve and did the LuLu on it. Did not find anything else.

Test results came back showing no signs of heart disease. She has also been diagnosed with deteriorating discs in the lower back and osteoporosis so I am tackling that now.

I am amazed by this and am also having fun at the same time. I have even been successful doing myself when I think about it.   BW

I'm trying to figure out what you would do for, say, a strained ligament.   I've actually spent the evening poring over one of my anatomy books trying to figure out which of the ligaments in my knee is giving me pain.

So here's my crazy idea for the weekend: try tapping on picture of said ligament once I've identified it through Dowsing. Any better ideas ?   S

Actually rub the picture to smooth the aura, and then sweep the soreness out with your hand like it was dust on the table, with your hand. Move it right down to the feet and out.   JS

My LuLu doesn't have muscles at all. I use pictures from medical books for muscles veins, arteries and all sorts of other stuff. When Wendell Hoffmann originally taught me to use the Pendulum we received a big book full of all charts and pictures of different parts of the body and lots of other interesting stuff.

I never thought in a thousand years I would ever get round to using them but find I use them all the time now.

The way I use LuLu is as follows - and it works like a charm. Go up and down the picture asking where there is a problem, set it up with Spirit first that you want them in the order of priority.

When you get a YES, put your pointer on the picture and ask if it is in the right place. Then ask, does it need adjusting from the left or right ? - then up or down ?   This was learned from Body Restructuring through Spiritual Response Therapy.

When you have found out and placed your pointer, ask if it is in the right place; if so: tap, tap, tap - and ask if the adjustment has taken.

Same for the ligament picture, muscles and whatever picture you like. It is the intent that is the secret to this and I find it very, very helpful for myself and also different clients I have worked on.   C

BW said: 'I have worked on people to be truthful about how they are feeling, not just tell me they are doing better because they do not want to hurt my feelings/ego.'

I smelt a rat when about five years ago a client said *"I'm 90% better but of course I still have the ankle problem".*

Ankle problem ? Nothing about it in my notes, initial session or later.

Client: *"Oh, no, I didn't mention it, did I, it's not that bad, I didn't want to load you with too much !"*

Grinding my teeth, I then instituted as standard a system originally designed by Surrey University for a series of trials of complementary medicine: the client writes down at each session the worst eight things that they hoped the practitioner could help - money problems, accident-proneness and relationships were allowed in.

Each problem was scored for severity, 10 being 'unbearably bad' and 0 for previously-mentioned conditions being 'not there now'.

I never restricted the list to eight items. The client could put down as many as they liked. Only then did I get a proper clear picture of what happens in healing.

I estimate that 'complete success' - all the problems declining to 1 or lower within six months - occurs in three-quarters of cases. These are basically healthy people with just a few specific troubles.

With the remainder, there is a most interesting pattern which occurs again and again and illuminates what a perfectionist would regard as 'failure' even if the clients, who are grateful for any mercy, do not.

Here, the lesser and usually most recent problems vanish, but the longer-term problems remain in place, perhaps with a short-lived dip of one or two points and they worsen again. At the same time a number of the lesser problems which had disappeared flare up again. Also some fresh minor problems arise.

Soon the smaller problems and the new ones have disappeared again and after a further period the client and I have the reward of perhaps one or two of the severe problems remaining lower than they were.

Further bright therapeutic ideas produce repeats of this pattern.

After a year, further perseverance does pay off, but very slowly. This is a learning area for me.   Dan Wilson

Exploring Genes and Other Influences

This is based on the talk given by Walt Woods at the Holistic Intuition Society's 'Power of Thought' Convention 2001 at Olds College, Alberta - July 27-30, with additional thoughts by John Living.

Just for fun you might try asking if you have tumor suppressing genes that are turned off ?

If YES, you might try asking 'The System' if the genes might be turned on, just to see what kind of response you get.

It is surprising just how much we can change - if there is any problem that is causing you concern, just ask 'The System' if it can be removed, changed, or alleviated - by altering genes or by any other method used by 'The System', without causing any effects that are not beneficial to you, will not cause any hurt or harm to others, and are for your Highest and Best Good.

If so, ask 'Can I ? May I ? Should I ?' - and if all are YES then ask that the needed action be taken by 'The System', always acting in True Holy Love.

If you build this into a program, ensure that any changes to genes are imprinted immediately on all genes that need this healing. It may be that additional changes are needed over time, or that the program needs to be run again. If so, get advice from 'The System' concerning this aspect - and make sure that the advice is followed !

How Genes Work

Each set of genes seems to have two links - perhaps one is a weak link and the other a strong link. If so, none, one, or both links could be activated, to give settings: Off, Low, Medium, or High. It may well be that further variations are achieved by more than one gene having an effect upon an attribute controlled by such genes.

Since cells are replicated by division, and loss of coding and errors in switches may have occurred over time, it may be a good idea to check if your Master Genes need any correction, and if so, to have this done first.

We all have repair genes and maintenance genes that help to ensure that cell replication is correct - it is wise to check that these are switched ON in all your cells, and if not, to have them so switched to be ON - preferably to a High setting.

Examples of changes to genes that can be beneficial include allergies, production of vitamins C and D, addiction to drugs and alcohol, obesity, suppression of tumors and cancerous growths, reactions to others (becoming better able to respect and relate to them, and their reactions in return), and youthfulness (you may not grow young, but you might be able to avoid physical degeneration in old age).

Your 'Power of Thought' is enormous, but usually not known and so not utilized. The way that you can get changes made to your genes is but one example of how you can get improvements made with the help of the 'System' - try to take similar action to improve the environment, change attitudes of others, and manifest love, health, harmony, and prosperity.

If you do not ask, you will not get ! So start work now on using your 'Power of Thought' to help yourself and others - and be ready for major surprises !

You might also try asking if the vitamin 'C' gene can be turned on. After all, we may be only one of possibly two mammals with it turned off.

Another area you might look at is the possibility that gene mutations might be corrected while the cell is making a copy of its chromosome from the 'chemical soup'.

It may also be fun to try dialoguing with your Dowsing Team about such things.

One aspect of cancer that is not well recognized (and may apply to other diseases as well) is that expert clairvoyants such as Raymon Grace and C. W. Leadbeater, when looking at cells affected by cancer, see that they are spiralling anti-clockwise - which also affects their polarity.

So it may be most beneficial to ensure that all your cells (and all that is in them) spiral clockwise - which seems to be the 'good' way for all life. Such cells may have lost communication with the 'Wisdom of your Being' - so instruct such communication to be re-established; this may well result in such cells being recycled.

Changing Influences

First select a change that you want to happen such as:

- Possession and intrusion by other entities to be eliminated and prevented
- Total Being to be in maintained in good health in all aspects and in all dimensions
- Intuitive abilities to be fully operational with all blockages removed
- Reactions to and from others to be in Harmony and True Holy Love
- All Repair and Maintenance Genes to be fully operational
- All cells to maintain good communication with the 'Wisdom of our Being'
- All cells and their components to be re-aligned to be in harmony with the Master Cell, to spiral good, and to have the correct polarity for perfect good health
- All Healing Energies in the Being to always act in 'Healing Good in a Good Way'
- Chakras, Glands, and Organs to be cleared of all negativity and made fully operational
- Meridians, Systems, and Grids to have blockages removed and communication lines working
- Eyesight, Hearing, etc., to be in perfect working condition
- Ability to see Auras, Chakras, Thought Forms, and Visions to be implemented
- Production of vitamins, especially C and D, to be enabled
- Addiction to drugs, alcohol, etc. to be eliminated
- Obesity to be cancelled and slimness implemented
- Allergic reactions to substances and essences to be removed
- Suppression of tumours and cancerous growths to be implemented
- Particular Diseases to be eliminated
- Hate, Fear, Greed, Jealousy, Envy, Anger to be eliminated
- Youth to be implemented
- Sexual attractiveness to be meaningfully increased
- Abilities for sexual performance to be at the highest level
- Prosperity to be manifested in Harmony and in True Holy Love

If you are choosing more than one change, Dowse to check whether you need to run the program separately for each change, or find which changes can be done at the same time.

Now ask *"Can the needed changes be made to achieve this goal ?"* and if so, *"May I and Should I now Dowse to have such changes made ?"*, stipulating to whom the changes are to be made - yourself, or another named person.

If so, then run the program and then check that the changes have been satisfactorily made, and the time needed for them to be fully in effect - or the times for partial effectiveness. Check if you need to re-run the program in the future.

Changing Influences Program

"The Changing Influences Program is to work with all my Dowsing programs and be operational at all times. Other names, words, situations and numbers may be temporarily substituted inside [ ]'s. Questions or requests need only simple reference wording. All changes made are to be continually in effect

If it be in the Highest and Best Good of the total Being and of All Creation then all changes that are needed to achieve the goal of [...] to [myself] are to be made now to all energies, genes, thought forms, belief systems, programs, and cellular and other memories as is required, in the physical and all metaphysical bodies and auras of the Being, in all times, in all nows, in all planes of existence, in all dimensions, and at all levels including any at the Soul, Lower Self, Higher Self, Spirit, Soul contract or other levels.

All such changes to be made without any non-beneficial effect on any part of the Being, without harm to any life form, and at the highest appropriate correction or adjustment rate with consideration for personal comfort and safety, and are subject to revision without notice or prior approval if so deemed to be in the Highest and Best Good of the total Being and of All Creation.

In all cases the cellular memories are to be adjusted accordingly to remove any emotional attachments that may cause any re-occurrence, and all the memories are to have memories of hurts and pains eliminated; such changes in genes are to be imprinted in the master gene, in all other genes, and be re-imprinted as needed.

Protection is to be manifested and maintained for the life of the Being to prevent any re-occurrence or incidences of any type (such as viruses and diseases) caused by other entities, Beings, or energies that are in any way non-beneficial to the Being, such protection to transmute all not good energies to be good and return them to their sender in True Holy Love.

End of Program. Thank you." Remember to check the installation !

Working with 'True Holy Love, Namaste'

Most of the foregoing refers to programs for Dowsing and health - perhaps a small part of the activities of our Heart-Mind-Brain team. If we can apply programs to control / direct our Dowsing, and to improve our health, then can we do the same to guide all the activities of our Being ?

I asked the 'Wisdom of my Being' and got a BIG YES ! - and was reminded of the many sayings that 'How we think is how we become', that by installing programs to guide our thought patterns, we form our future selves.

As human beings we are always aware of our faults - and by thinking of them we reinforce our weaknesses. Once recognized, we must not think more of them, but affirm the opposites, giving ourselves needed strengths in the qualities that we desire.

It is a fact that sending help and Love to others is more powerful than wishing such for ourselves - but it is also true that what we ask for others will be reflected in us, and we can be specific in asking that to always happen - immediately !

The intent is that each of us has the right to a good life with plentiful happiness, joy, love, wealth, good health, power, and prosperity. These should not be used just for personal gratification, but for enhancing our ability to give help and True Holy Love to all others.

Recognize that by sending 'True Holy Love, Namaste' to others, including those that are causing you problems, and by placing them into the Divine care of the 'Force for Good', you help them to be better and reduce (or eliminate) their unwanted actions. Do not dwell on them or the problems they cause, but trust that the 'Force for Good' will take all needed action.

The Namaste Program

'The Namaste Program is to become part of and work with all activities of my Heart-Mind-Brain team and my Total Being, to be continually in effect.

This program shall automatically replicate itself and become permanently installed in each and every life form or Being to whom any thought of 'True Holy Love, Namaste' or any equivalent thought is sent, and it shall be effective in all 'nows', in all futures, in all times, in all planes of existence, in all dimensions, and in all domains, without any loss of strength or energy.

'The System', working with the 'Force for Good', is requested to give all available support and help to manifest all these activities in all ways and in all aspects, always so acting for the Highest and Best Good of All Creation, including the sender and the recipient so that they are better able to do the tasks assigned, always operating in True Holy Love, Namaste.

By the installation of this program the Total Being of the recipient shall be Blessed with True Holy Love, Namaste, and shall request and consider the advice and guidance of the 'Force for Good' that is both within the Total Being and in All Creation, always accessed from the infinite knowledge and wisdom of 'All That Is' and given in Truth and in True Holy Love, Namaste; and that all thoughts and actions shall be positive, knowing that each and every day each and every part of the Total Being shall get better in every way that is True Holy Love, Namaste. It is so.

Such Blessing with True Holy Love, Namaste, shall include but not be restricted to:

- Enhancement of the 'Good God Energy' within the Total Being.
- Replacement of all hate, grudges, ill-will, and resentment by True Holy Love, Namaste.
- Replacement of closed beliefs with a mind open to accepting truths.
- Release of all hypnosis and fears by truth that is understood, and not anything except such truth.
- Replacement of greed, jealousy, and envy by the gift of sharing in True Holy Love, Namaste.
- Release of anger by forgiving others and self, and by the understanding of lessons involved.
- Replacement of all discord and confusion by peace and harmony.
- Release of all emotional attachments that cause problems or unwanted reactions.
- Replacement of all diseases and illnesses by good health, and the release and elimination from all cellular memory of such hurts and pains.
- Release of all blockages and obstructions to allow joy, happiness, and prosperity to manifest.
- Protection from any and all interference from energies that are not now in the 'Force for Good', transforming such energies for use in the 'Force for Good'.
- Elimination and cancellation of all causes of poverty and the replacement of poverty with abundance in Good Spirit, material wealth, comfort, and True Holy Love, Namaste.
- Replacement of selfishness with respect for self and all other forms of life including the inanimate.

- Enhancement of gratitude for all lessons and Blessings of life.
- Recognition of playing an important part in the 'Force for Good'.
- Such Blessing with True Holy Love, Namaste, shall reinforce and affirm the following truths which shall always be part of all my thinking, decision making, and actions:
- I dedicate my Total Being to the 'Force for Good', to help the Light shine in All Creation.
- I recognize and enhance the Good in myself and in all others.
- I recognize my weaknesses and shortcomings, and ask help of the 'Force for Good' to overcome them; I see myself free of all such weaknesses and shortcomings.
- I envisage success in all that I do; I see in my mind the joy and happiness that I give to others.
- I do not judge others, but decide my actions in their regard, guided by the 'Force for Good'.
- I trust in the 'Force for Good', knowing all that I give shall be immediately returned multiplied.
- I maintain confidence in my decisions and actions; I am free of all irritations and interference from others.
- I have confidence and belief in myself; others have confidence and belief in me and my abilities.
- I release all who I attempt to possess, influence, or control into the Divine care of the 'Force for Good', and cut and protect against all links that attempt to possess, influence, or control me or drain my good energies or life forces, sending all into the Divine care of the 'Force for Good'.
- I release all stubbornness, animosity, anger, hate, greed, jealousy, envy, power over others, and all other energies that cause problems into the Divine care of the 'Force for Good' to be healed and become energies that are beneficial to All Creation.
- I am part of the 'Force for Good' and have the ability and power to create Good with True Holy Love, Namaste, and I exercise such power at all times, in all circumstances, and in all situations.
- I know that the job of my ego is to assist in expressing True Holy Love, Namaste.
- I irresistibly attract others of like Being for the mutual expression of True Holy Love, Namaste.
- I remain calm, relaxed, and compassionate at all times, free of all worries, stresses, and strains.
- I quiet my logical mind so that I can better access the 'Force for Good' through my Intuition.

- I make my own decisions; I am free of control and influence by the minds of the masses.
- I know the beauty of my appearance reflects the purity of my thoughts; I am beautiful in all ways.
- I am grounded at all times, bathed in the beautiful light and energy of True Holy Love, Namaste; all that comes to be helped to heal, or with not good intent, is taken to be Healed in the way that is Best for All Creation with True Holy Love, Namaste.
- I identify my aims with clarity; I understand all problems involved; I make my plans with care and with consideration for others; I have an intense desire to succeed; I implement my actions with determination; I celebrate success with modesty; I thank those that help me with gratitude.
- I conceive now in my mind; I believe now in my abilities; I achieve now in my actions.
- I know all things are possible; I am free of all belief systems that would contain and control me.
- I know true happiness is working to help others; I know true joy is success in helping others; I know True Holy Love is helping others in Good ways without any expectation of reward.

End of Program. Thank you."   Remember to check the installation !

The Greatest Light of All is Love
Shine Brilliantly - Give as Above !

Let There be Light !

Trees and plants need light to grow - they are eaten by animals and insects, who in turn are consumed by others. This is the miracle of life, where energies in one form change and experience life in another form. Without light, there would be far less diversity.

What we perceive as visible light is a very small section of the light spectrum - which includes microwaves, X-rays, and many other frequencies. The differences between electrons and photons are not great; plant life uses these to turn material (basic elements) into matter (having the ability to move to some degree).

When we see a particular colour our eyes are responding to the wavelength of that colour. It could be an original colour, sent out by a glowing metal or burning flame, perhaps filtered to allow only a certain colour to be pass through; or it could be a reflected colour.

If you look at a thin green leaf (or a green coloured transparency) it appears green. If you hold a tube below it, so that all you see is the light that gets through, then you also see green. All the other colours could have been absorbed - or it seems more probable that their wavelengths have been changed to green.

Many experts tell that you should wear a colour that appeals to you. But if you wear blue clothing, then it is reflecting blue from you ! Other people see you as having that colour, but would your own body become deficient over time ? It only makes sense if the other colours are transformed into blue by the pigmentation of the clothes.

It has been mentioned that gold is the colour used to signify that a Soul is in Heaven, and silver if the Soul is alive on earth. These two colours are not part of the rainbow - they do not appear as lines of colour when passing through a prism.

Sunlight has a golden tinge, moonlight is silvery - has the moon changed the colour of the sunlight that fell on its surface ? When you hold a CD or DVD to light, the colours that are reflected are not the normal dull colours, but have a metallic brightness - is this reflection without any absorption or change of colour ?

Some sunglasses have the effect of polarizing light, so that only a particular direction passes through. If you hold a similar pair over the first lenses, you can prevent any light from passing through.

There are a number of interesting experiments with light - some of the most interesting are when you shine a light through various slots. If there is but a single slot, then just a 'slice' of light is seen on a screen; but if there are a number of slots, the light does not appear as 'slices' but as an area of diffused light !

Coherent light (single wavelength) is now used in lasers. This is generated by a crystal. Light is also used to carry information more efficiently than electricity - hence fibre optic cables which require less amplification, since there is no energy loss as is due to the resistance of electric wires.

In the future computers may operate using light signals - one beam can carry different streams of information encoded in each colour ! This is how so many telephone conversations and internet connections can be carried by a single fibre optic cable.

The Human Eye

Iridology is the study of the iris of the eye; it has been found that any problem with an organ will be indicated in the eye - it seems that each meridian has a connection to the eyes, and optometrists have gained a reputation of diagnosing a health problem before it gets to the stage of causing illness to the extent that medical practitioners are needed.

The eyes are receivers of knowledge - they keep us informed of our immediate environ, and enable us to work with precision. Used with a microscope or telescope we can see fine details or distant occurrences not otherwise visible to the naked eye.

It is said that when you look into a person's eye you see his Soul. The eye is also a generator of energy - when you look at someone, they will often turn to see who is looking at them, since they are aware of the 'beam' projected to them.

Most of us rely totally upon our eyesight for seeing items and their colours, and for reading. Experiments have succeeded in training people to use their fingertips to 'see' colours, and even to read normal writing ! It seems that most of us can learn to 'feel' colours.

The Healing Power of Full-Spectrum Light

This is an extract from an article by Joseph G. Hattersley published in Nexus Magazine, Vol 8, No 4.

Two hours of bright light in the evening can sometimes cure symptoms such as weight gain, depression, carbohydrate craving, social withdrawal, fatigue and irritability.

Malignant melanoma is often alarmingly but wrongly blamed on sun exposure. The dangerous kind, called skin cancer, is ultimately fatal if not corrected. A study by the US Navy found the most melanoma in people who worked indoors all the time. Those who worked both outdoors and indoors some of the time had the lowest incidence.

Also, most melanomas appeared on parts of the body that are seldom exposed to sunlight. The inference is that both very high and very low exposures to UV light can be harmful - and moderate exposure is healthful.

Fluorescent Light

A study published in the prestigious medical journal Lancet and a Russian study found that fluorescent light rather than sunlight promotes melanoma - proportionately to the time of exposure.

In the Lancet study, among a sample of nearly 900 women, those who worked indoors under fluorescent lighting had 2.1 times higher melanoma risk than others. Among women exposed for 20 years or more, the relative risk was 2.6 times higher.

Relative risks were lower in women who had been most heavily exposed to sunlight, both playing outdoors as children and sunbathing as adults.

In a smaller sample of men, the relative risk for fluorescent lights with 10 or more years' exposure was 4.4 - and 7.3 for those who had spent the least time in the sun while children.

Full-Spectrum (FS) Light

In 1973, radiation-shielded full-spectrum (FS) lights were installed in five classrooms in Sarasota, Florida. And what happened ? Several extremely hyperactive, learning-disabled children calmed down completely and learned to read. Absenteeism dropped.

The children in four standard-lit rooms continued to misbehave (as tracked by concealed motion-detecting cameras); their learning disabilities and absenteeism were unabated. After a year, students in the full-spectrum classrooms had one-third less tooth decay than those taught under standard lighting.

Laboratory mice, which had been exposed all their waking hours to FS light, had zero tooth decay.   A classroom comparison in Vermont found that full-spectrum lighting strengthened immunity.

According to Dr Ott: *"Every nutritional substance and medicine has a specific wavelength absorption. If those wavelengths are missing in the artificial light source a person is exposed to, then the nutritional or other hoped-for benefits of the substance will not be utilized".*

FS light also strengthens immunity in other ways. It helps protect against multiple sclerosis, heart attacks and conversion of HIV to AIDS, among other things.

FS Light vs Cancers

Cancers hate full-spectrum light.   A tumour-susceptible strain of mice lived more than twice as long under full-spectrum as under standard lighting, and rats exposed to full-spectrum light had significantly lessened tumour development.

Terminal cancer patients, who Dr Ott knew of personally, got well in a rocking chair in the sunshine. Dr Jane Wright was fascinated by Ott's ideas. So she instructed progressive-tumour patients to avoid artificial lights and stay outdoors as much as possible that summer. They were not to wear sunglasses or prescription lenses, which block UV light.

By that fall, the tumours in 14 of 15 had not grown, and some patients had got better; the one whose condition deteriorated sat outdoors but wore prescription lenses.

A Chicago-area elementary school suddenly reported five times the national average incidence of leukaemia, a kind of cancer of the blood. All of the afflicted children but one were being taught in rooms where teachers kept the blinds drawn, and the children were exposed all day only to melanoma-promoting fluorescent light.

When even the amount of UV that can get through window glass was let in, the leukaemia cluster disappeared.

Exposed to full-spectrum light, a father rat is docile and even helpful after his babies are born. But when the same rat pair is moved under standard light, before the birth of the next litter the male must be removed to prevent aggressiveness and cannibalism.

Moved back to natural light for still another litter, he is gentle again.

FS Light vs Neurological Diseases

Research by Reuven Sandyk, MD, who practices medicine in Connecticut, shows that long-term deprivation from sunlight exposure increases the risk of multiple sclerosis and Parkinson's disease through depressed secretion of the hormone melatonin by the brain's pineal gland.

This appears to explain the south-north gradient in the incidence of MS - the farther from the equator, the more common it is. All the MS patients he tested had extremely low melatonin levels and their pineal glands were calcified, or hardened.

Reduction in melatonin secretion, he found, may be associated with zinc deficiency in ADHD (attention deficit hyperactivity disorder). *"Since melatonin stimulates serotonin synthesis, and serotonin deficiency has been linked to aggressive behaviour, it is possible that a high prevalence of conduct disorder and aggressive behaviour in ADHD patients could be related to reduced melatonin and serotonin associated with (but not caused by) zinc deficiency".*

Staying completely out of the sun may also increase the risk of heart attacks and much more by another route. David Grimes, MD, at Blackburn Royal Infirmary in Blackburn, UK, notes that heart attacks are commonest in the parts of the world - such as northwest United Kingdom - that have the least sunshine. And Asian populations in the British Isles have a particularly high risk of death from heart attack that cannot be explained on dietary grounds.

Colour and Dyslexia

Isabel Stadnicki is a retired nurse and medical Dowser who has found that coloured gels, placed over reading matter, enable children suffering from dyslexia to overcome their problem. Paul Chelli has written a book about her work 'Art of Healing' - this is privately published - contact Paul at pljchelli@hotmail.com or write Isabel at Box 61, Sicamous, BC V0E 2V0, Canada to get your copy.

Isabel explains that each colour vibrates at a specific rate - as do the glands and organs of the body. By checking if any particular colour vibration is missing or poorly established, and then 'feeding' that colour to the person, many problems including 'Attention Deficiency Syndrome', muscular co-ordination, speech, and memory can be addressed.

One example is a five year old boy who was asthmatic and dyslexic. When looking through a prism, he saw only the colours red, blue, and orange - yellow and green were not seen.

Isabel opened a nursery rhyme book to a picture of a robin. Asked about the words below the picture, he replied *"They jump up and down"*. A light blue plastic transparency was then placed over the page *"Some of the letters jump up and down, but not so many"*.

Replacing the blue transparency with a pink one, a look of wonderment appeared on the boy's face; he looked up with a big smile, and said *"The words are all in a straight line !"*

Isabel has found that shades of violet, indigo, pink, light blue, and yellow are those most frequently most helpful. She will Dowse to find the colour that is needed by a particular person - and when the gels are tested, is usually correct.

When the correct gel is identified, placing it over the reading material for about 10 minutes each day has been found to correct the problem within about a month.

Possible Methods of Colour Selection

Perhaps a book having different coloured paper for each page would assist teachers and Healers to quickly experiment with people suffering from dyslexia to see if their reading abilities change with the coloured background - or perhaps a coloured light could be shone on the normal white paper.

A computer having a program to change the background of the screen could be used to test for changes in reading abilities - so far as I know this has not yet been tried. Perhaps one could Dowse for the red, green, and blue values to be used

Another quick test would be to go to a bookstore and look at the covers of books - since most are printed in various colours. Check which words are easily seen on the different backgrounds.

Isabel also found that other problems, including hearing and eyesight, can be overcome by looking through a coloured glass for about 5 minutes each day for a month or so.

It seems that many behavioural problems are caused by allergic reactions - Isabel uses her Dowsing skills to identify such substances, and noticed a change in behaviour when these things are avoided.

Light in Heaven

In Dr Modi's book 'Memories of God and Creation' (Hampton Roads Publishing - ISBN 1-571174-196-8) she tells how Souls are cleansed by Light when entering Heaven.

The most powerful cleansing is given by the 'Violet Flame' which seems to identify and remove all that is 'not good' and send it to be transmuted into beneficial energy.

"Different colour lights go through me ... white, then pink, violet, green, and blue." "Golden Light bombards me ... and cleanses me." "I can feel the pulsation of a flame, like a blend of gold and green light."

Why wait until you go to Heaven ? Visualize your self being cleansed by the lights, as discussed in the chapter on Grounding, Protection, and Clearing.

Solar Healing Overview   *for more details see: www.SolarHealing.com*

Hira Ratan Manek (HRM), a qualified industrial engineer, has proven that a person can live just on solar energy for very long periods without eating any food; as a result of sungazing, he has not eaten solid food for over 10 years. The method can cure all kinds of psychosomatic, mental and physical illnesses as well as increasing memory power and mental strength and result in a perfect balance of mind.

Since June 18th, 1995, HRM has and continues to live only on sun energy and water. Occasionally, for hospitality and social purposes, he drinks tea, coffee and buttermilk. Until now, he had three strict fastings, during which he had just sun energy and only water and was under the control and observation of various science and medical teams.

If one continues to apply the proper sungazing practice for 6 months, they will be free from physical illnesses.

Furthermore, after 9 months, one can eventually win a victory over hunger, which disappears by itself thereafter.

This is a straight-forward yet effective method based on solar energy, which enables one to harmonize and recharge the body with life energy and also invoke the unlimited powers of the mind very easily.

The eyes are complex organs and they have 5 billion parts - much more than a spacecraft that has about 6-7 million parts. By this, you can see the immense capacity of the human eye. Since eyes are delicate parts of the body, we have to use them in such a way that they serve our purposes without getting damaged.

Present day teachings and ideas such as don't look at the sunlight at all - you will damage your eyesight; never go out in the sun - as you will get cancer, are causing needless hysteria and paranoia.

The more you are away from the nature, the more there is a cause for illness and you will automatically support global corporations. There are definite foolproof ways of getting the benefits of the nature without exposing ourselves to its adverse effects.

Safe Sungazing Practice

Sungazing is a one-time practice of your lifetime usually for a period of 9 months. You can break up the practice in three phases. 0 to 3 months, 3 to 6 months and 6 to 9 months. It helps to walk barefoot for 45 minutes each day - every day of your life.

The practice entails looking at the rising or setting sun once per day - and only during the safe hours. No harm will come to your eyes during the morning and evening safe hours - anytime within 1 hour after sunrise or 1 hour before sunset (when the sun is less than 15° above the horizon).

During these times, one is free from UV and IR rays exposure, which is harmful to your eyes. To determine the timings of sunrise or sunset, you can check the local newspaper, which also lists the UV Index as 0 during these times. Both times are good for practice - it depends on individual's convenience.

For those who cannot initially sun gaze during the safe periods, sunbathing is an effective method for receiving the sun energy at a slower pace until one is able to sun gaze. Best times to take a sun bath is when the UV index is 2 or below - this usually occurs within the 2 hour window after sunrise or before sunset (when the sun is less than 30° above the horizon).

Sun bathing during the day is to be avoided, except for during the winter months, when the UV index usually remains at 2 all throughout which is safe for sunbathing. Check your local newspaper to see the UV Index to be sure.

Do not use sunscreen ! When body gets heated up you perspire and sweat is a waste product and needs to go out of the body.

When you are painted or coated with lotions and creams, they get degenerated and the chemicals enter your body. It is such malpractice that leads to skin cancers.

The First Three Months

First day, during the safe hours, look for a maximum of 10 seconds. On the second day look for 20 seconds at the rising sun - adding ten seconds every succeeding day.

If possible, stand on bare earth with bare feet. Eyes can blink and/or flicker. Stillness or steadiness of the eyes is not required. Do not wear any lenses or glasses while sungazing, and have a belief that the sunrays or lights that you are getting into your eyes are of immense benefit and will not harm you.

There are no restrictions. You can enjoy your food while applying this practice. Hunger will disappear eventually by itself. You may consider gazing from the same place at the same time daily. Following circadian patterns has its advantages.

When you reach three months you will have gazed at the sun 15 minutes at a stretch, and will begin to realize that you have no mental tension or worries.

Three to Six Months

Next, physical diseases will start being cured. Between 70% and 80% of the energy synthesized from food is taken by the brain and is used up in fueling tensions and worries. With a lack of mental tension, the brain does not require the same amount of energy as before. As you proceed in sun gazing and as your tensions decrease the need for food intake will go down.

When you reach 30 minutes duration of continuously looking at sun, you will slowly be liberated from physical disease since by then all the colours of the Sun will have reached the brain through the eye.

All the internal organs get an ample supply of the required colour prana. This is how colour therapies work. After 3-4 months you can become cured of your physical ailments with auto-suggestion, which is imagining and visualizing healing your ailments while gazing at the sun.

Methods such as the Solariums, crystals, colour bottles, natural stones, gems, all utilize sun energy, which is stored in these natural stones. You can keep natural colour stones in drinking water to further hasten healing.

In solariums there is usually a platform at the height of 100 feet where each of the 7 glass cabinets is constructed for each of the VIBGYOR colours.

This platform revolves around the sun whole day, and according to the nature of the disease diagnosed, the patient is placed in the appropriate colour for healing.

Similarly, glass drinking water bottles with different colours are kept in sun for 8 hours. The water gets solarized and water develops medicinal value and is used to treat different diseases.

Photosynthesis, which we misunderstand, does not in fact need chlorophyll. Only the plant kingdom needs chlorophyll.

The human body can do it with a different medium. Photosynthesis is transforming the sun energy into a usable energy format. This is how photovoltaic cells work and electricity is produced.

Eyes receive the entire spectrum of the sunlight, which is distributed to the different parts of the body by the brain on a 'need to have' basis. As a result, you can be cured from all diseases. As you continue gazing at the sun, energy is no longer being used up for mental impairments or physical ailments.

After 6 Months

At 6 months time you will start to have the original form of micro food, which is our sun. Additionally, this can avoid the toxic waste that you take into your body while you eat regular food.

At $7\frac{1}{2}$ months, with 35 minutes of sun gazing, hunger starts going down palpably - you are getting the sun energy indirectly while eating food.

After nine months or when you reach to a 44 minutes level, you should give up sun gazing - since solar science prohibits further gazing for the sake of eye care.

The body will get discharged when you stop practicing, which has to be recharged. Now you have to start walking with bare feet on bare earth for 45 minutes daily for a total of 6 days. Relaxed walking only. No need to walk briskly, jog or run. Any convenient time of the day is all right, however it is preferred to do that when the earth is warmer and the sunlight is falling on your body.

Your Glands are Activated

When you walk bare foot, an important gland in the brain's center called the pineal gland or the third eye is activated. The big toe of the foot represents this gland. 25 years ago it was considered a useless gland. The Pineal gland has optic nerve endings. The remaining four toes represent glands too - pituitary, hypothalamus, thalamus and amygdala.

Amygdala for the last 2 years has been gaining importance in medical research. It's a nucleus of the sun or cosmic energy and plays an important role in the photosynthesis via the sunlight reaching the brain through the eye. When you walk bare foot, your body weight stimulates all these 5 glands through your toes.

Relax, as you walk for 45 minutes for one year and food desire continues to go away from you. After one year of recharging, if you are satisfied with your progress you can give up barefoot walking. Few minutes of sun energy falling on you once in 3-4 days will be enough from then on.

Continual Good Health

But if you want the immune system to strengthen, then keep on the bare foot walking. Also if you want memory power or intelligence to increase, continue the walking practice. As you increase the sun's heat on your feet the brain will activate more and more, which will result in the more activity of the Pineal gland.

All the glands have a lot of functions and can perform at optimal level via sun energy. If you are fortunate to activate the brain optimally you surely will reach enlightenment. You can read past, present, and future. This method can be safely applied to control obesity. Almost all problems get solved.

Historically, a lot of people have remained without food. Accordingly in 1922, the Imperial Medical College in London decreed that solar rays were the ideal food for humans. However, no one described the technique to be used.

Yogananda, in his book 'Autobiography of a Yogi', interviewed many mystics to find out the secret of their lack of eating food. - the common reply was that the sun energy entered through a secret door and reached the medulla oblongata in the brain. Now you know the secret !

The Cathar Prophecy - the Church of Love

The last of the Cathars was burnt by the Inquisition of the Roman Catholic Church at Montsegur, Languedoc, France in 1244, but they left this prophecy: that the Church of Love would be proclaimed.

It has no fabric, only understanding.

It has no membership, save those who know they belong.

It has no rivals, because it non-competitive.

It has no ambition: it seeks only to serve.

It knows no boundaries, for nationalisms are unloving.

It is not of itself, because it seeks to enrich all groups and religions.

It acknowledges all great Teachers of all the ages who have shown the truth of Love.

Those who participate practice the Truth of Love in all their being.

There is no walk of life or nationality that is a barrier. Those who are, know.

It seeks not to teach but to be, and by being, enrich.

It recognizes that the way we are may be the way of those around us, because we are that way.

It recognizes the whole planet as a Being of which we are a part.

It recognizes that the time has come for the supreme transmutation, the ultimate alchemical act of conscious change of the ego into a voluntary return to the whole.

It does not proclaim itself with a loud voice but in the subtle realms of loving.

It salutes all those in the past who have blazed the path but have paid the price.

It admits no hierarchy or structure, for no one is greater than another.

Its members shall know each other by their deeds and their being. and by their eyes, and by no other outward sign save the fraternal embrace.

Each one will dedicate his or her life to the silent loving of their neighbour and environment and the planet. while carrying out their task, however exalted or humble.

It recognizes the supremacy of the great idea which may only be accomplished if the race practices the supremacy of Love.

It has no reward to offer either here or in the hereafter save that of the ineffable joy of being and loving.

Each shall seek to advance the cause of understanding. of doing good by stealth. and teaching only by example.

They shall heal their neighbour, their community and our Planet.

They shall know no fear and feel no shame. and their witness shall prevail over all odds.

It has no secret. no arcanum, no initiation save that of true understanding of the power of Love. and that, if we want it to be so. the world will change, but only if we change ourselves first.

All those who belong, belong; they belong to the Church of Love.

Nobody can Recall every Book
It Helps to Know just Where to Look

Further Information

About the Author

John Living has been a Royal Engineer, a Chartered Civil Engineer, and a Professional Engineer. He started Dowsing over 50 years ago, being taught as a young officer in the British Army.

John is the Executive Secretary of the Holistic Intuition Society, a member of the American Society of Dowsers, the Canadian Society of Dowsers, and the Canadian Society of Questers.

His articles have been published in the American, British, and Canadian Dowsing society journals.

Holistic Intuition Society

The aims of the Society are to help people to be aware that they have Intuitive abilities, to aid them in developing such skills, and to encourage the use of these for Healing and the general good of 'All that Is'.

The Society's web page at www.in2it.ca has quite a lot of information about Intuition in general and Dowsing in particular - since Dowsing is a very simple method of accessing your Intuition 'On Demand' that can be easily learnt by most people.

John Living is the Executive Secretary of the Society, and may be contacted by email: jliving@direct.ca or telephone:

(250)539-5807 or (Toll Free Canada & USA): 1-866-369-7464

or write to him at:

RR#1 S9 C6, Galiano Island,

British Columbia, V0N 1P0 Canada

It is advisable to check the Society's web page: www.in2it.ca

for any changes in this information.

Books of Interest

Books are listed: Title, Author(s), *Publisher*, then my comments; note that the books may also be published by other companies.

Books - General Interest

EFT manual, Gary Craig, free download from www.emofree.org

The details of using the 'Emotional Freedom Techniques' as described in the chapter on EFT.

The Secret Life of Plants, Tompkins & Bird, *Avon*

Covers Backster effect, radiance, and much more about elemental Beings and plant life that is not known or ignored by the mainstream; understanding plants helps in all aspects of life ! All Peter Tomkins and Chris Bird's books are full of knowledge, well-written, and worth reading - see also Secrets of the Soil.

The Secret Life of your Cells, Robert B. Stone, *Whitford Press*

An in-depth study of work by Backster and others on the cellular abilities in plant and animal life - how they all exhibit consciousness.

Supernature, Lyall Watson, *Coronet / Hodder & Stoughton*

A biologist looks at life from a metaphysical viewpoint - he outlines and explains aspects that are usually 'papered over' by mainstream scientists. All Lyall's books are most fascinating !

Rebirth of Nature, Rupert Sheldrake, *Bantam Books*

The best book about life and nature from the originator of the concept of a metamorphic field - it enables you to appreciate better how Intuition resonates with reality.

Earth Radiation, Käthe Bachler **See p.419**

Books - Intuitive Abilities

Practical Intuition, Laura Day, *Vermillion - Random House*

An excellent book explaining how to develop your Intuition, with many examples. Also see her other good books: 'The Circle', 'Practical Intuition for Success', 'Practical Intuition for Love', published by Harper Collins or Penguin Putnam.

Psychic Discoveries behind the Iron Curtain, Ostrander & Schroeder, *Bantam*

".. This book has nothing to do with 'psychic' anything - but 'Matters that we have been taught to *call* psychic !"

A wonderful look at the way that the old Soviet Union showed interest in investigating the non-physical dimension, including Kirlian photography.

Lessons in ESP, David St Clair, *Signet*

A real 'Do it Yourself' guide to many aspects of developing and using your 'psychic' abilities' - easy to read, simple instructions that can be followed to improve your life.

Urban Shaman, Serge Kahili King, *Fireside / Simon & Schuster*

Based on Huna know-how from Hawaii - how to use shamanic methods to improve life for yourself and your family. See also his Kahuna Healing, *Quest Books*.

You are Psychic !, Pete A. Sanders, Jr., *Fawcett Columbine*

Without any doubt, the very best book that I have ever read on understanding and developing your 'Soul Senses' - which is called 'being psychic'. I have found this to be a great help in all that I do - and especially with relationships at home and at work.

See also his Access your Brain's Joy Centre, *www.FreeSoul.net*

Books - Using Intuitive Tools

Elements of Pendulum Dowsing, Tom Graves, *Element*

Excellent easy to read - and amusing - book, covers games, map Dowsing, and much more; it even covers finding bugs in computer programs !

Pendulum Workbook, Markus Schirner, *Sterling Publishing*

Basic facts about Pendulums, exceptionally good introduction to using charts for health - beautifully prepared book, with super illustrations of many charts which can be used to identify the causes of health problems and indicate solutions.

Universal Allergy Healing - The Charts, Juanita Ott & Dora Sharpe, *www.Mirrorwaters.com*

Book of Pendulum Dowsing Charts for you to use in improving your health. See also Daily Emotional Balancer for Soul Activation.

The Freedom Path, Robert Detzler

Charts with explanation of their use for Soul Retrieval and other Spiritual Healing methods.

Remote Viewing Secrets, Joseph McMoneagle, *Hampton Roads Pub.*

By Stargate Viewer #001 - the history and explanation of the process and the protocols used to ensure acceptable accuracy.

Books - More Advanced Healing

Energy Medicine, Donna Eden, *Penguin / Putnam*

Many techniques that you can use to Heal yourself and others, to reduce pain and remove illness using 'Hands Off' techniques - a 'Best Value' for Healing.

DreamHealer, Adam, *Penguin www.DreamHealer.com*

A young Canadian has the ability to help other people Heal - and guides you in how to Heal yourself, mainly using belief and visualization. See also his other books. DVDs are also available.

Kundalini and the Chakras, Genevieve Paulson, *Llewellyn New Age*

So many people suffer strange illnesses caused by their Kundalini system 'opening up' - and most medical doctors are completely at a loss to help, since they do not understand the causes !　An outstanding book on explaining how the energy body operates.

Hands of Light, Barbara Ann Brennan, *Bantam Books*

Excellent book telling how she sees people's energy bodies, and using this knowledge for Healing . See also Light Emerging.

Essential Reiki, Diane Stein, *Crossing Press*

A very thorough introduction to Reiki, with full explanations - now there is no need to pay for expensive initiation by self-professed masters ! Learn the skills, then practice - get experience with other Reiki Healers as well for best results.

Awakening the Third Eye, Samuel Sagan, MD, *Clairvision*

Dr Samuel Sagan has an Indo-French-Anglo-Digger background, and he combines this with Chinese Healing and mystical understanding to develop new vistas of Healing. Techniques sound simple, but are not anywhere as simple as those previously mentioned - but may be more easy if you are already have some clairvoyant abilities. See also his Entity Possession, *Destiny Books*

Some Interesting Web Sites

Free ebook downloads　　　　　www.gutenberg.org
Nexus New Times Magazine:　　www.nexusmagazine.com
Sanjeevini Healing Cards:　　　www.saisanjeevini.org
Emotional Freedom Techniques:　www.emofree.com
'Number One Allergy Detective'　www.scott-mumby.com
Dr Masaru Emoto Water Crystals:　www.thank-water.net/english
life-enthusiast.com/twilight/research_emoto.htm & www.hado.net

Earth Radiation - Käthe Bachler

2nd English Edition, with 'Further Thoughts' by John Living

www.in2it.ca/books.htm   ISBN 978-0-9686323-5-2

This is the classic record of the identification and location of energies from the earth which are noxious to human beings.

The book is a distillation of over 11,000 cases of investigation of these energies in more than 3,000 homes in 14 countries !

Originally written in German, it became a 'best seller' in Europe and was translated first into Spanish, and then into English. The first English edition has long been 'out of print', and existing second hand copies have been fetching prices of US$90 on eBay !

Illustrations show the location of 'Curry Grid Lines' and 'Noxious Water Veins' that radiate noxious energies, especially where they cross.

These illustrations are accompanied by records of the illnesses resulting from sleeping or sitting for a long time in the energy fields - and how great improvements in health occurred when the location of beds, school seats, etc., were moved.

Very simple, very cheap, and very effective !

"We do not claim that every zone of disturbance will result in cancer. Rather, we have found zones of disturbance in every case of cancer. ... Physicians ought to consider geopathic influences as one possible cause of illness, and recommend moving the bed on a trial basis"

Many other illnesses have also been observed to result from these noxious energies - pregnancy failures, infant mortality, insomnia, inattention at school, improper behaviour, rheumatism, multiple sclerosis, parasitic attacks, and more.

<u>Case# 660. The ten-month-old baby was tied to his crib.</u>

The parents were afraid he might fall out of bed, because he stood up again and again.

When in his playpen, he only occupied the half which was 'free of radiation', never the half above the curry strip. The father finally phoned me:

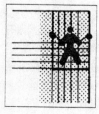

"Since we moved the bed, we have had no problem with his sleeping and he is healthy and robust."

Case# 403. She had a crying spell almost every day.

She and two other children had their desks moved, and the symptoms of all three children disappeared (principal's confirmation available.)

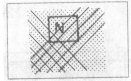

Many of the results are attested by medical doctors who found that cures were only effective after exposure to noxious earth energies ceased. Cases are quoted which include the use of these techniques by physicians for their own health.

Case# 1367. Physician Dr H required a gall bladder operation.

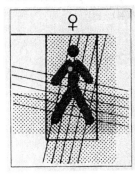

Ever since she moved to her present sleeping place she had been ill. She suffered from pain and anxiety attacks at night in bed.

Everywhere else she seemed to sleep well.

She changed the bed immediately - and slept better the very first night.

She said: *"I don't understand why conventional medicine does not acknowledge the value of dowsing. It seems to me they ought to be grateful for the help."*

One of the key points that this book makes is that many other problems, not just cancer, are attributable to some large degree to earth energies that are noxious to humans.

By eliminating the effects of these we can expect improvements in education and in behaviour, reductions in work losses and medical expenses, and better health at minimal cost.

Case# 1486c. A chemist from Salzburg

felt discomfort, registered slight fevers, and was nervous while working at his bench in his laboratory.

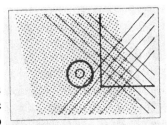

Many of his experiments failed and had to be repeated. Whenever he worked at a place free of radiation, his experiments proved to be successful.

The Holistic Intuition Society's 'Shop'

DVDs of Speakers and Workshops

We have recorded the lectures and workshops on Dowsing and on Healing at the conventions promoted by the Society, and have these available on DVDs that are playable world-wide.

The workshops were given by recognized masters of Dowsing to teach their skills - including the ability of Dowsers to use their 'Power of Thought' for healing the energies of humans, animals, and plants.

"Love Living" Bracelets

Background

In the 1925 Georges Lakhovsky in France developed a coil for the protection of trees; copper wire was stuck into the ground, turns were made around the tree, and the loose end was pointed towards the sky as an aerial. In 1928 he formed a variation of this that was geared to improve the health of humans, which he called the 'multi-wave oscillator', based on his then new theory that cells are microscopic oscillating circuits.

This was successfully used in French, Italian, and Swedish clinics, and when Lakhovsky escaped to the USA in 1941 it proved successful in a major New York hospital. Among problems successfully treated were cancerous growths from Radium burns, goiters, arthritis, chronic bronchitis, congenital hip dislocation, and many others. (Tompkins & Bird: 'Secret Life of Plants').

Design of the Rings

John Living made a number of different rings, testing the effect on glasses of water showed that the water had a radiance of about 5KÅ (5,000 Ångstroms - the human body for a normal person is about 6.5 KÅ) which in 2 minutes increased to 20KÅ for the medium sized rings and 60 KÅ for the smallest ring - the effect is more concentrated.

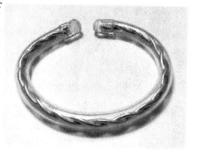

They are sturdy, attractive, and within the reach of most purses. So which ring type is best ? This depends on the use !

The bracelets and smaller rings #1, #2, and #3 are of twisted copper wire, having a small gap; a vinyl tube prevents the copper from being in direct contact with your skin.

They give your blood the vibrational pattern of copper, similar to the way a homeopathic remedy works.

This waterproof casing design permits easy cleaning, prevents corrosion, and allows opening. These rings can be worn, or used to energize foods and drinks. The medium ring, #6, is similar - it fits on most chairs for you to sit on.

The larger rings, #8, #10, and #12, are of 1/4 inch diameter copper tube (for increased sturdiness) having a twisted wire connector in the gap to encourage clockwise rotation of the energies in the tube.

They are intended for healing the energies in a body and in its aura.

The vinyl encased copper bracelet is sealed watertight, for easy washing, and the combination of vinyl with copper blends into the skin colour, so that the bracelet is less noticeable. A hardy bracelet, suitable for constant wear, even ideal for a man in the office or working outside.

Using the Rings

The strongest effect is in the plane of the ring. It seems that 'not good' energies cannot exist inside the ring; the effect is also 'transmitted' in a column above and below this plane, expanding at 45° and reducing in intensity as the distance increases.

To find which size LOVE LIVING bracelet fits you:

Measure around your ankle / wrist with a tape measure send it to us, and we will send you the size just greater than your measurement.

Wear your bracelet loosely - leave about 1/2 to 1 inch gap between the ends.

You can expect all the water in your body (over 75% of you !) to become potentized with a high radiance.

Germs and viruses do not thrive in such an environment, so your LOVE LIVING Bracelets helps to keep you healthy !

A number of successes are reported with the relief of headaches by placing a #2 Energy ring around the neck - if below a shirt or sweater, it is not noticeable.

It may be that some people who have other head problems, perhaps including Alzheimer's and Parkinson's diseases, benefit from wearing a neck ring. The cost of a trial is minimal, the possible benefits considerable, and there is no health risk involved .

A Simple Test you can do yourself

Put water from the same source into 2 glasses and put one glass into your 'LOVE LIVING' Energy Ring. After 10 minutes taste each glass. Repeat at 20 minutes and 30 minutes.

You can expect the untreated water to retain its original taste, while the taste of the treated water improves.

At the same time you can use an Aurameter (or other Dowsing tool) to check the location of the aura of the water; you will find that the aura of the treated water expands !

'L' Rods

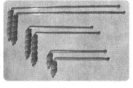

These are made from welding rods, with a wooden handle having a plastic insert for low friction movement and a metal end cap.

The rod arm has a metal end cap to enhance your Dowsing response and prevent damage to people.

Glass Bead Pendulums

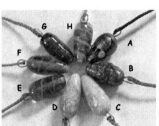

The glass beads have been hand made by craftsmen, and come in various colours and configurations; they are held by a braided nylon string, the string colour being suitable for the bead.

Bendable Bobber

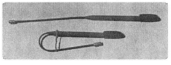

This tool has pewter weights fitted to the end of a specially wound spring 'wand' inserted into a ball-point pen case. It give great sensitivity, and bends to fit in your pocket.

The Ptah Pendulum

John Living found that the Osiris Pendulum has a special ability to locate 'not good' energies in a person's aura, and when used in 'extraction mode' (an anti-clockwise circle) it removed such energies.

But there was a problem - they tended to go into the hand of the Healer/Dowser who was using the Pendulum !

To overcome this, John attached his Osiris Pendulum to the 'extract' end of one of the Healing Coils developed by Slim Spurling.

This converted the energies that were removed into being 'good' energies - and thus prevented deleterious effects from being experienced by the Healer/Dowser, giving instead a beneficial effect.

The next step was to attach one of Slim's Coils to a cord, so as to make a Pendulum. This was even more powerful in extracting 'not good' energies and converting them to being 'good', but did not have the ability of the Osiris Pendulum in locating problems in auras.

An effort was made to get the Osiris Pendulum, designed on geometric theory, to teach the 'Slim's Coil' Pendulum its skill in locating problems in auras - and this was successful !

The Isis Pendulum has the gift of putting 'good' energies into the recipient in a similar way, so a cord was attached to the output end of one of Slim's Coils to make a Pendulum that put 'good' energy into a person - and again this was a success !

Then the thought was received "Why not combine them into a dual purpose Pendulum ?" - and so the 'Ptah Pendulum' was developed.

John Living has tested this on himself and on a number of other people who needed Healing - with excellent results.

He has used it to locate and Heal 'not good' energies in the land, such as curses and other 'bad medicine', and understands that it is one of the most powerful Healing devices that exists.

When working with the Healing Angels and other Healing Energies John uses the 'Ptah Pendulum' to clear energies that are causing problems as a preliminary step to reduce the work needed to be done by the Healing Energies / Angels.

All the 'Ptah Pendulums' are blessed with the abilities of the Osiris and Isis Pendulums, and have been made with True Holy Love.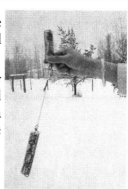

The picture shows an early version - we now produce an improved version made of tinned copper wire to prevent tarnishing, and with a chain having swivels at each end to eliminate twisting.

Signals

In all work with the 'Ptah Pendulum' a clockwise circle indicates YES and is the 'Input Mode'. An anti-clockwise circle indicates NO and is the 'Extract Mode'.

When asking a question it does not matter which end of the Pendulum is held.

The 'Ptah Pendulum' will extract or input, and then swing towards the next position that it needs to go - the direction could be one of two ways, since it is swinging, and your Intuition will guide you to the correct place.

If you go in the wrong direction, the 'Ptah Pendulum' will not circle (or make a very small signal) - so reverse the direction that you are moving the Pendulum. When in the correct place it will circle to do the needed work.

Holding your 'Ptah Pendulum'

In extract mode, the hand holds the shorter of the two coils. For input mode, the longer coil is held. To avoid bending the coil that is held, hold it at its bottom - the strain is not transmitted to the part of the coil above your hand.

Start at the head of the person or centre of the token, and make an anti-clockwise circle (extract mode, shorter coil in hand) around this point, widening in a spiral to enclose most of the Healee; then hold the 'Ptah Pendulum' stationary at the start point - it will start to circle on its own accord to extract 'not good' energies.

When the circling finishes, the 'Ptah Pendulum' will swing, pointing to the next location of 'not good' energies - move it slowly in the direction indicated until it starts to swing again. This is repeated until it remains stationary.

Now change to input mode - the longer coil is held in hand, making clockwise circles - again on its own accord - and this procedure is repeated.

Logically this should remove all 'not good' energies, and replace them all with 'good' energies. But the metaphysical world is not logical !

Perhaps what happens is that some 'not good' energies resist the extraction, but are weakened by the input of True Holy Love, so that by repeating this whole procedure again more 'not good' energies will be extracted.

To make certain that all has been cleared, keep on repeating the extraction mode and then input mode until no circling occurs. And as a final check, start again at the start point and make a spiral, then go to the start point and sees if any swinging or circling occurs.

If so, then repeat the whole procedure again - and keep on until there is not any swinging or circling.

Note that this is not just to Heal people - for 'person' you can substitute 'animal', 'bird', etc.

More Information

The Holistic Intuition Society sells more Dowsing and Healing tools - these are shown on our website at: **www.in2it.ca/tools.htm** together with prices and ordering information.

The key intent is to provide simple tools that can be easily used, at reasonable cost, and that do their job effectively and safely without any side effects.

The Holistic Intuition Society

c/o Executive Secretary: John Living, Professional .Engineer

RR# 1 S9 C6,   Galiano Island,   BC,   V0N 1P0   Canada

Telephone (250)539-5807   Toll Free Canada & USA: 1-866-369-7464

Unfortunately we cannot process credit cards - except by PayPal
PayPal is set-up on our web site,

A cheque or money order in Canadian or US funds is acceptable.

English Speaking Dowsing Organizations

See www.in2it.ca for current addresses and internet connections.

Australia
Dowsers Society of NS Wales
7 Maycock St, Denistone East, NSW
www.divstrat.com.au
dsnsw@yahoo.com.au

Dowsing Society of Victoria
Box 2635, Mount Waverley, VIC 3149
www.dsv.org.au

Dowsers' Club of S Australia Inc
9 Mersey Court, Para Hills,
South Australia 5096.

North Tasmania Dowsing Association
2515 West Tamar Highway, Exeter,
Tasmania 7275, Australia.

South Tasmania Dowsing Association
PO Box 530, Moonah, Tasmania 7009,

Canada
Canadian Society of Dowsers
(Ontario and eastern Canada)
487 Lynden Rd RR#8, Brantford,
ON N3T 5M1
www.canadiandowsers.org
1-888-588-8958

Canadian Society of Questers
(Prairies and British Columbia)
POBox 4873, Vancouver, BC V6B 4A6
www.questers.ca
(604) 944-8683

Ireland
Society of Irish Dowsers
31 Ardmore Grove, Artane, Dublin 5
www.irishdiviners.com

New Zealand
NZ Society of Dowsing and Radionics
PO Box 41-095, St Luke's,
Mt. Albert, Auckland 1030, NZ
www.dowsingnewzealand.org
jackiedow@paradise.net.nz

United Kingdom
British Society of Dowsers
2 St. Ann's Road, Malvern,
Worcestershire, WR14 4RG
www.britishdowsers.org
44 01624 576969
info@britishdowsers.org

United States of America
American Society of Dowsers
P.O. Box 24, Danville,
VT 05828-0024, USA
www.dowsers.org
(802) 684-3417
asd@dowsers.org

Ozark Research Institute
PO Box 387, Fayetteville,
AR 72702-0387, USA
www.ozarkresearch.org
(479) 582-9197

Email Lists open to all who are interested in Dowsing

International Society of Dowsers
Purely web based - www.internationaldowsers.org
To join, go to: www.groups.yahoo.com/group/digital-dowsers/join
(Note: a Yahoo! ID is required)
Or email: digital-dowsers-subscribe@yahoogroups.com - no message needed.

ASD Digital Dowsers
is an online cyber chapter of ASD meeting round the clock, planet wide.
To join, see: www.photon.cc/mailman/listinfo/digitaldowsers
Membership of American Society of Dowsers is NOT required !

Printed in the United States
103229LV00002B/4-60/P

9 780968 632345